W0227841

ENVIRONMENTS
AS THERAPY FOR
BRAIN DYSFUNCTION

ADVANCES IN BEHAVIORAL BIOLOGY

Editorial Board:

Jan Bures	*Institute of Physiology, Prague, Czechoslovakia*
Irwin Kopin	*National Institute of Mental Health, Bethesda, Maryland*
Bruce McEwen	*Rockefeller University, New York, New York*
James McGaugh	*University of California, Irvine, California*
Karl Pribram	*Stanford University School of Medicine, Stanford, California*
Jay Rosenblatt	*Rutgers University, Newark, New Jersey*
Lawrence Weiskrantz	*University of Oxford, Oxford, England*

Recent Volumes in this Series

A Continuation Order Plan is available for this series. A continuation order will bring delivery of each new volume immediately upon publication. Volumes are billed only upon actual shipment. For further information please contact the publisher.

ENVIRONMENTS AS THERAPY FOR BRAIN DYSFUNCTION

Edited by

Roger N. Walsh
Stanford University Medical Center

and

William T. Greenough
University of Illinois, Champaign

PLENUM PRESS • NEW YORK AND LONDON

Library of Congress Catalog Card Number 76-1116

ISBN 978-1-4684-3083-7   ISBN 978-1-4684-3081-3 (eBook)
DOI 10.1007/978-1-4684-3081-3

Proceedings of a workshop series at the Winter Conference on Brain Research
held in Steamboat Springs, Colorado, January, 1975

© 1976 Plenum Press, New York
A Division of Plenum Publishing Corporation
227 West 17th Street, New York, N.Y. 10011

All rights reserved

No part of this book may be reproduced, stored in a retrieval system, or transmitted,
in any form or by any means, electronic, mechanical, photocopying, microfilming,
recording, or otherwise, without written permission from the Publisher

Preface

At the 1975 Winter Conference on Brain Research a series of workshops were held to discuss the role of the sensory environment in the etiology and therapy of brain dysfunction. The participants represented a broad range of disciplines ranging from basic neuro-science through human development psychology. They were linked by a common belief that the role of the sensory environment in brain dysfunction had received insufficient attention. Each had made contributions to this question in their own respective disciplines and it was hoped that this meeting would provide an opportunity for cross fertilization and synthesis.

From these workshops this book evolved. Its production would have been impossible without the help of many people. Anna Taylor's flexibility allowed the holding of a larger than normal workshop, while the authors bore up well under editorial pressure to meet deadlines. Linda Coleman and Phyllis Straw provided excellent support from Plenum while Therese Linden gave editorial assistance. Valarie Munden, Rosemary Schmele, and Estelle Hoffman did an excellent job of typing. RNW was supported by a Fellowship from the Foundations' Fund for Research in Psychiatry. As always, our families provided continuous support and encouragement. To all these people and more we say thank you.

Roger N. Walsh
M.D., B.Med.Sc., Dip.Psychol., Ph.D.

William T. Greenough, Ph.D.

CONTENTS

INTRODUCTION

Over the past few decades, the plasticity of the brain in response to environmental stimulation has become widely recognized. The impact of the sensory environment on the developing -- and to a lesser extent, the adult -- brain has been demonstrated at anatomical, biochemical, and physiological, as well as behavioral, levels. There has been a growing realization that the effects of experiential deprivation upon brain function can be as profound as those brought about by physical damage, and conversely, that certain types of stimulation may sometimes augment development.

The past few years have likewise seen a reawakening of interest in the phenomena and mechanisms of plasticity or return of function following damage to the brain. Clinically, a number of disciplines have emerged based on the tenet that such recovery is possible and that it may be increased by appropriate intervention. However, it must be noted that in many areas clinical research sophisticated enough to adequately test these tenets, or to indicate the optimal intervention, has yet to be performed. At the level of basic research, interest has been spurred by a number of findings. The once popular belief that recovery is greater in younger than older animals has been questioned by a number of experimental findings. Likewise beliefs in the rigid localization of function have faltered in the face of demonstrations of apparent functional sparing if brain damage is sequential with adequate interpolated delays between stages. Paradoxically, some of the experimental variability and failures of replication of brain damage effects have provided useful food for thought in suggesting that the brain damaging and recovery processes may be susceptible to modification by a number of factors. Finally, evidence for functional, although often abnormal, growth following damage to the adult nervous system has provided a basis for theorizing at the biological level concerning the mechanisms of post-traumatic recovery at the behavioral level.

Despite the temporal and conceptual parallels between these two fields, there has been only limited convergence. Environment has been taken as a given in most empirical studies of brain damage

1

etiology and recovery, and this lack of control may partially
account for the previously mentioned variability and failures of
replication of brain damage effects. Indeed, this belief in the
unimportance of environment appears to have functioned as a self-
perpetuating fallacy through biased experimental design and interpretation. For example, as both Richardson, and Levine and Wiener
note in their chapters, malnutrition probably rarely occurs without
concomitant deprivations, yet the failure to appreciate the potency
of these other variables, has led to inadequate controls and purely
nutritional interpretations of findings.

The aim of this series of workshop sessions held at the Eighth
Annual Winter Conference on Brain Research was to examine the role
of sensory environment in the etiology of and recovery from brain
damage. As the potency of environmental variables to effect long-
lasting behavioral changes has been better appreciated, it has become
apparent that some, if not many, of the behavioral changes long
attributed solely to nonsensory brain damaging factors may actually
also reflect the effects of concomitant uncontrolled sensory variables. One of our primary aims was therefore the identification
of these variables and the nature of their effects of their interaction with nonsensory variables. Similarly for the recovery process we were interested first in knowing how much of the recovery
is dependent upon sensory stimulation. Second, if environmental
variation can affect recovery, then does the environment exert
qualitatively and quantitatively similar effects on damaged and undamaged brains; or is the effect a more specific interactive one
such that the damaged brain benefits more or less than the undamaged,
such that the effect can perhaps be attributed to modification of
the recovery process itself? Third, how specific is the therapeutic
effect? That is, will sensory stimulation effect generalized increments in performance or will the behaviors which are enhanced be
specific to the type of stimulation and the nature and localization
of the brain damage? This question became particularly relevant
when we noted the wide variability with which therapies of the
sensorimotor type were applied across different types of brain damage syndromes, being common following such injuries as trauma and
stroke but rare following others such as malnutrition. This seemed
to reflect both the nature of the deficit (being common where motor
or discrete functions, e.g. speech, were affected, but rare where
the deficit was more generalized) and the availability of alternative nonsensory medical therapies, e.g. in malnutrition. Certainly
the disparity across brain dysfunctions in the use of behavioral-
environmental therapy suggests arbitrary assumptions as to the therapeutic potential and/or the need for environmental input. More
importantly such therapy may represent an overlooked potential for
rehabilitation in a number of clinical situations. Further questions
of interest to this workshop concerned the nature of neural responses
to therapeutic environments and their relationship to behavior, an
assessment of the relevance, generalizability, and limitations of

animal models and an examination of the general problems and
caveats of therapy outcome research.

To consider these questions we brought together specialists
from an unusually broad array of clinical and experimental disciplines in order to maximize cross fertilization and to derive
general principles. While the participants were chosen as representative of diverse areas, few of the viewpoints represented
are orthodox restatements of the well-worn line, and several authors
presented controversial -- even radical -- suggestions. For
example, Levine and Wiener suggest that the effects of malnutrition
on behavioral capacity (at least in animal models) are vastly over-
rated. In a similarly controversial vein, Hunt attacks the traditional view of cognitive development as a homogeneous process,
citing increasing evidence in his research that specific sensory
input results in specific developmental responses in human infants.
One point upon which the participants certainly agreed is that the
interaction of environment with environmentally or physically based
brain dysfunction is becoming a dynamic and changing field. As we
wrote our chapters, and even as we have revised them since we met,
new findings both supported and questioned various phases of our
understanding. In addition, the exposure of the participants to
areas far different from their own broadened both their interests
and the range of research which was relevant to their views and
conclusions.

Within this framework, two additional caveats guided our
selection of participants. First, we limited our study to syndromes
in which objective evidence existed that the brain was actually
damaged or physically underdeveloped. The evidence for detectable
neuropathology could come from human clinical work, from parallel
experimental work in animal models, or from both. Hence, such
psychiatric disturbances as schizophrenia, depression, autism, etc.,
were eliminated, even though there are many who attribute these
syndromes to some form of organic brain dysfunction. Second, we
avoided the area of the aphasias and related language disorders
following brain damage since therapy for these syndromes is a subject which has already filled numerous books, although parenthet-
ically it should be noted that we could find very few controlled
outcome studies in this important clinical area.

The style which we have attempted to achieve in this book is in
part a reflection of the diversity of interests and background of
the participants. Those participants from the human-oriented and
clinical realms tended to be less familiar with the terminology and
everyday concepts of those from the biological areas and vice versa.
Hence, we attempted both to speak and to write in a way which could
be easily followed by all participants. As a result, the chapters
in this book are meant to be readily comprehensible to either clinical or research professionals whether or not they have a background

in the area of any individual chapter.

In assembling the book, we have classified the participants
and their chapters in two main topic areas: those using animal
models in their research and reviews, and those whose primary focus
is in the human clinical area. This classification is not easy in
all cases. Several of the authors who focused upon human data drew
heavily from animal research for theoretical background, while the
authors of chapters based upon animal data could hardly avoid discussing the human syndromes which the experiments attempted to
model. Hence, the ordering and grouping of chapters is somewhat
arbitrary and reflects the apparent closeness of the final products
from a theoretical point of view as well as from the viewpoint of
the subject of the research.

The animal model section begins with a discussion of the
effects of the pre-, inter-, and postoperative environment on
behavioral recovery following that most traditional of physiological
psychology techniques, the brain lesion. By adopting a developmental perspective Greenough, Fass, and DeVoogd derive some interpretations and viewpoints of recovery not common either to the more
therapeutically-oriented clinical field or to the more functionally-
oriented localization research. They argue that the experience an
animal has prior to the lesion appears to be at least as important
to its postlesion performance as is any rehabilitative effect of
experience after the lesion. Moreover, they point out that the
relationship between the nature of the pre- or postlesion experience
and the behavior whose recovery is facilitated is, in the literature,
relatively specific. Those few instances in which the effects of
experience on recovery of function appear to be generalized may
involve either mitigation of the emotional trauma an animal experiences when subjected to the altered sensory state associated with
brain damage, or learning processes not at all unique to the damaged
brain.

Levine and Wiener survey the literature on effects of perinatal
malnutrition in the rat on open field behavior and use this as a
model to point out the methodological and conceptual deficiencies
which have plagued the animal malnutrition field. They point out
that the age at which malnutrition has been induced, the method of
induction, and behavioral testing procedures have all been varied
widely without apparent appreciation of the major effects which
these variations may exert on the behaviors under investigation.
From these widely varying experimental procedures have come equally
varying findings which make it almost impossible to derive broad
general principles. However, they suggest that the long-lasting,
deleterious effects of malnutrition per se may have been over-
estimated and that many of the effects long thought due to it may
actually reflect variations in the physical and social sensory
environment, and perhaps especially altered maternal-infant inter-

action.

Davenport focuses upon neonatal hypothyroidism, another source of generalized brain damage, in which behavioral deficits appear to be more clear-cut. Davenport reports that the deficits produced by the early hypothyroid state can be considerably attenuated if the animals are exposed to a period of environmental complexity during development. Moreover, the degree to which the deficit is alleviated appears to be a function of the relative complexity of the inter-polated environment. Davenport also presents evidence from related syndromes which support his notion that learning deficits associated with various sources of generalized brain damage can be alleviated by exposure to a complex sensory environment, that the damaged brain responds more than the undamaged one, and that there are remarkable similarities in "normalization" across different syndromes.

Sackett, in his discussion of the effects of the early environment on behavioral development in infra-human primates, questions the the degree to which results from one such species can be generalized. Sackett finds that the pronounced syndrome of abnormal behavior which has been detailed following postnatal isolation in the rhesus monkey is much less noticeable under identical conditions in the closely related macaque, the pigtail monkey. Moreover, even within the rhesus population, the syndrome is considerably less pronounced in the female than in the male. Sackett suggests that the validity of this syndrome as a model of the etiology of various human behavioral abnormalities should be seriously re-examined.

In their discussion of primate models of human psychopathology, Morrison and McKinney address more general problems of animal models for human disorders. Criteria for models are presented and used to evaluate various primate behavioral abnormalities induced by the social environment or through pharmacological manipulations. Both the precipitating conditions and the effects of therapies are major criteria for the acceptability of a model, Morrison and McKinney note, and both may involve a complex interplay of biological and environmental variables. Rarely do the various primate syndromes meet all the criteria necessary for acceptance as equivalent to human psychopathology, and Morrison and McKinney urge restraint in affixing clinical labels and generalizing across species.

Walsh and Cummins review the effects of therapeutic environments on brain anatomy, physiology and chemistry and then speculate on mechanisms which may mediate some of these effects. They note that most research has been limited to recovery from sensorily induced dysfunction and that there are marked differences between unilateral and bilateral sensory deprivation. In general, recovery from the latter is relatively good, even in older animals, at least for the rodent. However, where deprivation is unilateral then it

appears that competition for postsynaptic sites causes suppression
of the deprived side such that recovery may be limited. They introduce the concept of a "function limiting factor" suggesting that in
both normal and recovering brains the level of function and development will be limited by the availability of a specific factor, either
chemical or sensory. A knowledge of the nature of this particular
factor, they suggest, would guide therapeutic approaches and possibly raise the therapeutic ceiling. Finally they point out that
much of the therapeutic sensory input appears to be self-generated
by the behavior of the recovering animal and suggest that perhaps
one of the major tasks facing therapists is the identification and
design of environments which are optimally reinforcing to these
behaviors.

        J. McV. Hunt opens the human behavior section with an histor-
ical and conceptual review of intellectual development and early
intervention and points out how a variety of fictions (unsupported
fallacious but widely held beliefs) have retarded both scientific
investigation and social implementation in these areas. The notion
that genetic and experiential factors interact in the development
of the organism is far from a new one, but it is only within comparatively recent times that it's been fully accepted and its
effects in the domain of child-rearing and educational practice
are only now being truly felt. Hunt describes how the social and
political climate of the sixties led to the premature initiation
of a widespread early intervention program, "Head Start", and the
repercussions of its failure. He then moves on to a criticism of
normative developmental scales and describes the advantages of an
individualized developmental assessment scheme based upon the work
of Piaget in which the infant's progress is monitored along a series
of ordinal scales. Recent results of Hunt's research with institutionalized children indicate that the rate at which a child pro-
gresses along these scales can be greatly modified by various aspects of the rearing environment and that the scales, which range
from measures of motor development to indices of cognitive abilities,
appear to reflect processes which may be independently affected by
environmental manipulations. Finally, through a comparison of differentially reared children he derives an estimate of the range of
intellectual response to environmental extremes and suggests that
the potential for environmental modification may exceed current
estimates.

        In a striking parallel to the animal research of Davenport,
and Levine and Wiener, Richardson describes the interaction between
malnutrition and the enriching aspects of the human environment.
Given the general finding that an episode of acute malnutrition
requiring hospitalization was associated with impaired intellectual
and general school behavior performance, Richardson examined the
degree to which various aspects of the home environment contributed
to this dysfunction. The striking finding is that the effect of

severe malnutrition upon later school performance depended upon the quality of the home environment. If that environment was suffi- ciently stimulating, very little effect of the malnutrition episode was seen in later behavior. These findings suggest the potential for therapy in an area where its use has been virtually nonexistent and support Richardson's statement that we must move towards cor- relational and ecological models of nutritional dysfunction.

In the following chapter, Beckwith reviews evidence for the therapeutic effect of the caretaker for the "at risk" infant. Here the particular source and extent of brain damage or dysfunction may be less clear-cut, although behavioral assessment of infants exposed to perinatal hazards such as prematurity strongly suggests a biolog- ical deficit in nervous system function. However, these behavioral deficits may be transient or greatly attenuated in infants later exposed to certain ameliorative environmental situations, such as a high socioeconomic status home. Beckwith describes progress in assessment of, and the range of individual differences in, infants' responsiveness to various types of sensory stimulation and charac- teristics of the infant-caretaker interaction. These may mediate the effects of broader psychosocial variables such as social class and provide a process understanding of their effects.

Ann Lodge continues the discussion of infant brain dysfunction produced by perinatal hazards, touching upon a broad range of assess- ment techniques against which the effects of therapeutic interven- tion can be measured. New physiological and more precise behavioral assessment techniques have allowed more precise descriptions of the syndromes associated with various forms of perinatal trauma. A limited number of studies suggest that differential emphasis should be placed on various aspects of the environment, depending upon the syndrome involved. Lodge also notes the peculiar sensory environ- ments which so often characterize traditional hospital nurseries and draws attention to the unusual stimulation to which "at risk" infants are exposed in the course of medical treatment.

Gerald Senf concludes the human behavior section with a dis- cussion of the methodological problems involved in the assessment of outcome following intervention in abnormal populations. One major difficulty is identification of homogeneous subject popula- tions when the etiology of the disorder is unknown. Assumptions of subject population homogeneity and comparability to other experi- mental populations are perhaps more common in these areas than is really justified. Furthermore, the traditional approach of treating subjects as an homogenous group, to be compared with another suppos- edly homogenous control group treats individual variation as "error". But yesterday's error variance is often today's independent variable and in a striking generalization of Richardson's plea for correla- tional designs in examining malnutrition, Senf argues for the greater power and informational value of multivariate correlational analyses as opposed to the traditional univariate sample-control comparisons and points to the need for a greater concern in the measurement of both intervention and outcome variables.

In the final chapter Isaacson provides an overview of the conference and attempts to synthesize the major themes, as well as to highlight some of the more novel and provocative aspects. In particular, he emphasizes the dangers of oversimplification and overgeneralization. All stimulation is not equivalent and certain types and quantities may be detrimental. Likewise stimulation produces diverse effects and studies which examine only a limited range of areas may draw erroneous conclusions, especially since univariate criteria of behavioral impairment are sometimes of dubious validity.

Viewed as a whole, this workshop series reveals a number of recurrent themes and explodes a number of psychobiological myths. Beyond the central theme that the importance of the sensory environment has been considerably underestimated in the etiology of and recovery from brain damage, it is apparent that there is a need for a re-examination of the data concerning the effects of brain damage per se. For example, the beliefs that increased experience prior to a brain lesion reduces recovery, that neural responses to therapeutic environments are too small for detection, or that a single acute episode of malnutrition or perinatal trauma inevitably leads to behavioral deficits can no longer be sustained. Rather the physiological and behavioral outcome can only be assessed and predicted within a broader ecological framework.

Another recurring aspect of our discussions involved the status of our assessment procedures in both clinical and research aspects of brain dysfunction. While several participants described advances in evaluative techniques, it became clear that there was a continuing need for both greater breadth and precision in the identification, classification, and post-rehabilitative analysis of human and animal subjects. A similar view emerged with regard to the analysis of therapeutic procedures. At the present time one of the research frontiers in this area lies in identifying the precise stimuli and processes within the individuals' environment which are most influential. This becomes all the more important in view of another theme: that the input-output relationships are likely to be quite specific. That is, specific sensory experiences and training seem to elicit specific behavioral responses and there is limited evidence for generalized recovery effects, although it must be noted that this may in part reflect the limited range of behaviors sampled by researchers. This re-emphasizes the importance of precise neuropsychological assessment of individual syndromes so as to predict the most appropriate therapeutic input.

Perhaps one of the most important themes is the extent to which

lack of attention to environmental variables has retarded and confused the study of behavioral effects of brain damage. Environmental effects have been falsely attributed to nonenvironmental
agents, resulting in false attribution of results, reduced exper-
mental sensitivity, overgeneralization, nonreplicability of findings and diminished clinical effectiveness. It is apparent that
we must move towards an ecological model of brain dysfunction and
that such a move represents an important and expanding direction
for future research and therapy.

Roger N. Walsh
Department of Psychiatry and
    Behavioral Sciences
Stanford University School of
    Medicine
Stanford, California 94305

William T. Greenough
Department of Psychology and
    Neural and Behavioral Biology
    Program
University of Illinois
Champaign, Illinois 61820

THE INFLUENCE OF EXPERIENCE ON RECOVERY FOLLOWING BRAIN DAMAGE IN RODENTS: HYPOTHESES BASED ON DEVELOPMENT RESEARCH[1]

William T. Greenough, Barry Fass,[2] and Timothy J. DeVoogd

Department of Psychology and Neural and Behavioral Biology Program
University of Illinois at Urbana/Champaign
Champaign, Illinois 61820

Our contribution to this workshop series is primarily a review of existing literature rather than a presentation of new experimental data. Our central concern is whether experience plays a role in recovery of behavioral function following demonstrable -- usually experimentally-induced -- brain damage. For the most part, this discussion is restricted to data from rodents and closely assumed species. The discussion focuses upon parallels between interactions of the environment with the developing brain and interactions of the environment with the damaged brain.

Aside from interpretations based upon newer evidence of axonal growth in the damaged mammalian brain, surprisingly little theoretical progress has been made on recovery of function mechanisms since Lashley reviewed the subject in 1938. At that time theorists had attributed the return of functions lost after brain damage to one or more of three classes of mechanisms: gradual dissipation of trauma or of some form of imbalance brought about by the lesion (e.g., "diaschisis"; Monakow, 1914); "spontaneous" or intrinsically-determined structural reorganization of the remaining tissue

1 Preparation of this manuscript was partially supported by Grant No. HD 06862 from the National Institute of Child Health and Human Development, by NSF Grant BMS 75 08596, and by Grant No. US PHS MH 10715, National Institute of Mental Health. We are indebted to R. L. Isaacson, M. R. Rosenzweig, E. Satinoff, D. G. Stein, and R. Walsh for their comments on this chapter.

2 Now at Clark University, Worcester, Massachusetts.

associated with a function; and "vicarious functioning" which
included both intrinsic and experience-dependent take-over of
function by areas not normally subserving that function (e.g.,
Fritsch and Hitzig, 1870).

Lashley believed that recovery of function was inversely
related to the amount of tissue removed within various functionally
defined systems, although this could be modified by pre- and postlesion experience. The one condition under which Lashley felt this
relationship might not apply was when the lesion had occurred in
early infancy. The apparent capacity of young animals to recover
more fully than adults from equivalent lesions was attributed either
to greater relative dependence on "lower centers" or to the influence
of experience, restoring both specific behaviors and general capacities during the period of growth. This view remains a popular one,
although the data are controversial (see, for example, Isaacson,
1975; Teuber and Rudel, 1962; Goldman, 1974).

A popular explanation for superior infant recovery, stemming
from the primate research of Kennard (1936, 1938) and Tsang's
(1937a,b) work with rodents, has been that the infant brain is more
"plastic" than that of the adult. Hence, following damage to the
young brain, functions normally carried out by the damaged regions
are more easily assumed by the remaining tissue. The adult brain,
"hardened" by maturation and experience, has lost this multipotential quality, and hence, function cannot be so easily assumed
by the undamaged areas.

A detailed analysis of more recent literature led Isaacson
(1975) to conclude that greater recovery of function in infants is
not a general principle. Many of the earlier positive studies did
not adequately control for differences in lesion extent and recovery
time. Apparent recovery also may vary with the assessment task used
(Nonneman and Isaacson, 1973). When these variables are equated the
most common result is, according to Isaacson, no age difference.
When dissimilarities are found, they may favor the infant- or the
adult-lesioned subjects, depending upon the type of damage and the
assessment procedure. Isaacson points out that recovery of function
is a complex process which depends not only upon the experimental
procedures but also upon the genetic and experiential background of
the organism.

While Isaacson invokes experience as a determinant of the
effects of brain damage, he does not review the data bearing upon
this issue. We will expand upon experience-recovery interactions
in this chapter, keeping in mind Isaacson's caveat that apparent
recovery may depend upon the assessment procedure. Many of the
studies described below have employed only one measure of behavioral
recovery, and this measure has often closely related to the experience manipulation that was being examined. Since experiments using

multiple or different assessment techniques have often indicated
that a relatively specific relationship may exist between experience
and the functions recovered, the univariate assessment experiments
may overestimate the potential for experience-facilitated recovery,
although they do maximize the probability of detecting an experience
effect (see chapter by Senf, this volume).

It should also be noted that we differ from Isaacson in the
criteria used to assess recovery of function. Isaacson emphasizes
the asymptotic or final level of behavioral function reached by the
brain-damaged organism, in his discussion of infant versus adult
lesions. In order to be certain that all transient traumata associated with the lesion have subsided, he suggests assessing recovery
only when it is as complete as it is going to get. In examining
experience effects, however, we must also consider the rate of
recovery. This measure is important to studies of the effects of
experience and other manipulations on the brain-damaged organism,
for at least three reasons:

1. If recovery of function involves relearning the means, or
the learning of alternate means, of achieving some behavioral goal,
then the effects of experience or other manipulations may well be
more clearly seen upon a rate measure than upon final level of
recovery. That is, the rate at which relearning takes place may be
a function of experience available over a given period of time.

2. If recovery of function involves restructuring at a neurological level which is more easily accomplished (or accomplished in
some different manner) in a particular population (e.g., developing
organisms), then rate may be a more sensitive parameter with which
to detect underlying differences in the process.

3. The rate of recovery has both clinical and biological
significance. To the extent that our interest in this area reflects
a search for better means of rehabilitating brain-damaged patients,
one concern must be to get the maximum effect from a given invest-
ment of therapeutic effort. In the harsher world of nature, any
incapacitating or debilitating injury affects the probability of
survival; hence, the organism's ability to benefit from its
environment bears directly upon its likelihood of contributing to
the gene pool. Thus, characteristics which enhance rate of recovery,
such as the ability to benefit from experience, may be naturally
selected. Of course, the rate must be assessed carefully and completely, since, in at least some cases, functions which appear to
be spared by infant lesions can be lost with advancing age (Goldman,
1971; Hicks and D'Amato, 1970).

I. AN ENVIRONMENTAL MODEL

Both pre- and post-injury experience may be important in coping
with brain damage and in recovery from injury-associated trauma.
Teitelbaum (1967) has stressed the parallels between post-lesion
recovery and initial development of feeding and motor behavior. A
similar parallel can be drawn between the effects of experience on
recovery of function and the effects of experience on sensory and
social development. The critical or sensitive period hypothesis
(Scott et al., 1974; Denenberg, 1967) has been proposed to describe
many aspects of the effects of the environment on the development of
sensory, social, and emotional capacities. Basically, the critical
period hypothesis states that certain events must occur within
specified periods in development if the organism is to mature normally. If an event is denied, it may be difficult or impossible to
"make up" for the deprivation at a later time. Conversely, once the
event has occurred, later deprivation is often rendered less damaging.

This phenomenon is illustrated by recent research on sensory
and social development. For example, Hubel and Wiesel (1970; Hubel,
1967; see Walsh and Cummins, this volume) have examined the effects
of temporarily closing one eye in the young kitten. If closed
during the fourth and fifth weeks of life, the eye loses its control
over nerve cells in the visual cortex, and vision in that eye is
severely impaired. The impairment persists even if extensive experience with both eyes open is then given. As the age at which the
eye is closed increases, sensitivity to deprivation decreases until,
at about three months of age, the closure of an eye which has
previously had visual experience has essentially no effect on its
function.

A similar process appears to occur in the development of social
responsiveness in dogs. Scott et al.(1974) have summarized research
on the development of attachment to humans and other dogs. The
period between approximately the third week and the third month of
life appears crucial in the "primary socialization" process. If the
dog has experience with humans or other dogs during this period, it
can withstand a later period of social isolation without losing
social responsiveness. If the relevant experience is prevented
during this period, later socialization takes place very slowly
and with great difficulty if at all. Similar sorts of experiments
in rodents, primates, and other species reinforce the view that
experience at appropriate time points can be far more efficient in
promoting normal development than is later experience. Conversely,
whatever occurs during these early critical periods, whether or not
appropriate, appears to "set" the brain, such that in later functioning its range of response is limited by those experiences (e.g.,
Welch, 1965).

One view of the interaction between experience and brain damage (e.g., Rosner, 1970) suggests that passing such critical periods may reduce the ability of the brain to recover after damage by rendering the nervous system less plastic or multipotential (see, e.g., Lashley, 1938). This view is supported by studies on the effects of left hemisphere lesions upon language capacity in man. Lenneberg (1967) has reviewed this research and concludes that language can develop normally in the opposite cerebral hemisphere if the damage occurs sometime before puberty. After puberty, however, hemispheric roles appear to be irreversibly specified such that a lesion in the language controlling area of the left hemisphere results in an enduring disability. This result is highly dependent upon the location of the lesion, and the forced development of speech in the alternate hemisphere exacts "an intellectual price," in terms of other functions (Milner, 1974; Teuber, 1974a). Thus, this view holds that the brain may "rigidify" as age increases and critical periods pass, although this does not negate the role of experience in the adult.

Alternatively, since experience during critical periods can protect against environmental deprivation, it could also protect against functional loss or promote later recovery from brain damage (Hebb, 1949). This view would predict that the adult brain would be less susceptible than the infant brain to the behavioral effects of damage. Furthermore, in parallel with the critical period hypothesis, this view suggests that experience following brain lesions would be a less effective contributor to recovery of function than prelesion experience. The following sections examine the absolute and relative effectiveness of prelesion, postlesion, and interlesion experience upon recovery of function.

II. PRELESION EXPERIENCE

The available evidence indicates that prelesion experience can protect against behavioral loss when age and other factors are equal. The ways in which prelesion experience might facilitate recovery of function can be described in terms of three models. All three agree that the more similar prelesion experience is to a particular behavior, the less that behavior is impaired following a lesion. The models differ in the mechanisms by which this recovery or sparing is hypothesized to occur.

A. Knowledge of Environment

Hebb (1949) presented one early theoretical view. He suggested that many problem-solving aspects of behavior require the organism to perceive relationships within the environment and with respect to its own behavior. Experience tends to broaden the range of relationships with which the organism is familiar. The ability to solve problems within this range following brain damage may, therefore, be less diminished than that of the more naive brain-damaged organism who is forced to learn these relationships for the first time. On the basis of his broader theory of brain function, Hebb felt that more brain tissue might be required to establish a new memory than to preserve and utilize an old one. Hence, experience might allow the "sparing" of related behaviors following a brain lesion, whereas the learning of truly novel behaviors or relationships could be severely impaired.

Hebb was thus able to separate two components of "intelligent" behavior: a "knowledge," or familiarity, component dependent upon prior experience, and an experience-independent "potential," or capacity, component whose survival was related to aspects of the lesion. He demonstrated the importance of the knowledge component by comparing the maze learning of rats blinded in infancy with rats blinded in adulthood. The adult-blinded animals outperformed their infant-blinded counterparts because, according to Hebb, their visual experience had made them aware of environmental relationships never perceived by the early blinded animals.

Of course, the nature of the experience determines the extent of therapeutic facilitation. As Teuber and co-workers (Semmes et al., 1954; Weinstein et al., 1955) have observed, in brain-damaged humans only a relevant pre-injury experience can enhance post-injury task solving ability. If pre-injury experience is generalized and nonspecific, later performance is impaired (Weinstein and Teuber, 1957).

B. Multiple Representation

Hebb's view of the action of experience on the organism relates primarily to development of behavioral flexibility, or the ability of the organism to cope with a problem in different ways. Rosner (1970) conceives of the brain as organized into subsystems which process in parallel and/or serially various aspects of a given environmental situation. Here, any environmental situation would have many perceptual facets which, at a higher level, are organized into a coherent perception upon which to base behavioral output decisions. As these systems work in parallel, one might expect "cross references" to be established such that a particular configuration in one subsystem corresponds to a particular configuration in another modality (for example, visual information mapping to touch information). This sort of intermodal integration has been described by Held and Hein (e.g., 1963; Hein, 1972), who studied the establishment of relationships between visual, kinesthetic, and motor systems through experience. Thus, limb movements can be coordinated with the visual and somatosensory environment. To the extent that

experience is necessary for the establishment of subsystem equivalence (and certainly, for many behavioral situations, only through
experience could cross-modal equivalence be acquired), the subject
called upon to use a restricted set of subsystems would benefit by
the variety in its history.

C. Emergence Trauma

Finally, support exists for a third possible view of experiential effects on the organism. This view is similar to Fuller's
(1967) concept of emergence trauma (see also Hebb, 1949; Melzack,
1969; Welch, 1965) following restricted rearing, which was developed
to explain aberrant behavior patterns in mammals reared in sensory
and social restriction. These authors have suggested that exposure
to a sudden increase in the complexity of the stimulus array can
overload the information processing capacity of the organism, leading
to inappropriate behavioral responses and emotional reactivity.
Similarly, an organism that has lost a significant portion of its
central nervous system may be expected to have altered perceptions
of its sensory array and/or self and response capacity. This is a
type of postoperative trauma quite different in origin from that
usually suggested. Tower (1940), for example, describes emotional
overreactions to the inability to perform simple responses in
monkeys following lesions of motor neocortex. An array of past
experiences could allow this altered perception to appear more
"familiar," resulting in less reactivity and hence a greater potential for normal behavior.

This "familiarity" notion appears to be supported by some
research on regulatory and sensory system lesions. For example,
Singh (1973, 1974) examined the effects of specific prior experience
upon food intake in rats subjected to ventromedial hypothalamic
(VMH) lesions. VMH rats typically overeat and become obese when
presented with food available ad lib. (Hetherington and Ranson,
1940). However, these animals do not appear to be more "hungry"
than normal rats, since they eat less than normal rats if they must
work for their food, or if the food is made less palatable (Miller
et al., 1950; Teitelbaum, 1957). Since VMH animals appear to be
hyperreactive to their environment (Wheatly, 1944), Singh (1973,
1974) reasoned that they might overreact to unfamiliar aversive or
demanding situations associated with feeding. When Singh exposed
rats to bar pressing for food (1973) or to quinine-adulterated water
(1974) prior to surgery, the VMH animals performed almost identically
to controls within a few days after the lesion.

Data from visual neocortex lesion studies which provide some
support for all three of the mechanisms outlined above have been
presented by Cooper and his associates (Bauer and Cooper, 1964;
Cooper et al., 1972; Miller and Cooper, 1974). When visual neocortex

is removed, a preoperatively learned brightness discrimination is
lost and must be relearned (Lashley, 1935; Horel et al., 1966).
Bauer and Cooper (1964) attempted to simulate the loss of pattern
vision preoperatively by training rats wearing translucent eye
occluders on a brightness discrimination. Such animals, following
visual neocortex lesions, did not require the usual extensive re-
training on the brightness habit. Cooper et al. (1972) found some
transoperative loss of the brightness discrimination learned preoperatively with occluders when the lesions were quite large, but
this may reflect the inability of the occluders to perfectly mimic
vision after such lesions (Miller and Cooper, 1974). Taken with the
results of Singh, these findings would seem to support the importance of familiarity with the test stimuli, although there is no
indication of differential emotional reactivity in the reports.
However, Thompson (1965, 1969) has suggested that brightness discrimination may be mediated by subcortical structures. Cooper et
al. (1972) propose that the occluders force the subject to use these
centers in learning the task preoperatively and, since they are not
irreversibly damaged by the operation, the learning is retained.
This latter notion is compatible with Hebb's knowledge view. Moreover, it suggests that experience may play a role in establishing
equivalence among multiple subsystems in the brain.

     In the Singh and Cooper studies, the relationship between pre-
operative experience and postoperative test performance was quite
specific. Several other experiments similarly indicate that preoperative experience which closely approximates the postoperative
test can affect performance. Animals trained on a task before
surgery are often easier than nontrained animals to retrain after
the lesion (even though the particular habit, such as brightness or
pattern discrimination, may be temporarily or permanently lost).
LeVere and Morlock (1973) have shown that some vestiges of a preoperatively learned brightness discrimination are retained even after
lesions of visual neocortex. That is, if rats with occipital damage
are required to reverse their preoperatively learned brightness
choice, they perform more poorly than rats which are merely retrained
on that task.

     The degree to which specific training is retained postopera-
tively appears to vary with the amount of preoperative training
(Rosner, 1970). For example, Worthington and Isaac (1967) found that
rats trained to a stringent criterion of ten consecutive shuttle box
avoidances, using a light CS, relearned the avoidance more rapidly
after visual neocortex removal than did rats trained to a weak preoperative criterion of five out of ten avoidances. Similarly,
Lukaszewska and Thompson (1967) reported that preoperative overtraining on a pattern discrimination facilitated postoperative relearning following pretectal lesions. Weese et al. (1973) found that
overtraining facilitated retention of a tactile discrimination
following somatosensory cortical destruction. Protective effects

of overtraining have also been reported in monkeys (Chow and Survis, 1958; Orbach and Fantz, 1958) and in dogs and rats following amygdaloid lesions (Fonberg et al., 1962; Thatcher and Kimble, 1966), but are not universally found (e.g., Glendenning, 1972). While such studies emphasize the importance of "familiarity," they are generally also compatible with knowledge or multiple representation notions.

It is far from clear -- even unlikely -- in the above studies that preoperative training would affect performance if the test tasks were dissimilar from the preoperative experience. As such, they seem merely to reflect the survival of some preoperatively acquired memory. Somewhat more generalized influences of experience can be seen in experiments involving preoperative treatment effects on the lateral hypothalamic (LH) syndrome. In contrast to the hyperphagic VMH animal previously mentioned, the LH animal does not eat at all, and starves to death. Feeding will return in successive stages, however, if the animal is kept alive by force-feeding postoperatively (Anand and Brobeck, 1951; Teitelbaum and Epstein, 1962). In contrast to the hyperreactive VMH animal, the LH subject is somnolent and minimally responsive to his environment, a phenomenon which Marshall et al. (1971) have termed "sensory neglect." Several investigators have examined the effects of preoperative experience upon the feeding deficit. Powley and Keesey (1970) reported that preoperative starvation shortened the delay of postoperative feeding recovery and suggested that LH animals were regulating about a new body weight "set point." However, Glick and Greenstein (1972) have found that the experience of starvation, rather than the body weight level, is the more important preoperative determinant of postoperative weight loss. Moreover, Balagura et al. (1973) have shown that preoperative insulin administration which induces feeding in normal rats also facilitates recovery from LH lesions. These studies can be interpreted to support Hebb's knowledge view if one suggests that the CNS has "learned" to regulate over a broader range with experience and is hence more capable of regaining control under the extreme condition of loss of major components.

Finally, Harrell and Balagura (1974) have examined the effects of pre- and postoperative lighting conditions on motor deficits associated with the LH syndrome. While postoperative lighting made no difference, rats which spent the last five preoperative days in darkness were less impaired than constant light controls on measures of horizontal stabilization, waxy flexibility (i.e., catalepsy), and ability to step down from a platform. This experiment may, however, reflect an additional deficit in the light-reared rats, since chronic lighting over such a period produces irreversible retinal degeneration in albino rats (e.g., Noell and Albrecht, 1971).

Perhaps the best evidence for a potentially nonspecific

relationship between preoperative experience and postoperative
recovery has come from studies in which rats have been housed preoperatively in complex environments. Such environments appear to
enhance the performance of normal unoperated animals on problem
solving and maze tasks (see e.g., Rosenzweig, 1971; Greenough, 1975);
therefore, the ideal result to demonstrate facilitation of recovery
is an interaction between environmental and surgical treatments.
Equivalent effects on operated and nonoperated animals would imply
an environmental effect independent of the recovery process (see
Davenport, this volume). Two studies have reported such results.
Donovick et al. (1973) reared rats in complex group cages or in
isolation from 25 to 85 days of age prior to ablation of much of the
septal region. Postoperatively, the isolates showed the usual
increased drinking and reactivity to taste qualities associated
with septal destruction, while the complex environment-reared rats
resembled unoperated controls. Similarly, the complex-reared septal
group showed an amount of exploratory behavior approaching that of
the unoperated complex-reared group. However, the complex rearing
had little effect on the ability to learn alternate choices in a
T-maze for water reward in either the operated or the control groups,
although both septal groups were severely impaired. More recently,
Donovick et al. (1975) manipulated the dietary experience of rats
from weaning until surgery at two months. Rats that had experienced
an array of food types and mild deprivation prior to septal lesions
differed from a standard-rearing septal group on fluid consumption
and exploration, but not on active avoidance measures. However, the
septal-experienced groups did not clearly parallel any other group
in the factorial design, and, to some extent, exhibited reduced
reactivity of the type which is expected under the emergence trauma
notion. These experiments suggest that generalized preoperative
experience may have generalized effects, although the alternation
results imply a limit to the generality.

An additional complex environment experiment similarly relates
relatively nonspecific preoperative experience and postoperative
ability and may support the familiarity and emergence trauma notions.
Hughes (1965) reared rats in complex group environments, group cages,
or isolation cages prior to hippocampal, neocortical, or sham lesions.
Complex rearing attenuated the effects of antero-dorsal hippocampal
lesions on Hebb-Williams maze learning. Both complex and group
housing conditions appeared to diminish deficits produced by postero-
ventral hippocampal destruction. A similar pattern emerged in the
case of subjects with neocortical lesions (neocortical damage
accompanied hippocampal lesions, and examination of Hughes' Fig. 2
suggests that the environmental effect on animals with postero-
ventral hippocampal lesions may be due entirely to this component).
While neocortically-damaged rats which had been reared in complex
and group environments did not differ from sham-operates from these
environments in maze learning ability, damaged rats which had been
reared in isolation committed nearly 50% more errors than did sham-

operated isolates.

Hughes' neocortical and sham groups suggest a true interaction between preoperative experience and behavioral recovery. A final experiment similarly suggests an interaction between the effects of complex environments upon brain development and the effects of lesions. Complex environments cause an increase in cortical weight, thickness, and neuronal dendritic branching which appears to be greatest in posterior dorsal neocortex in the rat (e.g., Greenough, 1975; Rosenzweig, 1971; Walsh and Cummins, this volume). Smith (1959) reared rats in complex or impoverished environments, adminis-tered anterior or posterior lesions, and examined maze performance. Complex environment rats were most debilitated, relative to non-lesion controls, by posterior neocortical lesions. In contrast, impoverished rats were impaired following anterior neocortical le-sions. Thus, destruction of the neocortical area most affected by complex environments appeared to produce the greatest effect in complex-reared animals, whereas maximal effects were produced by a different lesion site in animals not subjected to environmental complexity.

Taken together, these results suggest that appropriate pre-lesion experience can promote postoperative recovery, although the timing of most of the test periods does not permit us to determine whether rate or asymptotic recovery level (or both) is affected. There is some support for all three of the processes outlined above. Of these, the emergence trauma notion is not generally proposed as an explanation of such studies and might be tested by attempts to reduce emotionality with tranquilizing drugs. To the extent it has been examined, the relationship between prelesion experience and postlesion behavioral sparing or recovery often appears to be quite specific, but this may reflect both the limited test selection and the experimental emphasis on primary sensory neocortex lesions. Where less sensory-specific structures were damaged (hippocampus and septal region), generalized preoperative experience appeared to have positive effects. However, straight alley and maze per-formance may still be relatively similar to the complex environment, and a less related task, alternation, gave inconsistent results. It seems clear that a better understanding of the generality of pre-operative experience effects on recovery could be gained through use of multiple assessment procedures, including tasks which differ from the experiential manipulation.

III.   POSTLESION EXPERIENCE

In contrast to prelesion experience, in which the trans-operative survival of knowledge or capacity is at issue, postlesion experience may provide some insight into mechanisms underlying apparent recovery of function. Goldberger (1974; see also Rosner,

1970) has summarized modern formulations of historically proposed
mechanisms of recovery of function:

    1. Equipotentiality and mass action. The amount of remaining
tissue, at least within defined functional systems (e.g., visual
neocortex) is directly related to the level of ultimate recovery of
function. In the strict sense, reorganization (4, below) is not
required.

    2. Vicarious function. Take-over of function by an undamaged
system not originally performing that function. Related theories
imply some latent redundancy of functional capacity in the intact
nervous system. Again, reorganization is not required, but in
contrast to equipotentiality, the substitute system need not have
been a part of the system originally performing the function.

    3. Substitution. The development and/or the use of alternate
behavioral means to achieve a goal.

    4. Functional reorganization. Portions of the nervous system
which are not permanently damaged are actively altered to subserve
functions previously carried out by the damaged regions.

    These proposed mechanisms are not truly independent, except
when formulated in terms more limiting than those of their original
proponents. For example, some form of reorganization is common to
many theories of recovery, and Lashley (1929, 1938), who is credited
with equipotentiality, described situations in which all of the
others might play a role. In the strict formulation, however, it
would appear that postoperative experience should have minimal
influence upon recovery if equipotentiality or vicarious function
is involved. Potentially, postoperative experience has more influence over recovery involving behavioral substitution or reorganization depending, especially in the case of reorganization, upon the
requirements for extraorganismic feedback.

    Other mechanisms of postlesion behavioral improvement involve
dissipation of effects of the lesion per se. For example, Monakow's
(1914) concept of diaschisis posits that a brain lesion produces a
suppression or inhibition in the activity of certain undamaged
structures. This suppression causes aberrant behavior which becomes
less evident as the activity of the intact regions approaches preoperative levels. Related proposals include generalized CNS trauma
or "shock" following damage, which is similarly thought to dissipate
with time (see Isaacson, 1975). Such processes are usually separated
from those reviewed by Goldberger (1974), since the dissipation
involves a disinhibition of function rather than a recovery of
function lost when tissue which subserved or was involved in it was
destroyed. However, experience could affect such processes and, as
Isaacson (1975) notes, trauma could interfere with any influence of

experience upon other recovery mechanisms. Postoperative experience could similarly affect the emergence trauma described in the
preoperative section. In fact, if this form of trauma interfered
with either disinhibition or recovery of function, an experimental
remedy might be the use of transition environments to adapt the
subject to the postoperative perceptual alteration. This has been
done with some success in the rehabilitation of dogs and monkeys
socially deprived during development (Scott, 1968; Fuller, 1967;
Suomi et al., 1972).

The effectiveness of postlesion experience is implied or
assumed in the widespread use of therapy in cases of human central
nervous system pathology (for reviews, see Luria et al., 1969;
Gazzaniga, 1974). While clinical research is beyond the scope of
this review, arguments for the effectiveness of therapy in many
forms of human brain damage appear to be based upon evidence from a
limited number of controlled studies (but see Wepman, 1951), and the
issue remains controversial (Stern et al., 1971; Sarno et al., 1970;
Teuber, 1974b).

As previously discussed, a parallel can be drawn between the
timing of effective developmental experience and the timing of
therapeutic experience administered to brain-damaged organisms.
This parallel suggests that postlesion experience would usually
have less effect than prelesion experience upon recovery of function.
However, where recovery of function involves the learning of specific
behavioral substitutes, this need not apply. Indeed, Campbell and
Spear (1972) and others have noted that memory for specific tasks
improves with age during postnatal development. The parallel also
suggests that the sooner experience is given after surgery (paralleling closeness to a critical period), the more effective it might be
in contributing to recovery. In contrast, an emergence trauma
notion suggests that delaying exposure to any perceptibly radical
change in the environment might be beneficial as the organism adjusts
to perceptual alterations. (Clinical evidence exists in support of
both views -- see Wepman, 1951, and Iwanow-Smolenski, 1954 [skepti-
cally cited in Teuber, 1974b].)

Data from rodents have provided only limited evidence to support
the clinically-compatible view that postoperative experience is
equal or superior to preoperative experience in promoting recovery
of function, although recent reports suggest that this might reflect
the paucity of postoperative experience studies rather than the
absence of postoperative experience effects. Reports indicating
significant effects of postoperative experience upon the rate of
recovery (or level at a specific postoperative time) again suggest
that the relationship between effective experience and facilitated
test tasks may be relatively specific.

For example, DiCara (1970) has shown that experience with milk,

either before or after LH lesions, enhanced rats' recovery of feeding on milk compared with subjects which had no preoperative milk
experience and had the milk injected directly into the stomach postoperatively. This is presumably because the experienced animals had
become familiar with the liquid's taste. Gazzaniga et al. (1974)
reported that adipsic LH rats drank water to gain access to a running
wheel. However, the fact that their LH rats would run for 100 to 150
seconds per half-hour within a few days after the lesions contrasts
with other descriptions of LH animals (e.g., Marshall and Teitelbaum,
1974; Harrell and Balagura, 1974). (Interestingly, there was no
effect of prelesion experience with the drink-to-run contingency.)
Similarly, Chase and Wyrwicka (1973) found that cats preoperatively
trained to consume liquid for electrical stimulation of septum or
tegmentum continued to consume liquid for such stimulation following
LH destruction. Unlike the animals in the Gazzaniga et al. (1974)
study, aspects of the LH syndrome were well documented in these cats.
Whether generalized recovery of feeding was facilitated is not clear,
since nontrained controls were not run and none of the LH cats ate
dry food postoperatively. LH animals may be less capable postoperatively than others of learning such behavioral substitutes,
since Schwartz and Teitelbaum (1974) reported that LH animals retain
taste aversions learned preoperatively but are severely impaired in
learning them postoperatively.

Stricker and Zigmond (1975, in press) facilitated recovery from
intraventricular 6-hydroxy-dopamine injections with a postoperative
environment. This neurotoxin results in behavioral impairments
similar to those seen in LH rats. Stricker and Zigmond found that
these behaviors recovered more completely following exposure to a
mildly stressful environment than exposure to a more neutral environment. A final intriguing effect of "experience" on LH recovery is
described by Harrell et al. (1974) who found that one hour of daily
low-level electrical stimulation of the lateral hypothalamus through
the lesion electrodes shortened the feeding recovery period from an
average of 5.8 days for nonstimulated rats to only 2.4 days. This
suggests that an appropriate postlesion experience might simply
involve the activation of the affected area.

The VMH syndrome may also be amenable to postoperative experience. W. E. Wood (personal communication) found that VMH rats
gained weight less rapidly in the presence of running wheels or in
a complex environment. The animals showed an abrupt weight gain
when transferred to individual cages.

The VMH and LH studies provide preliminary evidence that basic
regulatory deficits may be ameliorated by postoperative experience.
While the bulk of these experiments report transient or situationally
dependent normalization of behavior, the DiCara (1970) and Harrell
et al. (1974) studies suggest altered rates of recovery, and the
Stricker and Zigmond (1975) experiment may indicate a higher final

level of functional return. Further work is needed to ascertain
the reliability of these findings. Recent results suggest that
recovery from damage to other limbic structures may be more amenable
to experience effects.

The septal lesion syndrome involves a transient increase in
reactivity to environmental change (e.g., Brady and Nauta, 1955),
for example, in the taste of liquids (Donovick et al., 1969).
Burright et al. (1974) found that the abnormal preference shown
by septal rats for palatable concentrations of saline and saccharine
was suppressed by postoperative experience with high, unpalatable
concentrations of these substances.

Septal lesions also enhance responding in a two-way shuttle box
(Krieckhaus et al., 1964; King, 1958). Johnson et al. (1972) found
that six days' handling following infant or adult septal lesions did
not affect rats' shuttle box acquisition. However, handling following infant lesions, but spread over the additional 83 days of recovery time allowed the infants before testing, resulted in more rapid
extinction, similar to that of controls. It is not clear whether
the age of the animal when handled or the distribution of handling
is the critical variable in this study.

Evidence indicating that distribution of handling is important
was provided by Gotsick and Marshall (1972; see also Glass and
Thomas, 1970). They found that postoperative handling of adult septal rats could either enhance recovery from the usual hyperemotion-
ality and rage behavior seen after such lesions or exacerbate the rage,
depending upon the distribution of handling. Excessive handling one
day after surgery prolonged the rage behavior, strongly suggesting
agonism of possible emergence trauma associated with the syndrome.
However, Seggie (1968) found that daily cage shaking reduced postoperative emotionality in septal rats, although daily handling was
more effective.

A final septal lesion experiment examined the effects of postoperative social housing conditions on shock-elicited aggression.
Ahmad and Harvey (1968) reported that higher than control levels of
aggressiveness persisted for up to 45 days in isolation-housed septal
rats while housing septal rats in pairs for 17 days eliminated
increased fighting. Irritability to handling was also reduced by
social housing.

Together, the septal lesion studies suggest that postoperative
experience can affect a comparatively general behavioral property --
reactivity to environmental change. The data cannot be easily
explained in terms of generalization of habituation to specific
stimuli, since a relationship is not always evident between the rate
of stimulus presentation and the degree of reduced reactivity. There
is a suggestion that the experience must be adjusted to the level

the animal can accept. Excessive stimulation may exacerbate traumatic reactivity to the environment, while understimulation may
prolong reactivity.

Postoperative pretraining has affected performance of rats with
lesions of the hippocampus in several studies. The role of postoperative pretraining with continuous reinforcement for every lever
press (CRF) on later training in which low rates of responding are
rewarded (DRL) has been a matter of some controversy. Ellen et al.
(1964) reported that rats given CRF training following small hippocampal lesions earned as many food pellets as controls. Schmaltz
and Isaacson (1966) found rats with larger lesions unable to learn
DRL when shifted from extended CRF pretraining, whereas nonpretrained
animals matched controls on the reward measure (although their response pattern differed from controls). More recently, Ellen et al.
(1973) have confirmed that a combination of large lesions and extended
CRF training is required to produce the DRL deficit. In a different
paradigm, Bauer (1974) reported that pretraining in a Y-maze without
cues interfered more with learning to respond to a brightness cue in
rats with hippocampal damage than in control rats. In both cases,
the expectation of the hippocampal rat was manipulated postoperatively, and, as noted by Kimble (1968), a characteristic of the
hippocampal rat is its inability to shift among hypothesis or
expectancies and to inhibit dominant behavioral tendencies.

A final experiment using the CRF/DRL hippocampal lesion paradigm provides some support for the emergence trauma notion outlined
under prelesion experience. Schmaltz and Isaacson (1968) reported
that postoperative peripheral blindness enhanced DRL performance of
hippocampal rats but impaired performance in controls. Postoperative emergence trauma associated with the loss of this central
attentional-inhibitory structure (Isaacson and Kimble, 1972) might
well be greater with the increased sensory load of vision. Hence,
blinding could reduce this sensory overload, allowing inhibitory
capacity to be concentrated on DRL performance. For controls, on
the other hand, blinding could have produced a traumatic perceptual
change which impaired their normally high level of performance.

Tests of postoperative lighting conditions upon recovery following visual neocortex damage have provided mixed results. Bland and
Cooper (1970) found postoperatively dark-housed rats inferior to
normal laboratory or complex environment housed rats on an 8:1
brightness discrimination, but not on light-dark or pattern discrimination (the latter was not learned by any group). Tees (1975)
reported no effect of either postoperative or preoperative dark-
rearing on acquisition or transfer of pattern discrimination in rats
given visual neocortex lesions in infancy or adulthood. Tees (in
press) did, however, find that the light-reared infant operates
improved with age and experience on visual cliff performance, while
dark-reared operates showed essentially no improvement. These studies

suggest that recovery facilitation within sensory systems may be quite task-dependent. Postoperative environmental effects fail to appear on tasks which are either too easy (light-dark discrimination) or too difficult (pattern discrimination) for the brain-damaged subjects.

Perhaps the most exciting postoperative experience study from a therapeutic or nonspecific reorganization viewpoint is that of Schwartz (1964). Rats which underwent posterior neocortical lesions at one day of age were reared for three months in stimulation "rich" or "poor" group environments, prior to maze training. The rich environment seemed to offset some effects of the lesion, such that the "rich/lesion" group made fewer errors than the "poor/sham" group, while the "poor/lesion" group made about 60% more errors than the "poor" controls, and the surgery by environment interaction was significant.

Will, Rosenzweig, and Bennett (in preparation) have replicated this finding. An enriched environment, which has been shown by this group to enhance maze learning and to increase neocortical weight in normal rats (e.g., Rosenzweig, 1971), improved maze learning and increased neocortical dimensions in rats which had sustained posterior neocortical lesions on postnatal day 1. These effects, in general, were seen in both males and females, with both large and small lesions, and whether the differential rearing extended from day 5 or day 25 to 65 days of age. Differences in sham operates were generally smaller than those in neocortically-damaged animals. Will, Rosenzweig, Bennett, Hebert, and Morimoto (in preparation) similarly found enriched environments to partially offset maze learning effects of lesions at 30 days of age. Environmental effects in lesion groups tended to be larger than in sham operates, and the environment by surgical treatment interaction was significant in one of two experiments.

Both Davenport and Richardson (this volume) discuss similar environmental effects following neonatal thyroid deficiency, malnutrition, and other insults. However, the complex environment effect does not appear to be universal. Bland and Cooper (1969) found no effects of postoperative environmental complexity upon pattern discrimination in rats decorticated in infancy or adulthood. Similarly, Isaacson (1975) cites unpublished work by Cornwell et al., in which postoperative rearing in a complex environment had no effect upon visual discrimination deficits produced by neonatal visual neocortex damage. The positive effects of complexity may be limited to maze-like tasks, again suggesting a degree of specificity between the experience and the recovery in behavior. Hence, as with preoperative experience, the effects of postoperative experience appear, at this point, to be restricted to cases where the measures used resemble the experience provided.

While many types of postoperative experience can affect
behavior after various lesions, there is little evidence that experience acts in a general way upon the mechanisms which mediate
recovery to promote the return of more normal behavior. Postoperative experience often exacerbates symptoms rather than alle-
viating them (e.g., Bauer, 1974; Gotsick and Marshall, 1972;
Schmaltz and Isaacson, 1966), either through the interaction of
brain dysfunction and learned patterns or, perhaps, through reactivity to the environmental manipulation. Complex environment
and other therapy studies suggest more generalized effects, but it
is not yet clear in such studies that the experience truly interacts with recovery in the brain-damaged animal, rather than merely
producing equivalent effects on operated and normal populations.
Statistical interactions may, of course, result from task ceiling
effects in the nonlesioned groups. Davenport, this volume, reports
complex environment effects which occur only in thyroid deficient
animals. This result may indicate a selective enhancement of
recovery, rather than a ceiling effect. The surprising effects of
brain stimulation in the Harrell et al. (1974) study offer some
evidence for a type of recovery process whose rate can be affected
by extrinsic input, and this is discussed with the data on drug
effects in a later section (see also the chapter by Walsh and
Cummins, this volume).

IV.   INTERLESION EXPERIENCE

Comparatively greater sparing or recovery of function often
occurs when bilateral lesions are spaced in time rather than made
simultaneously (see Finger et al., 1973). Although the mechanisms
underlying this serial lesion phenomenon are not well understood,
the hypotheses reviewed by Lashley (1938) and the others described
earlier in this chapter may account for the observed results.

CNS trauma or Monakow's (1914) concept of diaschisis could be
involved in the staged lesion effect. Successive unilateral
ablations might produce less trauma or inhibition than simultaneous
destruction of tissue. Furthermore, the interlesion interval (ILI)
may provide the time needed for a restoration of presurgical activity
so that, following the second lesion, the trauma or inhibition is not
as great as is the case in the one-stage preparation. Thus, following a postoperative recuperation period the animals with staged
lesions perform more"normally" than do those with simultaneous
ablations.

Alternatively, the mammalian CNS may possess greater capacity
to undergo reorganization when damage occurs in stages. This reorganization might be spontaneous, with remaining tissue assuming
control of behavior; in fact, it has been suggested (e.g., Gold,
1966; Fass et al., 1975) that the intact contralateral homologous

structure is important for recovery during the ILI. In the absence
of a homologous structure, the surrounding tissue becomes important
(see Teitelbaum and Epstein, 1962). It is also possible that reorganization is an active process which is triggered by the initial
unilateral destruction. According to this view, some area of the
brain not necessarily involved in controlling the behavior under
normal circumstances vicariously subsumes the function (e.g., Stein
et al., 1969). These reorganization processes could work together
to render the intact side ultimately less important in regulating
the behavior and thereby allow the organism to more rapidly and/or
fully return towards normal following the second operation.

In previous sections we have reviewed evidence for effects of
preoperative and postoperative experience on behavioral recovery.
Experience occurring between staged lesions confounds this preoperative versus postoperative distinction. If we consider ILI
experience to be postoperative, the relatively smaller amount of
physical trauma, diaschisis, or emergence trauma which might be
associated with a unilateral (versus bilateral) lesion might interfere less with any experiential effect (see Isaacson, 1975, and
Finger et al., 1973, for discussions of trauma interpretations of
the staged lesion phenomenon). Hence, staged lesion experiments may
magnify the consequences of experiential manipulations. Transient
disruption produced by the first lesion might reduce the effectiveness of ILI experience relative to pre-one-stage experience, but
the loss of structures on one side could allow experience to call
vicariously competent regions into play on the undamaged side.
Given this "dual potential" for an effect of interoperative experience, it is perhaps not surprising that some of the best evidence
for experiential facilitation of behavioral recovery comes from
this paradigm.

Most of the experiments to be discussed in this section
examined the effects of various interoperative experiences on the
retention of a presurgically learned habit. In some cases, it was
found that relatively nonspecific sensory stimulation was sufficient
to promote sparing; in others, a more directly relevant experience
was required. The other studies described here deal with the effects
of ILI sexual experience on copulation following two- and one-stage
bulbectomies. The influence of ILI experience on sparing of homeostatic regulatory responses (e.g., feeding) has yet to be explored.

In 1951, Stewart and Ades reported that monkeys subjected to
staged removals of the superior temporal gyrus (with an ILI of
seven days) retained a preoperatively trained auditory avoidance
response. They suggested that this behavioral sparing was mediated
by a spontaneous reorganization which had occurred between surgeries.
This stimulated other researchers to attempt to answer the question:
Are other behaviors spared as a consequence of "spontaneous" reorganization or is sensory stimulation required?

Meyer et al. (1958) studied this question in rats with spaced occipital neocortex ablations. When such animals were kept in total darkness throughout the 12-day ILI, there was no sparing of a pre-operatively learned light avoidance response. Operated animals housed in the light between surgeries retained the habit and, furthermore, did not differ significantly from light-housed sham operates. Thompson (1960), also employing rats with staged occipital lesions, examined postoperative retention following ILI practice on a preoperatively learned brightness discrimination. Animals allowed to practice showed considerable sparing compared to rats which were merely housed in light. Thompson suggested that sparing depended upon ILI practice, rather than mere visual experience.

Petrinovich and Bliss (1966) confirmed both the Meyer et al. (1958) and the Thompson (1960) results; that is, sparing of a black-white discrimination habit was observed in rats given practice on this task during the ILI and in those housed in the light. However, it was reported that the rats given practice had savings scores significantly superior to those of the subjects given visual stimu-lation. Petrinovich and Carew (1969) suggested that the light-housed animals of Thompson (1960) and Petrinovich and Bliss (1966) performed differently due to differences in lesion size, since rats with lesions that amounted to 20% of total neocortex required ILI practice for sparing to occur whereas the rats with 10% of their total neo-cortex damaged needed only to be housed in the light. More recently, Kircher et al. (1970) suggested that the type of ILI experience necessary for promotion of sparing depends upon the behavioral task used to test the animals. Again the relationship between experience and the behavior which is spared appears to be quite specific.

It should be noted that the studies described above can be interpreted in terms of the knowledge and emergence trauma theories presented in the Prelesion Experience section. The former hypothesis would suggest that in order to solve a light avoidance task, all that is necessary is detection of a sudden brightness change, which may be familiar to the damaged animal housed in normal light. For a bright-ness discrimination, more specific experience with relationships among different degrees of brightness might be needed. The Petrinovich and Carew (1969) finding is also consistent with this theory inasmuch as Hebb believed the experience-independent "potential" to depend upon aspects of the lesion, and extent of damage may be one of those aspects.

The emergence trauma notion is also compatible with the reports described above. Evidence of a more transient or less dramatic impairment following unilateral rather than bilateral lesions (e.g., Gold, 1966; Teitelbaum and Epstein, 1962) suggests that a unilateral lesion may alter an organism's perception to a lesser extent than does a simultaneous, bilateral removal of tissue. Once the animal is familiar with the distortions in its perception, the further

distortion produced by destruction of the contralateral homologue
may not be so traumatic. Experience during the ILI may familiarize
the unilaterally-damaged organism with a broader environmental range
such that the animal is less reactive following the second stage of
surgery. If the one-stage organism has a more abruptly altered
perception, then postoperative experience may, as noted earlier,
overload the system and exacerbate any emotional reaction. However,
since the experiments previously cited do not report comparable data
for one-stage animals, this interpretation of the effects of visual
or task-specific experience on sparing as applied to rats with
simultaneous occipital lesions is tentative.

The last theory proposed to account for the influence of prelesion experience on behavioral recovery posits multiple representation of environmental information across various subsystems within
and between various sensory modalities. Perhaps the best evidence
for this theory is that reported by Isaac (1964). In this study,
rats with staged occipital ablations were given ILI's of varying
durations and ILI experiences through varying sensory modalities.
When tested for retention of the preoperatively learned light avoidance task in which shock was accompanied by a buzzer, the animals
exposed to light and noise throughout a 12-day ILI showed greater
sparing than those exposed to light only, noise only, or neither.
Furthermore, the length of the ILI itself proved to affect the
degree of sparing; rats allowed 14 days were superior to those given
12 (both groups housed in darkness and quiet). Thus, Isaac concluded that multimodal sensory experience during the ILI promoted
more behavioral sparing than did unimodal. The effects of interoperative experience on brightness discrimination are similarly
interpretable in these terms if one posits that a representation of
"relative brightness" or "brightness shift" is more easily established in subcortical (or remaining neocortical) visually competent
tissue with the aid of undamaged neocortical visual tissue.

Two more recent studies shed light on the relationship between
experience and the behavioral task employed. Glendenning (1972)
demonstrated that sparing of a preoperatively learned brightness
discrimination depended upon further training between successive
unilateral occipital removals since additional training prior to
single stage surgery or the first of two stages had no effect. Dru
et al. (1975) found that rats allowed to walk around an environment
which had various patterns drawn on the walls for four hours daily
during the ILI showed retention of a presurgically trained pattern
discrimination. Groups of animals which were either transported
through the environment in a container, exposed only to diffuse
light, or housed in total darkness were considerably impaired on
the task when tested after the second occipital lesion. These results
are compatible with the Kircher et al. (1970) suggestion that sparing
is facilitated by a specific experience depending upon the behavioral
test employed.

The effects of ILI experience upon regulatory behavior have been examined in two experiments which interpolated sexual practice between staged removals of the olfactory bulbs. Simultaneous bulbectomy abolishes male mating behavior in mice (Rowe and Edwards, 1972) and hamsters (Murphy and Schneider, 1970). Rowe and Smith (1973) found that sexual performance in mice was not impaired if the ablations were spaced over a 30-day period, whether or not the animals were allowed to mate between surgeries. Experience did not facilitate recovery in the one-stage animals. In contrast, Winans and Powers (1974) were unable to promote sparing with two-stage bulbectomies in hamsters with or without interpolated mating.

The discrepancy between these studies may be due to the less extensive damage produced by the staged lesion procedure in the Rowe and Smith (1973) study. In at least some cases, staged lesions spared portions of the accessory olfactory bulbs, and Powers and Winans (1975) have reported that vomeronasal olfactory input via this structure can support male sexual behavior in the absence of olfactory epithelial input. Hence, it appears that neither staged lesions nor ILI experience cause sparing of this relatively "instinctive" behavior pattern. Studies of experiential effects on other regulatory systems -- particularly homeostatic behaviors such as feeding -- in the staged lesion paradigm would be of considerable interest. Fass et al. (1975) have reported more rapid recovery of feeding and weight gain following staged LH lesions (where ILI feeding experience, of course, occurred).

The results of the staged occipital neocortex ablation studies clearly suggest that interoperative experience may facilitate behavioral sparing or recovery. Furthermore, experience after the first stage lesion may have a greater effect than that same experience prior to the first (or a bilateral) lesion (e.g., Glendenning, 1972).

It should be noted that the staged lesion effect is not always obtained (e.g., Dawson et al., 1973; Isaacson and Schmaltz, 1968; LeVere and Weiss, 1973), a point we have glossed over in this review. Isaacson and Schmaltz (1968), for example, found that the impaired DRL performance following bilateral hippocampal lesions and postoperative CRF training (see Postoperative Experience) was not altered when the lesions were staged and both preoperative and interoperative DRL training was administered. This suggests that this behavior does not survive hippocampal destruction under conditions which, based upon the literature discussed above, might be those most likely to facilitate sparing. Differences among staged lesion and interoperative experience effects across experiments may reflect a number of procedural differences, the most important of which are the lesion location (and size) and the task used. Finger et al. (1973) have also attributed failures to interlesion interval duration, postoperative recovery period, species, and other factors.

Such negative results do not, of course, obviate the
positive findings described above. Interoperative experience clearly
seems to facilitate retention of visual discriminations, the requisite experience depending upon test task and lesion size. While the
results of these studies do not point clearly to a single interpretation of experiential effects, they add to the data which suggest
that passive reorganization or vicarious assumption of behavioral
capacity is not a complete description of the recovery process in
many cases. Even in positive staged lesion experiments in which no
specific ILI experience is provided (e.g., Stein et al., 1969), it
is quite possible that the stimulation available in the ILI environment plays a role in the enhanced recovery.

V.   A NOTE ON GENETIC FACTORS

The prelesion (and interlesion) experience data suggest that
animals' behavior after lesions depends upon its background prior
to the damage. This oversimplification points to an aspect of recovery of function which should be briefly mentioned: the role of
genetic differences. At the extremes, species differences in recovery of function after central nervous system lesions are obvious.
Most invertebrates and lower vertebrates are capable of regenerating
central nervous system axons and in some cases even nerve cell bodies
(Jacobson, 1970). In contrast, neuronal and axonal regeneration are
not characteristic of the adult mammalian central nervous system
(Clemente, 1964), although some growth of atypical axons appears to
occur when dendritic sites are vacated after lesions (e.g., Raisman,
1969; Lynch et al., 1973). Hence recovery of visual function following complete optic tract lesions in amphibians appears to be total
(Sperry, 1943; Jacobson, 1969), while the effects of the same operation in mammals are irreversible. Genetic differences in the response to damage among closely related organisms may be more subtle,
but evidence is accumulating to suggest their importance.

Differences among closely related strains and species in the
brain and behavioral response to environmental conditions during
development have been widely reported (e.g., Cooper and Zubek,
1958; Freeman and Ray, 1972; Henderson, 1970; LaTorre, 1968).
Similarly, sex differences in environmental impact upon development,
as well as in adult nonsexual behavior, are frequently reported
(e.g., Broverman et al., 1968; Freeman and Ray, 1972; Diamond et al.,
1971; Thor et al., 1974), and are described in this volume (see,
e.g., chapters by Sackett, McKinney). Henderson's (1968) caveat
against generalization of early experience results from one sex,
strain, or species is equally applicable to recovery of function
research.

A striking example of sex differences in response to lesions
has been reported by Goldman et al. (1974). Goldman et al. previously

showed that reversal and delayed response performance were spared
following orbital prefrontal neocortex lesions in infant rhesus
monkeys, but that impairments appeared as the subjects matured
(Goldman, 1971). Goldman et al. (1974) found that the onset of
impairment was much earlier in developing male monkeys than in
females, and suggested that orbital neocortex functions develop at
earlier ages in males.

Several reports suggest strain and species differences among
rodents following septal lesions (e.g., Deagle and Lubar, 1971;
Glass and Thomas, 1970; Sodetz et al., 1967). Differential effects
of brain lesions on male and female sexual behavior have been
reported on species ranging from Mantids (Roeder, 1963) to mammals
(Beach, 1940). Since sexual behavior in such species normally shows
dimorphism, differential effects might well be expected. However,
dimorphism in nonsexual behavior exists in many species (e.g.,
Broverman et al., 1968), and this alone could alter the effect of
behavioral substitution and other postlesion recovery mechanisms.
Sex differences in nonsexual behavior following lesions have been
reported in a number of studies, notably following ventromedial
hypothalamic damage. Singh and Meyer (1968) and Cox et al. (1969)
have reported that female rats overeat more and gain more weight than
do males. Milner (1970) describes an anonymous friend who was unable
to obtain the obesity effect in males. There is some evidence that
the sexes also differ in final weight levels following lateral hypothalamic damage (Cox and Kakolewski, 1970). In contrast, Gold (1970)
argued that no sex difference appears when initial weight is equivalent. Even in this study (using parasaggital knife cuts), however,
females gained in absolute weight at a rate 17% higher than that
of males during the first three weeks after the lesion. Gold's
conclusions are based upon comparisons between female weight gain
beginning three weeks after the lesion (when they reached a mean
weight equal to that of males prior to their lesions) and male
weight gain immediately after the lesion. Since both curves are
negatively accelerated functions, this comparison does not seem
appropriate.

Teitelbaum (1973; see also Stein, 1974) has reported sex
differences in recovery of delayed alternation performance following
staged frontal neocortical lesions in rats. Following staged lesions,
male rats showed recovery to nearly the level of male sham-operates,
while females which received staged lesions performed at the level of
single-stage females. Comparable poor performance was seen in single-
stage males and females, despite the fact that sham-operated females
were considerably better than males.

A host of additional studies indicating sex, strain, and species
differences in response to brain damage could be cited. Genetic
differences in response to experience, noted above, could obviously
affect recovery, although no clear patterns have as yet emerged.

The findings indicate that genetic factors must be taken into account in both therapeutic designs and experimental interpretations in recovery from brain damage, as well as in the array of recovery areas covered in this volume.

VI.   A NOTE ON DRUGS AND POSTOPERATIVE AROUSAL

Walsh and Cummins, in this volume, discuss possible contributions of arousal mechanisms to brain development and recovery of function. Various lesions can reduce apparent behavioral arousal and in some cases these effects can be transiently reversed by stimulant drugs or extrinsic stimulation (e.g., Glick, 1974; Herndon and Neill, 1973; Meyer et al., 1963; Wolgin and Teitelbaum, 1974). In other cases, drugs have appeared to aid long-term recovery.

An early experimental paper by Ward and Kennard (1942) summarizes prior clinical findings and reports that strychnine, carbaminol choline, and thiamine enhanced the rate of motor function recovery following unilateral ablation of motor neocortex in monkeys. Watson and Kennard (1945) further found that the anticonvulsant dilantin prevented carbaminol choline facilitation of recovery and that low doses of sodium phenobarbital retarded motor recovery.

A few more recent studies have also suggested that drugs may facilitate behavioral recovery. Cole et al. (1967) reported that administration of amphetamine to dark-housed rats between staged occipital neocortical lesions facilitated performance on a light avoidance task following the second lesion to about the same degree as did visual experience. They suggested that visual experience during this interval might facilitate recovery by increasing arousal. This notion is supported by Isaac's (1964) demonstration that auditory experience potentiated the facilitatory effects of visual experience during the interlesion interval. Glick and Greenstein (1974) reported that alpha-methyl-para-tyrosine, a nonstimulant drug which depletes brain catecholamines, facilitated recovery of feeding after lateral hypothalamic damage. Finally, the Harrell et al. (1974) report that electrical stimulation of the damaged LH similarly facilitated recovery emphasizes the importance of excitatory input.

The data on postoperative drug effects are not sufficiently extensive at this point to allow interpretation. If drugs do facilitate recovery, they may do so by acting directly upon the brain or through interaction with experience. Support for chemotherapeutic action at a brain level might come from the Berger et al. (1973) report that nerve growth factor promoted recovery of feeding after lateral hypothalamic damage. Stenevi et al. (1974) have reported that nerve growth factor facilitated the sprouting of central monaminergic neurons after lesions. However, Berger et al.

have also reported that the stimulation of feeding by norepinephrine following LH lesions is only transient, so the nerve growth factor results quite probably represent a process different from any facilitation reported after stimulant drug administration. Stimulant drugs could potentiate experience effects on behavioral recovery, as Bennett et al. (1973) suggest. They reported that amphetamines potentiated the effects of complex environments on rat brain development, and Peeke et al. (1971) have similarly reported drug-environment synergism with respect to later maze learning. In these cases, it is possible that the drugs increase behavioral arousal and hence the animals' interaction with their environment. However, Will et al. (in preparation) found no potentiation by meth-amphetamine of the effect of enriched rearing on behavioral recovery following neocortical damage. The use of drugs in recovery experiments would seem to demand further attention based upon these reports, as does the role of behavioral arousal in recovery, which is discussed by Walsh and Cummins in this volume.

VII. SUMMARY AND CONCLUSIONS

Our review has indicated that reasonable evidence exists for effects of preoperative, interoperative, and postoperative experience upon behavioral recovery following brain damage. Preoperative experiential and genetic background appears to be an important determinant of postlesion performance as Hebb (1949) and many others predicted and as researchers are currently pointing out with increasing frequency (e.g., Donovick et al., 1973, 1975; Isaacson, 1975; King, 1959). Moreover, preoperative experience may interact with specific types of lesions (e.g., Smith, 1959). A lesion may alter the gain on pre-existing behavioral tendencies (King, 1959), and prior experience may facilitate behavioral substitution, perceptual recognition, or emotional adaptation in the postoperative situation.

Like preoperative background, postoperative experience may ameliorate or exacerbate the behavioral consequences of brain damage. Unless we assume that postoperative experience operates only upon postoperative trauma or imbalance, the fact that post-operative and interoperative experience can play a role suggests that passive reorganization or takeover of function cannot account for all behavioral recovery. Likewise, unless all behavioral re-covery is due to recession of transitory dysfunctional influences, reorganization and/or the shifting of some control of behavior to alternate healthy tissue resources must certainly be involved. The still uncertain potential of stimulant drugs to enhance recovery may further point to both an active recovery process and a thera-peutic tool. The possibility that stimulants may increase post-operative trauma or imbalance must, however, be considered.

The possibility of postlesion emotional trauma resulting from perceptual alterations is rarely considered in the rodent litera- ture (but see Isaacson and Schmaltz, 1968), although it is mentioned in the therapeutic context (e.g., Eidelberg and Stein, 1974) and in association with certain psychiatric treatments (Gallinek, 1956). The apparent importance of emotional trauma to behavioral studies involving gross changes in environmental stimulation (Fuller, 1967; Malzack, 1969; Welch, 1965) strongly suggests that emotional factors not directly related to the effects of the lesion on brain function should be considered in interpretation of results, particularly when testing closely follows the operation. Moreover, this factor could be crucial to the evaluation of the role of experience in behavioral recovery from brain damage.

Finally, as we have noted throughout this chapter, the relation- ship between pre-, post-, and interoperative experience and its behavioral consequences appears to be relatively specific (see also Greenough, 1975; Hunt, this volume). For example, feeding experience may promote feeding recovery after LH lesions and visual experience may affect visual performance after occipital neocortical lesions, but effects of experience on a nonrelated process are rarely report- ed. To an extent, the apparent specificity may result from the expectations of the experimenters: Who would examine the effects of visual experience upon feeding recovery? Transient effects of sensory experience on the behavior of LH lesioned animals have, however, been reported (Wolgin and Teitelbaum, 1974), and an exam- ination of less specific experiential effects may well help to elucidate the mechanisms underlying behavioral recovery. Nonethe- less, both our developmental parallel and the specificity of exper- iential effects even when manipulations are confined to one sensory system (e.g., Dru et al., 1975; Petrinovich and Bliss, 1966) suggest that specificity may be the rule. Even if this is so, an under- standing of the process would be a far more than trivial contribution to both theory and therapy, and this certainly dictates further experimental exploration of the effects of experience on behavioral recovery.

REFERENCES

Ahmad, S.S., and Harvey, J.A. 1968. Long-term effects of septal lesions and social experience on shock-elicited fighting in rats. J. Comp. Physiol. Psychol. 66:596-602.

Anand, B.K., and Brobeck, J.R. 1951. Hypothalamic control of food intake. Yale J. Biol. Med. 24:123-140.

Balagura, S., Harrell, L., and Ralph, T. 1973. Glucodynamic hormones modify the recovery period after lateral hypothalamic lesions. Science 182:59-60.

Bauer, J.H., and Cooper, R.M. 1964. Effects of posterior cortical lesions on performance of a brightness-discrimination task. J. Comp. Physiol. Psychol. 58:84-92.

Bauer, R.H. 1974. Brightness discrimination of pretrained and non-pretrained hippocampal rats reinforced for choosing brighter or dimmer alternatives. J. Comp. Physiol. Psychol. 87:987-996.

Beach, F. 1940. Effects of cortical lesions upon the copulatory behavior of male rats. J. Comp. Psychol. 29:193-244.

Bennett, E.L., Rosenzweig, M.R., and Wu, S.Y.C. 1973. Excitant and depressant drugs modulate effects of environment on brain weight and cholinesterases. Psychopharm. (Berl.) 33:309-328.

Berger, B.D., Wise, C.D., and Stein, L. 1973. Nerve growth factor: Enhanced recovery of feeding after hypothalamic damage. Science 180:506-508.

Bland, B.H., and Cooper, R.M. 1969. Posterior neodecortication in the rat: Age at operation and experience. J. Comp. Physiol. Psychol. 69:345-354.

Bland, B.H., and Cooper, R.M. 1970. Experience and vision of the posterior neodecorticate rat. Physiol. Behav. 5:211-214.

Brady, J.V., and Nauta, W.J.H. 1955. Subcortical mechanisms in emotional behavior: The duration of affective changes following septal and habenular lesions in the albino rat. J. Comp. Physiol. Psychol. 48:412-420.

Broverman, D.M., Klaiber, E.L., Kobayashi, Y., and Vogel, W. 1968. Roles of activation and inhibition in sex differences in cognitive abilities. Psychol. Rev. 75:23-50.

Burright, R.G., Donovick, P.J., and Zuromski, E. 1974. Septal lesion and experiential influences on saline and saccharin preference-aversion functions. Physiol. Behav. 12:951-959.

Campbell, B.A., and Spear, N.E. 1972. Ontogeny of memory. Psychol. Rev. 79:215-236.

Chase, M.H., and Wyrwicka, W. 1973. Electrical stimulation of the brain as reinforcement of food consumption in aphagic cats. Exp. Neurol. 40:153-160.

Chow, K.L., and Survis, L. 1958. Retention of over-learned visual habit after temporal cortical ablation in monkey. AMA Arch. Neurol. Psychiat. 79:640-648.

Clemente, C.D. 1964. Regeneration in the vertebrate central ner-
    vous system. Int. Rev. Neurobiol. 6:257-301.

Cole, D.D., Sullins, W.R., Jr., and Isaac, W. 1967. Pharmacological
    modification of the effects of spaced occipital ablations.
    Psychopharm. (Berl.) 11:311-316.

Cooper, R.M., and Zubek, J.P. 1958. Effects of enriched and re-
    stricted early environments on learning ability of bright and
    dull rats. Canad. J. Psychol. 12:159-164.

Cooper, R.M., Blochert, K.P., Gillespie, L.A., and Miller, L.G.
    1972. Translucent occluders and lesions of posterior neo-
    cortex in the rat. Physiol. Behav. 8:693-697.

Cox, V.C., and Kakolewski, J.W. 1970. Sex differences in body
    weight regulation in rats following lateral hypothalamic
    lesions. Commun. Behav. Biol. 5:195-197.

Cox, V.C., Kakolewski, J.W., and Valenstein, E.S. 1969. Ventro-
    medial hypothalamic lesions and changes in body weight and
    food consumption in male and female rats. J. Comp. Physiol.
    Psychol. 67:320-326.

Dawson, R.G., Conrad, L., and Lynch, G. 1973. Single and two-stage
    hippocampal lesions: A similar syndrome. Exp. Neurol. 40:263-
    277.

Deagle, J.H., and Lubar, J.F. 1971. Effect of septal lesions in
    two strains of rats on one-way and shuttle avoidance acquisi-
    tion. J. Comp. Physiol. Psychol. 77:277-281.

Denenberg, V.H. 1967. Stimulation in infancy, emotional reactivity,
    and exploratory behavior, pp. 161-190. In D.C. Glass (ed.).
    Neurophysiology and Emotion. Rockefeller University Press,
    New York.

Diamond, M.C., Johnson, R.E., and Ingham, C. 1971. Brain plasticity
    induced by environment and pregnancy. Int. J. Neurosci. 2:
    171-178.

DiCara, L.V. 1970. Role of postoperative feeding experience in
    recovery from lateral hypothalamic damage. J. Comp. Physiol.
    Psychol. 72:60-65.

Donovick, P.J., Burright, R.G., and Lustbader, S. 1969. Isotonic
    and hypertonic saline injection following septal lesions.
    Commun. Behav. Biol. 4:17-22.

Donovick, P.J., Burright, R.G., and Swidler, M.A. 1973. Pre-
    surgical rearing environment alters exploration, fluid con-
    sumption, and learning of septal lesioned and control rats.
    Physiol. Behav. 11:543-553.

Donovick, P.J., Burright, R.G., and Bentsen, E.O. 1975. Pre-
    surgical dietary history and the behavior of control and
    septal lesioned rats. Devel. Psychobiol. 8:13-26.

Dru, D., Walker, J.P., and Walker, J.B. 1975. Self-produced loco-
    motion restores visual capacity after striate lesions.
    Science 187:265-266.

Eidelberg, E., and Stein, D.G. (eds.). 1974. Functional recovery
    after lesions of the nervous system. Neurosciences Research
    Program Bull. (Whole No. 12).

Ellen, P., Wilson, A.S., and Powell, E.W. 1964. Septal inhibition
    and timing behavior in the rat. Exp. Neurol. 10:120-132.

Ellen, P., Aitken, W.C., Jr., and Walker, R. 1973. Pretraining
    effects on performance of rats with hippocampal lesions.
    J. Comp. Physiol. Psychol. 84:622-628.

Fass, B., Jordan, H., Rubman, A., Seibel, S., and Stein, D. 1975.
    Recovery of function after serial or one-stage lesions of the
    lateral hypothalamic area in rats. Behav. Biol. 14:283-294.

Finger, S., Walbran, B., and Stein, D.G. 1973. Brain damage and
    behavioral recovery: Serial lesion phenomena. Brain Res. 63:
    1-18.

Fonberg, E., Brutkowski, S., and Mempel, E. 1962. Defensive con-
    ditioned reflexes and neurotic motor reactions following
    amygdalectomy in dogs. Acta Biologiae Experimentalis (Warsaw)
    22:51-57.

Freeman, B.J., and Ray, O.S. 1972. Strain, sex, and environment
    effects on appetitively and aversively motivated learning
    tasks. Devel. Psychobiol. 5:101-109.

Fritsch, G., and Hitzig, E. 1870. Über die electrische Erregbarkeit
    des Grosshirns. Arch. Anat. Physiol. Wiss. Med. 37:300-332.

Fuller, J.L. 1967. Experiential deprivation and later behavior.
    Science 158:1645-1652.

Gallinek, A. 1956. Fear and anxiety in the course of electro-
    shock therapy. Amer. J. Psychiat. 113:428-434.

Gazzaniga, M.S. 1974. Determinants of cerebral recovery, pp. 203-216. In D.G. Stein, J.J. Rosen, and N. Butters (eds.). Plasticity and Recovery of Function in the Central Nervous System. Academic Press, New York.

Gazzaniga, M.S., Szer, I.S., and Crane, A.M. 1974. Modification of drinking behavior in the adipsic rat. Exp. Neurol. 42:483-489.

Glass, J.D., and Thomas, G.J. 1970. Effects of cortical ablations upon recovery from the septal syndrome in hooded rats. Physiol. Behav. 5:879-882.

Glendenning, R.L. 1972. Effects of training between two unilateral lesions of visual cortex upon ultimate retention of black-white discrimination habits by rats. J. Comp. Physiol. Psychol. 80:216-229.

Glick, S.D. 1974. Changes in drug sensitivity and mechanisms of functional recovery following brain damage, pp. 339-372. In D.G. Stein, J.J. Rosen, and N. Butters (eds.). Plasticity and Recovery of Function in the Central Nervous System. Academic Press, New York.

Glick, S.D., and Greenstein, S. 1972. Facilitation of survival following lateral hypothalamic damage by prior food and water deprivation. Psychon. Sci. 28:163-164.

Glick, S.D., and Greenstein, S. 1974. Facilitation of lateral hypothalamic recovery by postoperative administration of a-methyl-p-tyrosine. Brain Res. 73:180-183.

Gold, R.M. 1966. Aphagia and adipsia produced by unilateral hypothalamic lesions in rats. Amer. J. Physiol. 211:1274-1276.

Gold, R.M. 1970. Hypothalamic hyperphagia: Males get just as fat as females. J. Comp. Physiol. Psychol. 71:347-356.

Goldberger, M.E. 1974. Recovery of movement after CNS lesions in monkeys, pp. 265-338. In D.G. Stein, J.J. Rosen, and N. Butters (eds.). Plasticity and Recovery of Function in the Central Nervous System. Academic Press, New York.

Goldman, P.S. 1971. Functional development of the prefrontal cortex in early life and the problem of neuronal plasticity. Exp. Neurol. 32:366-387.

Goldman, P.S. 1974. An alternative to developmental plasticity: Heterology of CNS structures in infants and adults, pp. 149-174. In D.G. Stein, J.J. Rosen, and N. Butters (eds.). Plasticity and Recovery of Function in the Central Nervous

System. Academic Press, New York.

Goldman, P.S., Crawford, H.T., Stokes, L.P., Galkin, T.W., and
    Rosvold, H.E. 1974. Sex-dependent behavioral effects of
    cerebral cortical lesions in the developing rhesus monkey.
    Science 186:540-542.

Gotsick, J.E., and Marshall, R.C. 1972. Time course of the septal
    rage syndrome. Physiol. Behav. 9:685-687.

Greenough, W.T. 1975. Experiential modification of the developing
    brain. Amer. Scientist 63:37-46.

Harrell, L.E., and Balagura, S. 1974. The effects of dark and
    light on the functional recovery following lateral hypothalamic
    lesions. Life Sci. 15:2079-2088.

Harrell, L.E., Raubeson, R., and Balagura, S. 1974. Acceleration
    of functional recovery following lateral hypothalamic damage
    by means of electrical stimulation in the lesioned areas.
    Physiol. Behav. 12:897-899.

Hebb, D.O. 1949. Organization of Behavior. John Wiley & Sons,
    New York.

Hein, A. 1972. Acquiring components of visually guided behavior.
    In A.D. Pick (ed.). Minnesota Symposia on Child Psychology,
    Vol. 6. University of Minnesota Press, Minneapolis.

Held, R., and Hein, A. 1963. Movement produced stimulation in the
    development of visually-guided behavior. J. Comp. Physiol.
    Psychol. 56:872-876.

Henderson, N.D. 1968. The confounding effects of genetic variables
    in early experience research: Can we ignore them? Devel.
    Psychobiol. 1:146-152.

Henderson, N.D. 1970. Brain weight increases resulting from
    environmental enrichment: A directional dominance in mice.
    Science 169:776-778.

Herndon, J.G., and Neill, D.B. 1973. Amphetamine reversal of
    sexual impairment following anterior hypothalamic lesions in
    female rats. Pharmacol., Biochem., Behav. 1:285-288.

Hetherington, A.W., and Ranson, S.W. 1940. Hypothalamic lesions
    and adiposity in the rat. Anat. Rec. 78:149-172.

Hicks, S.P., and D'Amato, C.J. 1970. Motor-sensory behavior after
    hemispherectomy in newborn and mature rats. Exp. Neurol. 29:

416-438.

Horel, J.A., Bettinger, L.A., Royce, G.J., and Meyer, D.R. 1966.
    Role of neocortex in the learning and relearning of two visual
    habits by the rat. J. Comp. Physiol. Psychol. 61:66-78.

Hubel, D.H. 1967. Effects of distortion of sensory input on the
    visual system of kittens. The Physiologist 10:17-45.

Hubel, D.H., and Wiesel, T.N. 1970. The period of susceptibility
    to the physiological effects of unilateral eye closure in
    kittens. J. Physiol. 206:419-436.

Hughes, K.R. 1965. Dorsel and ventral hippocampus lesions and
    maze learning:Influence of preoperative environment. Canad.
    J. Psychol. 19:325-332.

Isaac, W. 1964. Role of stimulation and time in the effects of
    spaced occipital ablations. Psychol. Rep. 14:151-154.

Isaacson, R.L. 1975. The myth of recovery from early brain damage.
    In N.R. Ellis (ed.). Aberrant Development in Infancy.
    Lawrence Erlbaum Associates, Potomac.

Isaacson, R.L., and Kimble, D.P. 1972. Lesions of the limbic
    system: Their effects upon hypotheses and frustration. Behav.
    Biol. 7:767-793.

Isaacson, R.L., and Schmaltz, L.W. 1968. Failure to find savings
    from spaced, two-stage destruction of hippocampus. Commun.
    Behav. Biol. 1:353-359.

Iwanow-Smolenski, A.G. 1954. Gründzuge der Pathophysiologie der
    höheren Nerventätigkeit. Akademie Verlag, Berlin.

Jacobson, M. 1969. Development of specific neuronal connections.
    Science 163:543-547.

Jacobson, M. 1970. Developmental Neurobiology. Holt, Rinehart &
    Winston, New York.

Johnson, D.A., Poplawski, A., Bieliauskas, L., and Liebert, D.
    1972. Recovery of function on a two-way conditioned avoidance
    task following sptal lesions in infancy: Effects of early
    handling. Brain Res. 45:282-287.

Kennard, M.A. 1936. Age and other factors in motor recovery from
    precentral lesions in monkeys. Amer. J. Physiol. 115:138-146.

Kennard, M.A. 1938. Reorganization of motor function in the cere-
    bral cortex of monkeys deprived of motor and premotor areas in
    infancy. J. Neurophysiol. 1:477-496.

Kimble, D.P. 1968. Hippocampus and internal inhibition. Psychol.
    Bull. 70:285-295.

King, F.A. 1958. Effects of septal and amygdaloid lesions on
    emotional behavior and conditioned avoidance responses in the
    rat. J. Nerv. Mental Dis. 126:57-63.

King, F.A. 1959. Relationship of the "septal syndrome" to genetic
    differences in emotionality in the rat. Psychol. Rep. 5:11-17.

Kircher, K.A., Braun, J.J., Meyer, D.R., and Meyer, P.M. 1970.
    Equivalence of simultaneous and successive neocortical ablations
    in production of impairments of retention of black-white habits
    in rats. J. Comp. Physiol. Psychol. 71:474-480.

Krieckhaus, E.E., Simmons, H.J., Thomas, G.J., and Kenyon, J. 1964.
    Septal lesions enhance shock avoidance behavior in the rat.
    Exp. Neurol. 9:107-113.

Lashley, K.S. 1929. Brain Mechanisms and Intelligence. University
    of Chicago Press, Chicago.

Lashley, K.S. 1935. The mechanism of vision: XII. Nervous struc-
    tures concerned in habits based on reactions to light. Comp.
    Psychol. Monog. 11:43-79.

Lashley, K.S. 1938. Factors limiting recovery after central nervous
    lesions. J. Nerv. Ment. Dis. 88:733-755.

LaTorre, J.C. 1968. Effect of differential environmental enrichment
    on brain weight and on acetylcholinesterase and cholinesterase
    activities in mice. Exp. Neurol. 22:493-503.

Lenneberg, E.H. 1967. Biological Foundations of Language. Wiley, N.Y.

LeVere, T.E., and Morlock, G.W. 1973. Nature of visual recovery
    following posterior neodecortication in the hooded rat. J.
    Comp. Physiol. Psychol. 83:62-67.

LeVere, T., and Weiss, J. 1973. Failure of seriatum dorsal hippo-
    campal lesions to spare spatial reversal behavior in rats.
    J. Comp. Physiol. Psychol. 82:205-210.

Lukaszewska, I., and Thompson, R. 1967. Retention of an over-
    trained pattern discrimination following pretectal lesion in
    rats. Psychon. Sci. 8:121-122.

Luria, A.R., Naydin, V.L., Tsvetkova, L.S., and Vinarskaya, E.N.
     1969. Restoration of higher cortical function following
     local brain damage. In R.J. Vinken and G.W. Bruyn (eds.).
     Handbook of Clinical Neurology, Vol. 3. North-Holland,
     Amsterdam.

Lynch, G., Stanfield, B., and Cotman, C.W. 1973. Developmental
     differences in post-lesion axonal growth in the hippocampus.
     Brain Res. 59:155-168.

Marshall, J.F., and Teitelbaum, P. 1974. Further analysis of sens-
     ory inattention following lateral hypothalamic damage in rats.
     J. Comp. Physiol. Psychol. 86:375-395.

Marshall, J.F., Turner, B.H., and Teitelbaum, P. 1971. Sensory
     neglect produced by lateral hypothalamic damage. Science 174:
     523-525.

Melzack, R. 1969. The role of early experience in emotional
     arousal. Ann. N.Y. Acad. Sci. 159:721-730.

Meyer, D.R., Isaac, W., and Maher, B. 1958. The role of stimula-
     tion in spontaneous reorganization of visual habits. J.
     Comp. Physiol. Psychol. 51:546-548.

Meyer, P.M., Horel, J.A., and Meyer, D.R. 1963. Effects of dl-
     amphetamine upon placing responses in neodecorticate cats.
     J. Comp. Physiol. Psychol. 56:402-404.

Miller, L.G., and Cooper, R.M. 1974. Translucent occluders and the
     role of visual cortex in pattern vision. Brain Res. 79:45-59.

Miller, N.E., Bailey, C.J., and Stevenson, J.A.F. 1950. Decreased
     "hunger" but increased food intake resulting from hypothalamic
     lesions. Science 112:256-259.

Milner, B. 1974. Hemispheric specialization: Scope and limitations.
     In F.O. Schmitt and F.G. Worden (eds.). The Neurosciences
     Third Study Program. MIT Press, Cambridge.

Milner, P.M. 1970. Physiological Psychology. Holt, Rinehart &
     Winston, New York.

Monakow, C.V. 1914. Die Lokalisation im Grosshirn und der Abbau
     der Funktion durch korticale Herde. Excerpted in K.H. Pribram
     (ed.). Brain and Behavior. I. Mood, States and Mind. 1969.
     Penguin Books, Baltimore.

Murphy, M.R., and Schneider, G.E. 1970. Olfactory bulb removal
     eliminates mating behavior in the male golden hamster.

Science 167:302-303.

Noell, W.K., and Albrecht, R. 1971. Irreversible effects of visible light on the retina: Role of Vitamin A. Science 172:76-79.

Nonneman, A.J., and Isaacson, R.L. 1973. Task dependent recovery after early brain damage. Behav. Biol. 8:143-172.

Orbach, J., and Fantz, R.L. 1958. Differential effects of temporal neocortical resection on overtrained and nonovertrained visual habits in monkeys. J. Comp. Physiol. Psychol. 51:126-129.

Peeke, H.V.S., LeBoeuf, B.J., and Herz, M.J. 1971. The effect of strychnine administration during development on adult maze learning in the rat, II: Drug administration from day 51-70. Psychopharm. (Berl.) 19:262-265.

Petrinovich, L., and Bliss, D. 1966. Retention of a learned brightness discrimination following ablations of the occipital cortex in the rat. J. Comp. Physiol. Psychol. 61:136-138.

Petrinovich, L., and Carew, T.J. 1969. Interaction of neocortical lesion size and interoperative experience in retention of a learned brightness discrimination. J. Comp. Physiol. Psychol. 68:451-454.

Powers, J.B., and Winans, S.S. 1975. Vomeronasal organ: Critical role in sexual behavior of the male hamster. Science 187: 961-963.

Powley, T.L., and Keesey, R.E. 1970. Relationship of body weight to the lateral hypothalamic feeding syndrome. J. Comp. Physiol. Psychol. 70:25-36.

Raisman, G. 1969. Neuronal plasticity in the septal nuclei of the adult rat. Brain Res. 14:25-48.

Roeder, K.D. 1963. Nerve cells and insect behavior. Harvard University Press, Cambridge.

Rosenzweig, M.R. 1971. Effects of environment on development of brain and of behavior. In E. Tobach (ed.). Biopsychology of Development. Academic Press, New York.

Rosner, B.S. 1970. Brain functions. In P.H. Mussen and M.R. Rosenzweig (eds.). Annual Review of Psychology, Vol. 21. Annual Reviews, Palo Alto.

Rowe, F.A., and Edwards, D.A. 1972. Olfactory bulb removal: Influences on the mating behavior of male mice. Physiol. Behav. 8:37-41.

Rowe, F.A., and Smith, W.E. 1973. Simultaneous and successive ol-
    factory bulb removal. Influences on the mating behavior of
    male mice. Physiol. Behav. 10:443-449.

Sarno, M.T., Silverman, M., and Sands, E. 1970. Speech therapy
    and language recovery in severe aphasia. J. Speech &
    Hearing Res. 13:607-625.

Schmaltz, L.W., and Isaacson, R.L. 1966. The effects of preliminary
    training conditions upon DRL performance in the hippocampecto-
    mized rat. Physiol. Behav. 1:175-182.

Schmaltz, L.W., and Isaacson, R.L. 1968. The effect of blindness
    on DRL-20 performances exhibited by animals with hippocampal
    destruction. Psychon. Sci. 11:241-242.

Schwartz, M., and Teitelbaum, P. 1974. Dissociation between learn-
    ing and remembering in rats with lesions in the lateral hypo-
    thalamus. J. Comp. Physiol. Psychol. 87:384-398.

Schwartz, S. 1964. Effect of neocortical lesions and early environ-
    mental factors on adult rat behavior. J. Comp. Physiol.
    Psychol. 57:72-77.

Scott, J.P. 1968. The process of primary socialization in the dog.
    In G. Newton and S. Levine (eds.). Early Experience and
    Behavior. C. C. Thomas, Springfield, Il.

Scott, J.P., Stewart, J.M., and DeGhett, V.J. 1974. Critical
    periods in the organization of systems. Devel. Psychobiol.
    7:489-513.

Seggie, J. 1968. Effect of somatosensory stimulation on affective
    behavior of septal rats. J. Comp. Physiol. Psychol. 66:820-
    822.

Semmes, J., Weinstein, S. Ghent, L., and Teuber, H.L. 1954.
    Performance on complex tactual tasks after brain injury in man:
    Analyses by locus of lesion. Amer. J. Physiol. 67:220-240.

Singh, D. 1973. Effects of preoperative training on food-motivated
    behavior of hypothalamic hyperphagic rats. J. Comp. Physiol.
    Psychol. 84:47-52.

Singh, D. 1974. Role of preoperative experience on reaction to
    quinine taste in hypothalamic hyperphagic rats. J. Comp.
    Physiol. Psychol. 86:674-678.

Singh, D., and Meyer, D.R. 1968. Eating and drinking by rats with
    lesions of the septum and the ventromedial hypothalamus. J.
    Comp. Physiol. Psychol. 65:163-166.

Smith, C.J. 1959. Mass action and early environment. J. Comp. Physiol. Psychol. 52:154-156.

Sodetz, F.J., Matalka, E.S., and Bunnell, B.N. 1967. Septal ablation and affective behavior in the golden hamster. Psychon. Sci. 7:189-190.

Sperry, R.W. 1943. Visuomotor coordination in the newt (Triturus viridescens) after regeneration of the optic nerve. J. Comp. Neurol. 79:33-55.

Stein, D.G. 1974. Some variables influencing recovery of function after central nervous system lesions in the rat, pp. 373-428. In D. G. Stein, J.J. Rosen, and N. Butters (eds.). Plasticity and Recovery of Function in the Central Nervous System. Academic Press, New York.

Stein, D.G., Rosen, J.J., Graziadei, J. Mishkin, D., and Brink, J.J. 1969. Central nervous system: Recovery of function. Science 166:528-530.

Stenevi, U., Bjerre, B., Björklund, A., and Mobley, W. 1974. Effects of localized intracerebral injections of nerve growth factor on the regenerative growth of lesioned central nora-drenergic neurons. Brain Res. 69:217-234.

Stern, P., McDowell, F., Miller, J.M., and Robinson, M. 1971. Factors influencing stroke rehabilitation. Stroke 2:213-218.

Stewart, J.W., and Ades, H.W. 1951. The time factor in reintegra-tion of a learned habit after temporal lobe lesions in the monkey. J. Comp. Physiol. Psychol. 44:479-486.

Stricker, E.M., and Zigmond, M.J. 1975. Recovery of function following damage to central catecholamine-containing neurons: A neurochemical model for the lateral hypothalamic syndrome. In J.M. Sprague and A.N. Epstein (eds.). Progress in Psychobiology and Physiological Psychology, Vol. 6. Academic Press, New York (in press).

Suomi, S.J., Harlow, H.F., and McKinney, W.T., Jr. 1972. Monkey psychiatrists. Amer. J. Psychiat. 128:927-932.

Tees, R.C. 1975. The effects of neonatal striate lesions and visual experience on form discrimination in the rat. Canad. J. Psychol. Rev. Canad. Psychol. 29:66-85.

Tees, R.C. Depth perception after infant and adult visual neo-cortical lesions in light- and dark-reared rats. Devel. Psychobiol., in press.

Teitelbaum, B. 1973. Sex differences in delayed alternation performance following single or multiple stage frontal lesions in rats. Paper presented at 81st Annual Convention of American Psychological Association in Montreal, Quebec, August 29.

Teitelbaum, P. 1957. Random and food-directed activity in hyperphagic and normal rats. J. Comp. Physiol. Psychol. 50:486-490.

Teitelbaum, P. 1967. The biology of drive. In F.O. Schmitt (ed.). The Neurosciences, A Study Program, Vol. 1. The Rockefeller University Press, New York.

Teitelbaum, P., and Epstein, A.N. 1962. The lateral hypothalamic syndrome: Recovery of feeding and drinking after lateral hypothalamic lesions. Psychol. Rev. 69:74-90.

Teuber, H.-L. 1974a. Why two brains? In F.O. Schmitt and F.G. Worden (eds.). The Neurosciences Third Study Program. The MIT Press, Cambridge.

Teuber, H.-L. 1974b. Recovery of function after lesions of the central nervous system: History and prospects. In E. Eidelberg and D.G. Stein (eds.). Functional Recovery after Lesions of the Nervous System. Neurosciences Research Program Bulletin, 197-200.

Teuber, H.-L., and Rudel, R.G. 1962. Behavior after cerebral lesions in children and adults. Devel. Med. Child. Neurol. 4:3-20.

Thatcher, R.W., and Kimble, D.P. 1966. Effect of amygdaloid lesions on retention of an avoidance response in overtrained and nonovertrained rats. Psychon. Sci. 6:9-10.

Thompson, R. 1960. Retention of a brightness discrimination following neocortical damage in the rat. J. Comp. Physiol. Psychol. 53:212-215.

Thompson, R. 1965. Centrencephalic theory and interhemispheric transfer of visual habits. Psychol. Rev. 72:385-398.

Thompson, R. 1969. Localization of the "visual memory system" in the white rat. J. Comp. Physiol. Psychol. Monog. 69:4, pt. 2.

Thor, D.H., Ghiselli, W.B., and Ward, T.B. 1974. Infantile handling and sex differences in shock-elicited aggressive responding of hooded rats. Devel. Psychobiol. 7:273-279.

Tower, S.S. 1940. Pyramidal lesion in the monkey. Brain 63:36-90.

Tsang, Y.C. 1937a. Maze learning in rats hemidecorticated in infancy. J. Comp. Psychol. 24:221-254.

Tsang, Y.C. 1937b. Visual sensitivity in rats deprived of visual cortex in infancy. J. Comp. Psychol. 24:255-262.

Ward, A.A., Jr., and Kennard, M.A. 1942. Effect of cholinergic drugs on recovery of function following lesions of the central nervous system in monkeys. Yale J. Biol. & Med. 15:189-229.

Watson, C.W., and Kennard, M.A. 1945. The effect of anticonvulsant drugs on recovery of function following cerebral cortical lesions. J. Neurophysiol. 8:221-231.

Weese, G.D., Neimand, D., and Finger, S. 1973. Cortical lesions and somesthesis in rats: Effects of training and overtraining prior to surgery. Exp. Brain Res. 16:542-550.

Weinstein, S., and Teuber, H.-L. 1957. The role of preinjury education and intelligence level in intellectual loss after brain injury. J. Comp. Physiol. Psychol. 50:535-539.

Weinstein, S., Teuber, H.-L., Ghent, L., and Semmes, J. 1955. Complex visual task performance after penetrating brain injury in man. Amer. Psychol. 10:408 (abst.).

Welch, B.L. 1965. Psychophysiological response to the mean level of environmental stimulation: A theory of environmental integration, pp. 39-96. In D.M. Rioch (ed.). Medical Aspects of Stress in the Military Climate. U.S. Government Printing Office, Washington, D.C.

Wepman, J.M. 1951. Recovery from Aphasia. Ronald Press Co., New York.

Wheatley, M.D. 1944. The hypothalamus and affective behavior in cats. Arch. Neurol. Psychiat. (Chicago) 52:296-316.

Will, B.E., Rosenzweig, M.R., and Bennett, E.L. Effects of differential environments on recovery from neonatal brain lesions, measured by problem-solving scores and brain dimensions. In preparation.

Will, B.E., Rosenzweig, M.R., Bennett, E.L., Hebert, M., and Morimoto, H. Relatively brief environmental enrichment aids recovery of learning capacity and alters brain measures after postweaning brain lesions in rats. In preparation.

Winans, S.S., and Powers, J.B. 1974. Neonatal and two-stage olfactory bulbectomy: Effects on male hamster sexual behavior. Behav. Biol. 10:461-471.

Wolgin, D.L., and Teitelbaum, P. 1974. The role of activation
    and sensory stimuli in the recovery of feeding following
    lateral hypothalamic lesions in the cat. Paper presented at
    the Eastern Psychological Association meetings, Philadelphia,
    April 18-20.

Worthington, C.S., and Isaac, W. 1967. Occipital ablation and
    retention of a visual conditioned avoidance response in the
    rat. Psychon. Sci. 8:289-290.

MALNUTRITION AND EARLY ENVIRONMENTAL EXPERIENCE:

POSSIBLE INTERACTIVE EFFECTS ON LATER BEHAVIOR

Seymour Levine and Sandra G. Wiener

Department of Psychiatry and Behavioral Sciences
Stanford University School of Medicine
Stanford, California 94305

I.   INTRODUCTION

The lack of adequate food supplies is a pressing problem for a considerable portion of the world's population. However, as yet researchers have not been able to isolate the specific effects of malnutrition during the early developmental years on later human mental function. As Richardson notes in this volume, human malnutrition rarely occurs under circumstances which are not detrimental in many other ways. In order to attempt a more controlled investigation of the mechanisms which may be involved in the influence of early malnutrition on later behavior, many investigators have turned to animal models. Most of the studies on biochemical changes in the brain under conditions of early malnutrition have used animals for obvious reasons. There now exists an extensive literature on the effects of early malnutrition on biochemical, physiological, and behavioral processes in animals.

It is our contention that there is an apparent lack of appreciation on the part of many investigators of the early environmental determinants of physiological and behavioral events. Thus, many of the animal malnutrition studies, as with most human studies, are difficult to interpret because of uncontrolled non-nutritional environmental factors. The purpose of this paper is to demonstrate that the existing animal models of malnutrition are confounded by a variety of environmental variables which may interact with early malnutrition to cause the behavioral differences which are observed in adulthood. In many instances the differences attributed to impoverished diets may not be related to malnutrition at all, but rather to one or another of the artifacts that result from the failure to control these psychosocial factors.

51

A review of the animal malnutrition literature reveals a remarkable set of inconsistencies with regard to both methodologies and results. These inconsistencies are disturbing in view of the sweeping generalizations about the effects of early malnutrition which have been made from animal models. When one examines carefully the approaches to the problem of using animal models in this field, there appear to be three relevant variables, all of which presumably can affect the subsequent outcome. The first is the age at which the malnutrition is begun and the length of time it is imposed. Malnutrition can be induced prenatally either at conception or during the second or third trimester of gestation. This can be accomplished by restricting the mother's intake of food or reducing the protein content of her diet. Such manipulations, while drastically altering the nutritional status of the mother, have an undetermined effect on the nutritional status of the fetus. Postnatally, malnutrition can be imposed for varying lengths of time during the suckling period or after weaning. Malnutrition has been imposed at each of these points in time and in any number of permutations and combinations. Since there have been few intensive investigations to determine the critical age at which malnutrition must occur to cause long-term effects, it is difficult to compare studies.

The second variable is the method used to produce malnutrition. Pups can be nutritionally deprived by altering the quality/quantity of the milk. The quantity of milk available to each pup can be reduced either by increasing the number of pups in the litter or by reducing the milk production of the mother. The quality of the pups' diet can be modified by artificially feeding a synthetic diet. The assumption that has been pervasive in the field is that all forms of protein-calorie malnutrition are the same. We hope to show in this review that the different methods of producing malnutrition can lead to different consequences.

The third, and perhaps the most critical variable, is the fact that the type of testing used to assess the consequences of early malnutrition has varied so markedly from laboratory to laboratory as to prevent any generalizations about the effects of early malnutrition on later behavior. Malnourished animals have been examined for changes in emotionality and/or learning by many different tasks. Unfortunately, the naive assumption has been made that learning is the same under all circumstances. Animals have been tested at a variety of different ages with little consideration being given to the experiences that intervene between the termination of malnutrition and the onset of testing. In many situations the animals have been tested while they are still malnourished. Under these conditions, the behavior may be affected by the physical debilitation of the animal, independent of any change in its intellectual functioning.

This paper will focus on an examination of the influence of **early** protein-calorie malnutrition on at least one aspect of behavior in the rehabilitated adult animal. Thus, the results of studies which only test the malnourished subject during infancy (Altman et al., 1971; Smart and Dobbing, 1971a,b; Sobotka et al., 1974) or before nutritional rehabilitation is begun while the adult is still malnourished (Cowley and Griesel, 1959, 1962, 1963, 1964) will not be discussed. The review will be limited to data reported for the rat, the species most frequently used as an animal model to determine the effects of malnutrition on physiology and behavior. The use of the rat as a model of human development has been discussed elsewhere (Dobbing, 1971, 1974) and will not be considered here. The material to be covered will also be limited to studies where malnutrition is imposed during the prenatal and/or early postnatal (preweaning) period. It is this perinatal period in the rat that several investigators (Dobbing and Sands, 1971; Dobbing et al., 1971; Winick and Noble, 1965, 1966; Winick et al., 1972; Zamenhof et al., 1968) have suggested is the critical period during which malnutrition causes irreversible deficits in brain cell number, even when nutritional rehabilitation is begun at weaning. Malnutrition begun after these early weeks of life does not appear to cause biochemical changes which cannot be reversed by subsequent refeeding. Thus, behavioral studies where the malnutrition is begun at weaning (Barnett et al., 1971; Griffiths and Senter, 1954; Mandler, 1958) or later (Rajalakshmi et al., 1965) will not be included. The biochemical changes found in the perinatally malnourished rat have received a great deal of attention. Given these deficits in the brains of early malnourished animals, it is easy to make the inferential leap from neurochemical deficits to functional deficits in behavior. It is our contention that such an assumption is tentative at best, and more likely erroneous under most circumstances.

II. TECHNIQUES FOR PRODUCING MALNUTRITION IN INFANT RATS

In the laboratory there have been a variety of methods used to produce perinatal protein-calorie malnutrition in rodents (Plaut, 1970). All methods attempt to limit the amount of milk available to the pup during the preweaning period. These methods include (a) removing the mother from the nest for several hours each day (Eayrs and Horn, 1955); (b) increasing the litter size to 15-20 pups per mother (Kennedy, 1957); (c) restricting the amount of control (high protein) diet available to the mother (Chow and Lee, 1964); (d) allowing the mother unlimited access to a low protein diet (Barnes et al., 1968); and (e) artificially feeding the neonate either mechanically by gastric infusion (Hofer, 1973; Messer et al., 1969) or manually by means of an intubation technique (Miller and Dymsza, 1963).

Separating the pups from the mother is a procedure which removes

not only the mother as a source of nutrition but also as a source
of social, thermal, and sensory stimulation. During the period the
pups are away from their mother they have been kept in the nest in
the home cage or in an incubator to maintain body temperature.
Slob et al. (1973), attempting to control for the missing non-
nutritive maternal components, allowed the pups to stay with a non-
nutritive mother substitute ("aunt"). The "aunt" was a virgin
female that showed the complete complement of maternal behavior
(except lactation) because of prior daily exposure to pups (Rosenblatt, 1967). It is interesting to note that Slob and his co-
workers found no effect on adult behavior from this technique of
producing early malnutrition compared to a nonseparated control
group. Unfortunately, there was no malnourished group which was
removed from the nutritive mother without the mother substitute,
to determine if there are behavioral consequences of this type of
nutritional deprivation. In fact, Rajalakshmi et al. (1967) reported
that mother-separated offspring kept in an incubator during separation did not differ from nonseparated controls on a visual discrimination task in adulthood. Thus, it is impossible to determine
if the replacement mother ameliorated behavioral deficiencies, or
whether these deficits ever existed in the first place.

The large versus small litter method also is subject to many
confounding variables which make it difficult to isolate the influence of malnutrition from other early psychosocial variables.
This method assumes that since there are more pups than nipples,
each pup will get less access to the milk source. However, variation in the individual body weights within a single litter suggests
that some pups are more successful in competing for the limited
number of nipples (Galler and Turkewitz, 1975). Thus, pup interaction and the effects of crowding in the nest may also be important determinants of later behavior. In addition, there is competition for the amount of maternal attention each pup gets. Seitz
(1954) observed that mothers assigned six pups behaved significantly
more maternally than mothers given litters of 12. Grota and Ader
(1969) found that given a choice, the mother of a litter of 12 rats
will spend up to 40% less time in the same cage with her litter
over a 24-hour period than will a mother of a litter of four pups.
Thus it appears that pups raised in large litters are deprived of
all aspects of maternal contact for a greater proportion of the day.

Limiting the amount of diet fed to the mother to some percentage of the normal intake of a lactating female is a method utilized
to decrease the amount of milk produced by the mammary glands
(Mueller and Cox, 1946). If the restriction of intake is begun
during pregnancy, prenatal effects of this nutritional deprivation
of the mother can be investigated. Nutritionally, this technique
is subject to criticism since the mother is subjected to a deprivation of all components of her diet -- protein, carbohydrates, fats,
vitamins and minerals. Thus, the exact dietary component responsible

for the effects seen in the pups cannot be determined. In addition, it would not be surprising to find that maternal behavior is disrupted in some manner under these conditions of food restriction. Anecdotal evidence was reported by Simonson et al. (1969) that "Restricted mothers are not, in general, good mothers. They are preoccupied by the search for food and are highly irritable." Smart and Preece (1973) noted that diet-restricted mothers displayed a daily pattern of nest occupation and desertion during lactation that was quite different from control mothers fed ad libitum. In addition, deficits in retrieval and licking behavior were also noted in these diet-restricted mothers. Stern and Levin (in press) have demonstrated that feeding lactating mothers only during their lights-on period can cause a shifting of the normal circadian rhythm of maternal behavior. Thus, this method also appears to disrupt the normal mother-infant relationship.

The next method to be discussed seeks to reduce the milk production of the lactating female by the unrestricted feeding of a diet which has been modified to lower its protein content without changing its caloric, vitamin, or mineral value. Control diets for pregnant and lactating rats have contained approximately 20-26% protein, while experimental diets have ranged from 8% to 14% protein. As with the last technique, the feeding of a low protein diet can be instituted during gestation to cause prenatal malnutrition. It was hoped that since the mother had free access to an isocaloric diet, her maternal behavior would be minimally disturbed by this method. However, recent reports by Fraňková (1971, 1974a), Massaro et al. (1974), and from our own laboratory (Levin et al., in preparation) indicate that this assumption is not valid. Fraňková (1971) reported that mothers fed a low protein diet took longer and retrieved fewer pups than control mothers. Massaro et al. (1974) demonstrated that mothers fed low protein diets spent more time in the nest with their litters during the lights-off period. Our laboratory found that the malnourished mothers spent more time in the nest in an active nursing posture during both lights-on and off, but spent less time licking their pups and were poorer retrievers than nondeprived mothers. Thus, a mother fed a low protein diet shows a change in her maternal behavior. The direction of this change cannot be easily classified as a deficit or an improvement since it depends on the specific behavior tested. It would be of interest to determine if these alterations in maternal behavior are due to the fact the mother is herself receiving a low protein diet or due to her raising a litter of small pups.

The last method, intragastric feeding, allows the experimenter to manipulate the diet of the newborn rat most precisely. In addition to limiting the quantity of milk, this technique permits the investigator to alter the protein:carbohydrate:fat ratio of the diet (Dymsza et al., 1964). However, this procedure suffers the disadvantage of being technically more difficult and time-consuming

for the investigator. Though artificially fed pups are often given
an "aunt" to perform non-nutritive maternal functions, the amount
of handling by the investigator required in this technique constitutes a major intervention into the early environment of the pup.

Thus it should be apparent that none of the above methods are
free from confounding environmental variables produced by changes in
the early social environment of the neonatal rat. Alterations in
the mother-infant environment of the rodent can produce extensive
behavioral changes in the adult (Denenberg et al., 1968; Levine and
Thoman, 1969; Thoman and Levine, 1969). It therefore becomes difficult to isolate the effects of the early malnutrition from the
effects resulting from the disruption of the normal mother-infant
environment.

III. OPEN FIELD BEHAVIOR OF PERINATALLY MALNOURISHED RATS

The behavior of early malnourished animals has been studied in
a wide variety of situations. Rather than attempting an extensive
review of the literature concerned with the later behavioral effects
of perinatal malnutrition during development, we will concentrate
on one behavioral testing situation, the open field. We believe
that the studies that have been conducted using this paradigm illustrate most of the problems that are prevalent in the area.

For several decades experimental psychologists have been using
the open field as a test to measure the response of organisms to
novel environments. The open field was originally developed by Hall
(1934, 1936, 1941) and was assumed to be a test for emotionality.
The open field usually consists of an arena of varying dimensions in
which the animal is either placed or required to enter. Emotionality in the rat was measured by the activity level and defecation
in response to an environment to which the animal had never been
previously exposed. Activity levels and defecation have proven to
be sensitive to many variables, including genetics (Broadhurst,
1969), early handling (Denenberg, 1969a; Levine et al., 1967), and
preshock (Levine et al., 1973; Stern et al., 1973). For reviews of
current perspectives on the use of the open field as a test of
emotionality, see papers by Denenberg (1969b), Archer (1973), and
Walsh and Cummins (1975).

Several investigators have used an open field to study the
behavior of the offspring of perinatally diet-restricted mothers.
In these studies the mothers were restricted during gestation and
lactation to 50% of their normal food intake. To determine the
relative effects of pre- or postnatal deprivation alone, the offspring were cross-fostered. [Changing the mother's diet at parturition is not recommended because of the delay between the diet
change and the subsequent reduction in milk supply (Miller, 1968).]

The pups were weaned onto an adequate diet, provided ad libitum, and tested as adults in the open field.

Simonson et al. (1971) compared the open field performance of prenatally malnourished to control diet offspring at 26 weeks of age. The prenatally malnourished subjects were less active (as measured by their longer latency to leave the entry square and smaller number of squares crossed) and defecated more frequently than control subjects. In a follow-up study (Hsueh et al., 1973) the relative importance of pre- and postnatal deprivation was investigated. Subjects which were deprived both pre- and postnatally were the least active and defecated the most when tested at 76 weeks of age. Subjects deprived only prenatally appeared to be more severely affected than those deprived solely postnatally, though both were significantly less active and defecated more than control subjects. Thus, these investigators concluded that perinatally malnourished subjects were more emotional.

Smart's results (1974), on the other hand, are directly opposite to those reported by Simonson and her co-workers (Hsueh et al., 1973; Simonson et al., 1971). With the exception that the mothers were diet-restricted at seven days of gestation rather than at conception, the technique for producing malnourished offspring was the same. Offspring of mothers both pre- and postnatally restricted were more active (number of squares crossed and frequency of rearing) and defecated less than controls when tested at 16 weeks of age. Thus, Smart concluded that perinatally malnourished subjects were less emotional.

Finally, Ottinger and Tanabe (1968), using a nutritional protocol similar to the above studies, found that neither the number of squares crossed nor the amount of defecation differentiated the subjects that had been malnourished (pre- or postnatally or both) from controls when tested at seven weeks of age.

Although the above open field results were obtained using the same method for producing perinatal malnutrition, a direct comparison of the experiments is difficult because of large variations in the parameters of the testing situation used in each study. For example, the age of testing varied from seven weeks of age (Ottinger and Tanabe, 1968) to 76 weeks of age (Hsueh et al., 1973). Thus, not only the age of the subject at testing varied but the amount of postweaning nutritional rehabilitation was different for each study. The amount of early handling of the subjects was often not reported (Ottinger and Tanabe, 1968; Smart, 1974) while in other cases, the subjects were part of a neuromotor development study which required that the animals be handled extensively for the first 55 days of life (Simonson et al., 1971).

The conditions of the open field test situation also differed

among studies. The size of the open field arena ranged from a
large square (122 x 122 cm) (Hsueh et al., 1973; Ottinger and
Tanabe, 1968; Simonson et al., 1971) to a rectangle not much larger
than the home cage (61 x 33 cm) (Smart, 1974). The time of day
that subjects were tested varied: animals were tested during their
lights-off period under dim red illumination (Smart, 1974) or during
their lights-on period under recessed white light (Simonson et al.,
1971). Further, the length, frequency and total number of trials
in the open field differed for each study: Ottinger and Tanabe
(1968) used a single three-minute trial on three consecutive days;
Simonson et al. (1971) used a single six-minute trial on 27 test
days (no intertrial interval reported); and Smart (1974) ran eight
ten-minute trials at hourly intervals on a single day. Since all
these factors are known to affect performance in the open field
(Archer, 1973; Walsh and Cummins, 1975) it is extremely difficult
to compare the studies directly.

The open field results obtained from studies using the technique of feeding the mother a low protein (isocaloric) diet to
produce perinatal malnutrition of the pups are no more consistent.
Fraňková and Barnes (1968) reported that perinatally malnourished
males (rehabilitated at weaning) ambulated and reared more when
tested at seven weeks of age but were less active at 12 weeks of
age as compared to offspring of mothers fed a high protein diet.
Hsueh et al. (1974) also reported that perinatally malnourished
subjects were less active and defecated more frequently when tested
at 14 weeks of life. However, Cowley and Griesel (1966) reported
that perinatally malnourished subjects, tested at ten weeks of age,
could not be differentiated from controls by measures of either
ambulation or defecation. Finally, Fraňková (1972) reported that
animals malnourished only during the suckling period and tested at
13 weeks of age did not differ in the amount of ambulation, but
reared less and were inactive for a higher percentage of the trial
than controls.

Animals which were malnourished during the suckling period and
for four weeks postweaning before nutritional rehabilitation have
been reported to ambulate less (Fraňková and Barnes, 1968), ambulate
less but rear more (Mysliveček et al., 1971), ambulate more (Levitsky
and Barnes, 1972), or exhibit no difference in ambulation from controls (Zimmermann and Zimmermann, 1972).

The open field results from the large versus small litters
technique are no more consistent than the other methods of producing
malnutrition. Pups raised in litters of 15-20 pups have been reported to ambulate less and defecate more (Seitz, 1954), rear less
(Fraňková, 1968), ambulate more and defecate more (Semiginovský et
al., 1969, 1970), or not differ in ambulation or defecation (Guthrie,
1968; Lát et al., 1960) from controls raised in litters of 6-10 pups.

IV. ENVIRONMENTAL INFLUENCES ON OPEN FIELD
BEHAVIOR OF MALNOURISHED RATS

Some investigators studied the influence of early extra stimulation, or conversely, reduced stimulation on the malnourished pup.
It is interesting to note that changes in the quality of the early
environment are capable of interacting differentially with the
nutritional history of the animal. However, again the lack of consistency in methodology makes a direct comparison of the results
nearly impossible.

Franková (1968) reported a series of studies in which malnourished pups were stimulated from days 3-28 of age. Stimulation
consisted of daily weighing, marking and gentling (for an unspec-
ified length of time per day), and twice-weekly exposure to an
environment outside the home for a six-minute open field test. Nonhandled subjects were minimally disturbed until testing at 90 days
of age in the open field. The pups were malnourished by either
restricting the food intake of the mother to 50% of normal during
pregnancy and lactation or increasing the litter size to 13-20 pups
per mother. Well-nourished subjects were progeny of unrestricted
mothers raising litters of nine pups. All subjects were weaned onto
a high protein diet.

Handling increased exploratory behavior, as measured by rearing,
of both malnourished and well-nourished subjects, though the handled/
malnourished animals still showed less exploration than handled/well-
nourished animals. However, when handled/malnourished animals were
compared to nonhandled/well-nourished subjects, there were no significant differences between the two. Thus, Franková concluded that
handling normalized the activity of nutritionally deprived animals.

Levitsky and Barnes (1972) reported the effects of stimulation
on pups raised by mothers fed a low (12%) protein diet during lactation and weaned at 21 days of age onto an even lower (3%) protein
diet for four weeks before rehabilitation on a high (25%) protein
diet. Well-nourished animals were offspring of mothers fed the high
protein diet during lactation and weaned onto this diet at 21 days
of age. Preweaning stimulation consisted of daily handling for three
minutes, and postweaning stimulation consisted of daily handling and
a one-hour "play" period in a box with toys and other animals five
days a week. An additional set of malnourished and well-nourished
animals were raised under control (nonenriched) environmental conditions. Under nonenriched environmental conditions the malnourished
animals, when tested at 17 weeks of age, were more active in an automated open field measuring horizontal activity. Handling abolished
this difference by reducing the malnourished animal's activity and
increasing the activity of the well-nourished subjects only slightly.
Thus, the malnourished/handled animals were not different from the
well-nourished subjects either handled or nonhandled.

At this point it is interesting to note that Fraňková (1968) reported that malnourished animals raised under control environmental conditions were less active and Levitsky and Barnes (1972) found them more active than well-nourished subjects. Despite this difference in direction of activity change, handling was capable of producing a malnourished subject not significantly different from a nonhandled/well-nourished subject. Fraňková (1974b) found that a similar amelioration of open field differences could be achieved when a nonlactating "aunt" was added to the home cage of malnourished subjects. These malnourished animals, when tested in the open field did not differ from well-nourished animals that were raised without an "aunt".

Both Fraňková (1971) and Levitsky and Barnes (1972) have also reported effects of early environmental isolation on malnourished animals. Fraňková (1971) found that offspring of mothers fed a low (8%) protein diet during lactation and weaned onto a high (25%) protein diet raised under control environmental conditions were less active than control progeny from mothers fed a high protein diet. Sensory deprived malnourished and control subjects were raised for their preweaning life in a darkened soundproof room with handling restricted to cage cleaning once a week under weak light. Sensory isolation produced a decrease in exploratory activity (duration of rearing) in the well-nourished animals to levels seen in malnourished/control environment animals. The malnourished sensory deprived animals exhibited the lowest levels of exploratory activity.

Levitsky and Barnes (1972) also reported the effects of early environmental isolation on malnourished and well-nourished rats (see above for nutritional protocol and control environmental conditions). Isolation consisted of minimal handling during suckling and individual housing in wire cages in lightproof sound-attenuated chambers for four weeks postweaning. Early isolated subjects were more active in the automated open field than subjects raised under control environmental conditions when tested at 17 weeks of age. A well-nourished/isolated animal's activity level was not different from a malnourished animal raised under control environmental conditions. In addition, they note that early isolation had a greater effect on the malnourished than the well-nourished subjects.

Again these two groups of investigators do not agree on the direction of the difference between malnourished and well-nourished animals raised under control environmental conditions. However, they do agree that early isolation or lack of stimulation of well-nourished offspring produces an animal with similar open field performance to that of a malnourished subject raised under control environmental conditions.

V. DISCUSSION OF OPEN FIELD RESULTS

After an examination of the open field results reported for perinatally malnourished animals, one is left in a state of confusion. On the basis of these studies one could conclude that early malnutrition causes a rat to become more emotional, less emotional, or that early malnutrition has no influence on emotionality. All the above conclusions may be correct but, in fact, be based on the specifics of the testing conditions. Many investigators in the field of malnutrition appear to be unaware of the sensitivity of the open field to the specifics of the testing situation. Factors such as the size of the arena compared to the home cage, the time of day that the animals are tested, the levels of illumination and noise, length and number of tests, etc. are known to affect the open field results (Archer, 1973). Activity scores measure both emotional reactivity and exploratory behavior. Denenberg (1969b) noted that activity scores from the first exposure to the open field should be interpreted differently from those on subsequent exposures. High activity on the first trial indicates high emotionality. With repeated testing the animals become habituated to the test procedure, and thereafter, high activity is indicative of low emotionality and a strong exploratory tendency. Very few malnutrition studies have been analyzed in this manner. Finally, crucial details of the early environment have often been omitted. It is important to specify all aspects of the pup's early environment since open field testing is sensitive to variations in the amounts of early handling and maternal stimulation.

What is apparent from the malnutrition studies reviewed is that it is impossible to make any sweeping generalizations about the emotional status of perinatally malnourished animals on the basis of open field data. The open field is particularly sensitive to early environmental variables. Since many of these studies fail to describe the specifics of the non-nutritive environmental conditions, it is possible that the influences attributed to early malnutrition may be more directly related to other environmental determinants or to an interaction of the malnutrition with these nonspecified environmental variables.

VI. CONCLUSION

Although there now exists a large literature on the effects of perinatal malnutrition on later behavior using an animal (rat) model, we find it difficult to arrive at any conclusion concerning the behavioral effects of early malnutrition in the rehabilitated animal. This review has limited its discussion to open field testing; however, similar conclusions could be reached after critically reviewing studies on the effects of early malnutrition on adult avoidance learning (Levine and Wiener, 1975) or maze testing (Levitsky and

Barnes, 1973). There appears to be little question that animals
that are still malnourished at the time of behavioral testing do
show a number of striking behavioral differences when compared with
nondeprived animals (Baird et al., 1971; Barnes et al., 1966;
Cowley and Griesel, 1959, 1962, 1963, 1964; Rajalakshmi et al.,
1965). Thus, it is important that results obtained from chronically
malnourished animals not be lumped together with those obtained from
animals malnourished only during the presumed critical perinatal
period for brain development. The studies which examine the behavior of rehabilitated animals do not present any clear or consistent
set of results which would support a generalization that there are
profound and permanent behavioral deficits as a consequence of early
malnutrition. A clear comparison of the studies in this field is
made difficult by the large variation in the techniques used to produce the malnutrition, the length and severity of the nutritional
deprivation, and the age and conditions under which behavioral testing takes place. We have suggested that the disruption of the
animal's early environment may, in part, be responsible for the
differences in later adult behavior that have been attributed to
malnutrition. It thus appears that the animal model of malnutrition
is far from free of contaminating psychosocial variables.

The supposition that malnutrition causes permanent mental retardation in humans is often stated as a proven fact. However, in
a review of the studies on human mental development of early malnourished children, Frisch (1970, 1971) concluded that there is
little conclusive evidence to support this supposition. A number
of recent studies (Christiansen et al., 1974; Ricciuti, 1974;
Richardson, 1972; Richardson et al., 1973; Richardson, this volume;
Stein et al., 1972) have demonstrated the importance of non-nutritional environmental factors in the study of the effects of early
malnutrition on later intellectual functioning in man. For example,
Richardson (1972; this volume) concluded that the primary factor
that resulted in lower IQ and poorer school performance in a group
of Jamaican children who were hospitalized for kwashiorkor was not
the malnutrition per se, but the environmental impoverishment which
occurred concomitantly with the malnutrition. A study on the adult
mental performance of babies born during the hongerwinter in the
Netherlands during World War II (Stein et al., 1972) reported that
starvation during pregnancy had no detectable effects on the adult
mental performance of surviving male offspring, but that the association of socioeconomic class with mental performance was strong.

It appears that although malnutrition is a major insult to the
developing organism, the organism has a remarkable resiliency and
following nutritional rehabilitation shows very few major changes
in later performance as a consequence of the early malnutrition.
It will be necessary to derive an animal model in which malnutrition
can be produced with a minimum of disturbance of other environmental
conditions. Only then will it be possible to determine whether or

not malnutrition during critical periods in development has any prolonged and permanent effects on the organism's behavior. Aside from possibly answering the above question, we are not sure that an animal model of malnutrition with optimal environmental conditions will represent anything which occurs naturally. Certainly in most human cases, malnutrition is closely associated with profound changes in other environmental variables. It may indeed be that early malnutrition and changes in other psychosocial determinants are inseparable and we should no longer think about a simplistic cause and effect relationship between malnutrition and behavior.

In conclusion, the evidence from animal models suggests that dietary rehabilitation can and does eliminate many of the behavioral deficits that are observed in the chronically malnourished animal. The inconsistencies in the literature may be the result of the lack of control of psychosocial variables that can also affect the development of behavior.

ACKNOWLEDGMENTS

This study was supported by Research Grant NICH&HD 02881 from the National Institutes of Health and Biosciences Training Grant MH-8304 from the National Institute of Mental Health. Dr. Levine is supported by Research Scientist Award K05-MH-19936 from the National Institute of Mental Health.

REFERENCES

Altman, J., Sudarshan, K., Das, G.D., McCormick, N., and Barnes, D. 1971. The Influence of Nutrition on Neural and Behavioral Development: III. Development of Some Motor, Particularly Locomotor Patterns During Infancy. Develop. Psychobiol. 4:97-114.

Archer, J. 1973. Tests for Emotionality in Rats and Mice: A Review. Anim. Behav. 21:205-235.

Baird, A., Widdowson, E.M., and Cowley, J.J. 1971. Effects of Calorie and Protein Deficiencies Early in Life on the Subsequent Learning Ability of Rats. J. Nutr. 25:391-403.

Barnes, R.H., Cunnold, S.R., Zimmermann, R.R., Simmons, H., MacLeod, R.B., and Krook, L. 1966. Influence of Nutritional Deprivations in Early Life on Learning Behavior of Rats as Measured by Performance in a Water Maze. J. Nutr. 89:399-410.

Barnes, R.H., Neely, C.S., Kwong, E., Labadan, B.A., and Fraňková, S. 1968. Postnatal Nutritional Deprivations as Determinants of Adult Rat Behavior Toward Food, Its Consumption and Utilization. J. Nutr. 96:467-476.

Barnett, S.A., Smart, J.L., and Widdowson, E.M. 1971. Early Nutrition and the Activity and Feeding of Rats in an Artificial Environment. Develop. Psychobiol. 4:1-15.

Broadhurst, P.L. 1969. Psychogenetics of Emotionality in the Rat. Ann. N. Y. Acad. Sci. 159:806-824.

Chow, B.F., and Lee, C.J. 1964. Effect of Dietary Restriction of Pregnant Rats on the Body Weight Gain of the Offspring. J. Nutr. 82:10-18.

Christiansen, N., Vuori, L., Mora, J.O., and Wagner, M. 1974. Social Environment as it Relates to Malnutrition and Mental Development, pp. 186-199. In J. Cravioto, L. Hambraeus, and B. Vahlquist (eds.). Early Malnutrition and Mental Development. Almquist and Wiksell, Stockholm.

Cowley, J.J., and Griesel, R.D. 1959. Some Effects of a Low Protein Diet on a First Filial Generation of White Rats. J. Genet. Psychol. 95:187-201.

Cowley, J.J., and Griesel, R.D. 1962. Pre- and Postnatal Effects of a Low Protein Diet on the Behaviour of the White Rat. Psychol. Africana 9:216-225.

Cowley, J.J., and Griesel, R.D. 1963. The Development of Second-Generation Low-Protein Rats. J. Genet. Psychol. 103:233-242.

Cowley, J.J., and Griesel, R.D. 1964. Low Protein Diet and Emotionality in the Albino Rat. J. Genet. Psychol. 104:89-98.

Cowley, J.J., and Griesel, R.D. 1966. The Effect on Growth and Behaviour of Rehabilitating First and Second Generation Low Protein Rats. Anim. Behav. 14:506-517.

Denenberg, V.H. 1969a. Experimental Programming of Life Histories in the Rat, pp. 21-43. In A. Ambrose (ed.). Stimulation in Early Infancy. Academic Press, New York.

Denenberg, V.H. 1969b. Open-Field Behavior in the Rat: What Does it Mean? Ann. N. Y. Acad. Sci. 159:852-859.

Denenberg, V.H., Rosenberg, K.M., Paschke, R., Hess, J.L., Zarrow, M.X., and Levine, S. 1968. Plasma Corticosterone Levels as a Function of Cross-Species Fostering and Species Differences. Endocrinology 83:900-902.

Dobbing, J. 1971. Undernutrition and the Developing Brain: The
    Use of Animal Models to Elucidate the Human Problem. Psychiat.
    Neurol. Neurochir. 74:433-442.

Dobbing, J. 1974. Prenatal Development and Neurological Development,
    pp. 96-110. In J. Cravioto, L. Hambraeus, and B. Vahlquist
    (eds.). Early Malnutrition and Mental Development. Almquist
    and Wiksell, Stockholm.

Dobbing, J., and Sands, J. 1971. Vulnerability of Developing
    Brain: IX. The Effect of Nutritional Growth Retardation on
    the Timing of the Brain Growth-Spurt. Biol. Neonate. 19:363-
    378.

Dobbing, J., Hopewell, J.W., and Lynch, A. 1971. Vulnerability of
    Developing Brain: VII. Permanent Deficit of Neurons in Cerebral
    and Cerebellar Cortex Following Early Mild Undernutrition.
    Exp. Neurol. 32:439-447.

Dymsza, H.A., Czajka, D.M., and Miller, S.A. 1964. Influences of
    Artificial Diet on Weight Gain and Body Composition of the
    Neonatal Rat. J. Nutr. 84:100-106.

Eayrs, J.T., and Horn, G. 1955. The Development of Cerebral Cortex
    in Hypothyroid and Starved Rats. Anat. Rec. 121:53-61.

Fraňková, S. 1968. Nutritional and Psychological Factors in the
    Development of Spontaneous Behavior in the Rat, pp. 312-322.
    In N.S. Scrimshaw and J.E. Gordon (eds.). Malnutrition,
    Learning and Behavior. M.I.T. Press, Cambridge, Massachusetts.

Fraňková, S. 1971. Relationship Between Nutrition During Lactation
    and Maternal Behaviour of Rats. Activ. Nerv. Sup. 13:1-8.

Fraňková, S. 1972. Effect of Early Dietary and Sensoric Reduction
    on Behaviour of Adult Rats. Activ. Nerv. Sup. 14:1-7.

Fraňková, S. 1974a. Effects of Protein Deficiency in Early Life
    and During Lactation on Maternal Behaviour. Baroda J. Nutr.
    1:21-28.

Fraňková, S. 1974b. Interaction Between Early Malnutrition and
    Stimulation in Animals, pp. 202-208. In J. Cravioto, L.
    Hambraeus, and B. Vahlquist (eds.). Early Malnutrition and
    Mental Development. Almquist and Wiksell, Stockholm.

Fraňková, S., and Barnes, R.H. 1968. Influence of Malnutrition in
    Early Life on Exploratory Behavior of Rats. J. Nutr. 96:477-
    484.

Frisch, R.E. 1970. Present Status of the Supposition that Mal-
    nutrition Causes Permanent Mental Retardation. Am. J. Clin.
    Nutr. 23:189-195.

Frisch, R.E. 1971. Does Malnutrition Cause Permanent Mental Re-
    tardation in Human Beings? Psychiat. Neurol. Neurochir. 74:
    463-479.

Galler, J.R., and Turkewitz, G. 1975. Variability of the Effects
    of Rearing in a Large Litter on the Development of the Rat.
    Develop. Psychobiol. 8:325-331.

Griffiths, W.J., Jr., and Senter, R.J. 1954. The Effect of Protein
    Deficiency on Maze Performance of Domestic Norway Rats. J.
    Comp. Physiol. Psychol. 47:41-43.

Grota, L.J., and Ader, R. 1969. Continuous Recording of Maternal
    Behaviour in Rattus Norvegicus. Anim. Behav. 17:722-729.

Guthrie, H.A. 1968. Severe Undernutrition in Early Infancy and
    Behavior in Rehabilitated Albino Rats. Physiol. Behav. 3:
    619-623.

Hall, C.S. 1934. Emotional Behavior in the Rat: 1. Defecation and
    Urination as Measures of Individual Differences in Emotion-
    ality. J. Comp. Psychol. 18:385-403.

Hall, C.S. 1936. Emotional Behavior in the Rat: III. The Relation-
    ship Between Emotionality and Ambulatory Behavior. J. Comp.
    Psychol. 22:345-352.

Hall, C.S. 1941. Temperament: A Survey of Animal Studies. Psychol.
    Bull. 38:909-943.

Hofer, M.A. 1973. The Role of Nutrition in the Physiological and
    Behavioral Effects of Early Maternal Separation on Infant Rats.
    Psychosom. Med. 35:350-359.

Hsueh, A.M., Simonson, M., Kellum, M.J., and Chow, B.F. 1973. Peri-
    natal Undernutrition and the Metabolic and Behavioral Develop-
    ment of the Offspring. Nutr. Rep. Intern. 7:437-445.

Hsueh, A.M., Simonson, M., Hanson, H.M., and Chow, B.F. 1974. Pro-
    tein Supplementation to Pregnant Rats During Third Trimester
    and the Growth and Behavior of Offspring. Nutr. Rep. Intern.
    9:31-44.

Kennedy, G.C. 1957. The Development with Age of Hypothalamic Re-
    straint upon the Appetite of the Rat. J. Endocrinol. 16:9-17.

Lát, J., Widdowson, E.M., and McCance, R.A. 1960. Some Effects of Accelerating Growth: III. Behaviour and Nervous Activity. Proc. Roy. Soc. (London) 153:345-356.

Levin, R., Wiener, S., Fitzpatrick, K., and Levine, S. Alterations in the Maternal Behavior of Malnourished Rats. (in preparation).

Levine, S., and Thoman, E.B. 1969. Physiological and Behavioral Consequences of Postnatal Maternal Stress in Rats. Physiol. Behav. 4:139-142.

Levine, S., and Wiener, S. 1975. A Critical Analysis of Data on Malnutrition and Behavioral Deficits. Advances in Pediatrics, Vol. 22. (in press).

Levine, S., Haltmeyer, G.C., Karas, G.G., and Denenberg, V.H. 1967. Physiological and Behavioral Effects of Infantile Stimulation. Physiol. Behav. 2:55-59.

Levine, S., Madden, J., IV., Conner, R.L., Moskal, J.R., and Anderson, J.C. 1973. Physiological and Behavioral Effects of Prior Aversive Stimulation (Preshock) in the Rat. Physiol. Behav. 10:467-471.

Levitsky, D.A., and Barnes, R.H. 1972. Nutritional and Environmental Interactions in the Behavioral Development of the Rat: Long-Term Effects. Science 176:68-71.

Levitsky, D.A., and Barnes, R.H. 1973. Malnutrition and Animal Behavior, pp. 3-16. In D.J. Kallen (ed.). Nutrition, Development and Social Behavior. DHEW Publication No. (NIH) 73-242.

Mandler, J.M. 1958. Effect of Early Food Deprivation on Adult Behavior in the Rat. J. Comp. Physiol. Psychol. 51:513-517.

Massaro, T.F., Levitsky, D.A., and Barnes, R.H. 1974. Protein Malnutrition in the Rat: Its Effects on Maternal Behavior and Pup Development. Develop. Psychobiol. 7:551-561.

Messer, M., Thoman, E.B., Terassa, A.G., and Dallman, P.R. 1969. Artificial Feeding of Infant Rats by Continuous Gastric Infusion. J. Nutr. 98:404-410.

Miller, S.A. 1968. Short Comments, pp. 229-232. In N.S. Scrimshaw and J.E. Gordon (eds.). Malnutrition, Learning and Behavior. M.I.T. Press, Cambridge, Massachusetts.

Miller, S.A., and Dymsza, H.A. 1963. Artificial Feeding of Neonatal Rats. Science 141:517-518.

Mueller, A.J., and Cox, W.M., Jr. 1946. The Effect of Changes in
    Diet on the Volume and Composition of Rat Milk. J. Nutr.
    31:249-259.

Mysliveček, J., Hassmannová, J., Semiginovský, B., and Fraňková, S.
    1971. Some Electrophysiological and Behavioral Parameters in
    Rats Reared on a Low Protein Diet. Activ. Nerv. Sup. 13:105-
    106.

Ottinger, D.R., and Tanabe, G. 1968. Effects on Offspring Behavior
    and Development. Develop. Psychobiol. 2:7-9.

Plaut, S.M. 1970. Studies of Undernutrition in the Young Rat:
    Methodological Considerations. Develop. Psychobiol. 3:157-167.

Rajalakshmi, R., Govindarajan, K.R., and Ramakrishnan, C.V. 1965.
    Effect of Dietary Protein Content on Visual Discrimination
    Learning and Brain Biochemistry in the Albino Rat. J. Neuro-
    chem. 12:261-271.

Rajalakshmi, R., Ali, S.Z., and Ramakrishnan, C.V. 1967. Effect of
    Inanition During the Neonatal Period on Discrimination Learning
    and Brain Biochemistry in the Albino Rat. J. Neurochem. 14:
    29-34.

Ricciuti, H.N. 1974. Assessing the Interaction of Nutritional and
    Socio-environmental Influences on Development, pp. 182-185.
    In J. Cravioto, L. Hambraeus, and B. Vahlquist (eds.). Early
    Malnutrition and Mental Development. Almquist and Wiksell,
    Stockholm.

Richardson, S.A. 1972. Ecology of Malnutrition: Non-nutritional
    Factors Influencing Intellectual and Behavioral Development,
    pp. 101-109. In Nutrition, the Nervous System and Behavior.
    Pan American Health Organization, WHO, Scientific Publication
    No. 251.

Richardson, S.A., Birch, H.G., and Hertzig, M.E. 1973. School Per-
    formance of Children Who Were Severely Malnourished in Infancy.
    Am. J. Ment. Defic. 77:623-632.

Rosenblatt, J.S. 1967. Nonhormonal Basis of Maternal Behavior in
    the Rat. Science 156:1512-1514.

Seitz, P.F.D. 1954. The Effects of Infantile Experiences Upon Adult
    Behavior in Animal Subjects: I. Effects of Litter Size During
    Infancy upon Adult Behavior in the Rat. Am. J. Psychiat. 110:
    916-927.

Semiginovský, B., Mysliveček, J., Springer, V., and Rokyta, R. 1969.

Testing of Emotionality in Animals with Different Levels of Nutrition. Activ. Nerv. Sup. 11:282-283.

Semiginovský, B., Mysliveček, J., and Žalud, V. 1970. Spontaneous Exploratory Activity in Rats with Different Nutrition in the Early Postnatal Period. Activ. Nerv. Sup. 12:158.

Simonson, M., Sherwin, R.W., Anilane, J.K., Yu, W.Y., and Chow, B.F. 1969. Neuromotor Development in Progeny of Underfed Mother Rats. J. Nutr. 98:18-24.

Simonson, M., Stephan, J.K., Hanson, H.M., and Chow, B.F. 1971. Open Field Studies in Offspring of Underfed Mother Rats. J. Nutr. 101:331-336.

Slob, A.K., Snow, C.E., and Natris-Mathot, E. de. 1973. Absence of Behavioral Deficits Following Neonatal Undernutrition in the Rat. Develop. Psychobiol. 6:177-186.

Smart, J.L. 1974. Activity and Exploratory Behavior of Adult Offspring of Undernourished Mother Rats. Develop. Psychobiol. 7:315-321.

Smart, J.L., and Dobbing, J. 1971a. Vulnerability of Developing Brain: II. Effects of Early Nutritional Deprivation on Reflex Ontogeny and Development of Behaviour in the Rat. Brain Res. 28:85-95.

Smart, J.L., and Dobbing, J. 1971b. Vulnerability of Developing Brain: VI. Relative Effects of Foetal and Early Postnatal Undernutrition on Reflex Ontogeny and Development of Behaviour in the Rat. Brain Res. 33:303-314.

Smart, J.L., and Preece, J. 1973. Maternal Behaviour of Undernourished Mother Rats. Anim. Behav. 21:613-619.

Sobotka, T., Cook, M.P., and Brodie, R.E. 1974. Neonatal Malnutrition; Neurochemical, Hormonal and Behavioral Manifestations. Brain Res. 65:443-457.

Stein, Z., Susser, M., Saenger, G., and Marolla, F. 1972. Nutrition and Mental Performance. Science 178:708-713.

Stern, J.M., and Levin, R. Food Availability as a Determinant of the Rats' Circadian Rhythm in Maternal Behavior. Develop. Psychobiol. (in press).

Stern, J.M., Erskine, M.S., and Levine, S. 1973. Dissociation of Open-Field Behavior and Pituitary-Adrenal Function. Horm. Behav. 4:149-162.

Thoman, E.B., and Levine, S. 1969. Role of Maternal Disturbance
     and Temperature Change in Early Experience Studies. Physiol.
     Behav. 4:143-145.

Walsh, R.N., and Cummins, R.A. 1975. The Open Field Test: A
     Critical Review. Psychol. Bull. (in press).

Winick, M., and Noble, A. 1965. Quantitative Changes in DNA, RNA,
     and Protein During Prenatal and Postnatal Growth in the Rat.
     Develop. Biol. 12:451-466.

Winick, M., and Noble, A. 1966. Cellular Response in Rats During
     Malnutrition at Various Ages. J. Nutr. 89:300-306.

Winick, M., Rosso, P., and Brasel, J.A. 1972. Malnutrition and
     Cellular Growth in the Brain. Bibl. Nutr. Diet. 17:60-68.

Zamenhof, S., van Marthens, E., and Margolis, F.L. 1968. DNA (Cell
     Number) and Protein in Neonatal Brain: Alteration by Maternal
     Dietary Protein Restriction. Science 160:322-323.

Zimmermann, R.R., and Zimmermann, S.J. 1972. Responses of Protein
     Malnourished Rats to Novel Objects. Percep. Motor Skills 35:
     319-321.

ENVIRONMENTAL THERAPY IN HYPOTHYROID AND

OTHER DISADVANTAGED ANIMAL POPULATIONS

John W. Davenport
Regional Primate Research Center
University of Wisconsin - Madison

I. Introduction

Bluntly stated, our ultimate concern in this chapter is whether mental deficiency can be alleviated by environmental stimulation. But since we will restrict our attention to sub-human studies bearing on this question, let us change the language at once from "mental deficiency" to "behavioral deficits," and let the implications of these studies for the understanding and treatment of human behavioral dysfunctions emerge under their own power. Our focus will be on the question of whether the environmental stimulation conditions which have produced many kinds of brain changes in rodent studies (e.g., Rosensweig et al 1972; Greenough 1975) also result in improved behavioral capacities, particularly those reflected by performance in learning situations. We will examine this question in normal animals of both rodent and primate species, but our major concern will be with animal populations which are disadvantaged in their neural development and adult learning capacities by hormonal abnormalities, undernutrition, genetic factors, or other detrimental conditions in early life.

With special attention to hypothyroid rats in our own research and comparisons with other types of disadvantaged animals, we will examine the following: How much can the behavioral deficits in such animals be offset by enrichment of the rearing environment? Are there lasting benefits? Since disadvantaged populations have "more room for improvement," do they benefit more than normal populations from enrichment? What sorts of abilities are enhanced? How does this depend on the type of disadvantage?

A. Experimentally-Induced Cretinism in Rats

Ideally, we would begin studying these questions in a good animal model of a well-known form of human mental deficiency, in controlled behavioral settings which can be counted on to reveal the disadvantaged animal's deficits in a quantitative manner, and under conditions which readily lend themselves to follow-up study of neural correlates. At the present stage of animal mental retardation research, probably no preparation fits these requirements better than the perinatally thyroid-deficient rat. Since the classic work by the English anatomist J.T. Eayrs showing maze learning deficits in neonatally thyroidectomized rats (Eayrs 1961), close parallels have been evident between the effects of early hypothyroidism in the rat and human cretinism, the hallmark of which is persisting intellectual impairment. Eayrs showed, for example, that when the rat's period of thyroid deficiency was restricted to the first two or three postnatal weeks (after which his thyroid ectomized rats were maintained on thyroid hormone replacement), enduring deficits in maze learning appeared in adulthood, but not when the hypothyroid state was induced after the neonatal period . Analogously, permanent IQ deficits in humans result from thyroid deficiency in infancy but probably not when the deficiency begins in later childhood or thereafter (Wilkins 1965).

In our laboratory we have extended this parallel by showing that, as in humans, the critical period of thyroid deficiency for the induction of adult learning disorders in rats includes a portion of the prenatal stage (Davenport et al 1976). We have also extended earlier studies showing other rat-human parallels in cretinism, e.g., physical growth deficits (drawfism) from long periods of hypothyroidism starting before birth (Hughes 1944; Davenport 1970), and delayed maturation of early motor capacities from briefer deprivation periods around the time of birth (Eayrs and Lishman, 1955; Wallock and Davenport, 1970; Davenport et al 1976). As in human infantile hypothyroidism, the degree of impairment shown in adulthood by early-hypothyroid rats varies with severity of the thyroid-deficient state near birth, and under the most severe conditions the adult impairment extends beyond maze learning to simpler tasks such as operant discrimination and single-alternation pattern learning (Davenport and Dorcey 1972; Davenport et al 1976). Some other recent data (Davenport and Hennies 1976), showing reduced emotionality in perinatal-hypothyroid rats, suggest that there may be additional parallels to human cretinism in the realm of personality traits. In general, the correspondences at the behavioral level seem good enough for us to assume that the study of neurological correlates of behavioral disorders in hypothyroid rats can shed considerable light on the nature of brain dysfunction in human cretinism, and a similar promise of applicability may hold for any therapeutic measures which successfully reduce behavioral deficits in cretinoid rats.

B. Therapeutic Implications of Neuroanatomical Findings

The types of neurohistological abnormalities which early thy-roid-deficient rats display add interest to the question of whether their behavioral disorders can be alleviated by environmental stimu-lation. Eayrs (1968, 1971) has shown, among other neuroanatomical defects, reduced axonal and dendritic densities in the cerebral cortex of neonatally thyroidectomized rats, resulting in greatly reduced synaptic connectivity. More detailed histological studies of cerebellar tissues by Nicholson and Altman (1972a, b) have also demonstrated reduced synaptogenesis in developing hypothyroid rats. The general indication from these studies and related neurochemical work (see Balazs 1971, for review) is that the cretinoid rat's cortex suffers not so much from a restriction in neuronal or glial cell numbers as from a gross underdevelopment in cell differentiation, particularly the elaboration of dendritic processes. Although more studies of this sort need to be performed with fully-adult animals, this effect and the resulting reduction in synaptic connectivity appear to represent an arrest, rather than mere delay, in neural development.

Continuing plasticity of the incompletely-developed neural processes has not been ruled out by the neurological studies, however, and similar studies of the effects of rearing environ-ments have shown brain changes from environmental stimulation which are opposite to those produced by early thyroid deficiency. Specifically, the experience-induced effects of increased dendritic branching (Volkmar and Greenough 1972; Greenough 1975), increased numbers of dendritic spines (Globus et al 1973), and increased synaptic size (as revealed in ultrastructural studies by Møll-gaard et al 1971, and West and Greenough 1972) in cortical neurons represent changes which contrast with demonstrated effects of early hypothyroidism and which could directly reverse those effects. In other words, it is entirely conceivable that the cretinoid rat's synaptic connectivity may be augmented to a significant extent by environmental stimulation of increased synaptogenesis or increased functioning of synapses already formed (Greenough 1975), even after the age of maximal rate of synaptogenesis (10 to 30 days in normal rats, according to Eayrs and Goodhead 1959). And from the standpoint that the cretinoid rat has "more room for improvement" than the normal rat at this neurohistological level, we may anti-cipate differential plasticity at the behavioral level, such that increasing the degree and variety of environmental stimulation could benefit performance in learning situations to a greater extent in hypothyroid than in normal rats.

This in fact turned out to be the basic finding in our studies to be presented below. From this finding we have gone on to examine

whether similar differential facilitation occurs in other types of
brain dysfunction in studies conducted elsewhere.

C. Varieties of Environmental Experience

        In the sections which follow we will be displaying many examples
in which normal and disadvantaged animals have been shown better
performance following enriched rearing than after more impoverished
rearing conditions. Largely as a matter of convenience, we will
usually describe such findings as "enhancement by enrichment" or
"reduction of deficit by enrichment", even though this verbal
convention may horrify those who prefer to emphasize the obviously
detrimental behavioral consequences of impoverishment.

        We take the view that a meaningful (albeit multidimensional)
continuum of degree, variety, and complexity of organism-environment interactions exists. Along this continuum various rearing
environments range -- from the total-isolation conditions that are
well-known in primate studies of social development (e.g. Harlow
et al 1965), through the standard isolation, social-control, and
enriched conditions that have been defined by Rosenzweig et al
(1972), to various "superenriched" environments which will be
illustrated. Perhaps all of these are more impoverished than
natural conditions in the field for a given species. For our
specific purposes here, however, when we refer to "improving
performance by enrichment" it should be understood that the performance difference thereby summarized, usually between enriched
and isolated animals, is simply an effect produced by moving along
the continuum of environmental complexity in either direction, and
in most cases could just as appropriately be described as a detrimental effect of impoverishment.

        II. Reduction of Learning Deficits in Hypothyroid Rats

A.   1972 and 1973 Enrichment Studies

        We conducted our first studies of environmental stimulation
effects in hypothyroid rats in 1972 and 1973. In this work, enriched (E) and isolated (I) conditions were defined as in the Berkeley studies by Rosensweig et al (1972) and administered to control
(C) and thiouracil-treated (T) rats for one month after weaning.

        In the first study (Gonzalez and Davenport 1972) we induced
hypothyroidism by feeding mash containing thiouracil (0.2% dose)
to pregnant Holtzman rats during the last 16 days of gestation
and the first 16 days after parturition. Control mothers received
untreated mash during the same period. At 30 days of age 55 offspring were weaned and littermates were randomly assigned to the

E and I conditions. The C and T rats in the E condition were housed separately in groups of 15 in Wahmann LC-27 gang cages (56 x 51 x 38 cm). These cages always contained a random selection of eight "play" objects from a pool of 25 objects and five of these were changed daily. The I rats were housed individually in translucent plastic nesting cages (46 x 25 x 15 cm) of the same type used for the initial rearing of the litters; these contained wood shavings but no play objects. Except during the rehousing at weaning, neither the E nor the I rats were handled until the 60th day, after which all rats were housed individually in standard (24 x 18 x 17.5 cm) cages having three opaque sides and wire mesh fronts and floors.

Behavioral testing began with tests of locomotion, following, grooming, and fighting behavior in open-field settings on Days 61-66. These tests, which were similar to those used by Levitsky and Barnes (1972) in revealing interactions of early malnutrition and environmental stimulation, failed to disclose any important group differences. At age 67 days of age we placed the rats on a daily food deprivation schedule in which body weights were held to approximately 85% of their Day 67 ad libitum weights.

On Days 70-92 we tested the rats in a symmetrical maze. This apparatus, described elsewhere (Davenport et al 1970), represents a modernized version of the Hebb and Williams (1946) "closed-field intelligence test" for rats. In comparison to many other learning tasks in our thyroid research program, it has proven to be the most sensitive test instrument, revealing persistent learning deficits in neonatally thyroxine- (Davenport and Gonzalez 1973) and triiodothyronine-stimulated (Davenport et al 1975) rats as well as in perinatal-hypothyroid rats. The symmetrical maze resembles the Hebb-Williams maze in having endboxes at two opposite corners of a field containing barriers, as illustrated in the insert diagrams of Fig. 1; with symmetrical patterns of barriers, the rat is confronted by the same problem regardless of the direction in which it is shuttling between the endboxes.

Our 1972 rats received the standard pretraining procedures including practice problems P-1 through P-4 (see Davenport et al 1970) and four test problems in the maze. The main finding was better performance by the E than the I hypothyroids. Error scores (Fig. 1) showed the usual large performance deficit from 0.2% perinatal thiouracil treatment (F = 124.6; df = 1, 47; p <.001) and a reliable drug-by-environment interaction (F = 4.55; df = 1, 47; p <.05). By a conservative t test of TE - TI differences (the environmental effect in the thiouracil-treated rats) with the C groups' scores excluded from the error variance, facilitation by enrichment was significant (p <.05) for total errors over the four problems and errors on problem T-9 (corresponding p values were <.10 and <.20 for problems T-6 and T-10, respectively). The re-

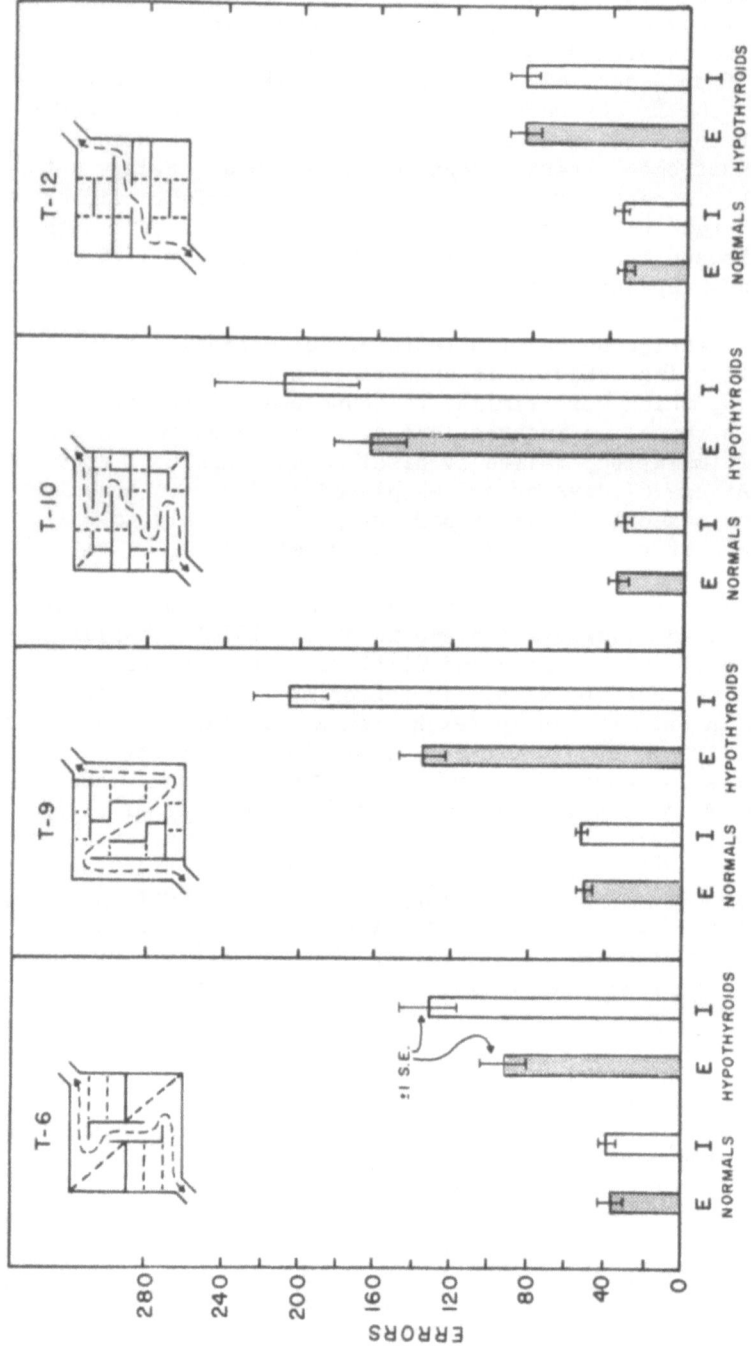

Fig. 1. Results of the 1972 enrichment study: mean errors to criterion on four test problems of the symmetrical maze series by the enriched (E, shaded bars) and isolated (I, open bars) normal and hypothyroid rats.

duction of the thiouracil-induced deficit by enrichment averaged 33% over the four problems, ranging from zero on problem T-12 to 46% on problem T-10, in terms of the total-error difference between the hypothyroid groups (TI - TE) divided by the hypothyroid-normal difference under I conditions (TI - CI). Interestingly, the E and I normal groups had virtually identical scores on all problems.

Our 1973 study did not confirm these positive results in the hypothyroid rats, however. With 47 newly-reared rats, the same control-thiouracil manipulation, and the same E-I treatments, means of errors per problem showed no environmental effect in either the thiouracil (TE: 144.6, TI: 137.9) or the control (CE: 52.1, CI: 53.2) rats over problems T-6, T-9, and T-10 in this second study. There were some differences between the 1972 and 1973 studies -- the open-field tasks were omitted and some apparatus features were changed in the second study -- but neither of these nor any other factors provided a reasonable explanation of the discrepancy. Since there was nothing freakish about the error scores in the over-all normal-hypothyroid difference in the 1973 study, we had no basis for disregarding its negative results -- until the next studies to be described.

B. 1974-75 Superenrichment Studies

In our latest work we have increased the differences between E and I treatments by employing a modified version of Kuenzle and Knüsel's (1974) "superenriched" environment. In their laboratory at Zurich, these researchers have devised a living-training apparatus large enough for 70 weanling rats at a time. It consists of two interconnected compartments containing play objects, sleeping boxes, shelves, ramps and a maze. The most distinguishing feature of Kuenzle and Knüsel's conditions is that approximately every three days the rats are confronted with a new learning problem, solution of which is required for access to food or water. Thus, besides the rats' interactions with each other and the physical objects in the apparatus, they receive the additional experiences involved in learning to shuttle between the compartments through tunnels, to discriminate visual stimuli on the tunnel gats which signify their direction of swing, to traverse the maze for food, and other tasks. Kuenzle and Knüsel present data showing that these superenriched conditions produce significantly greater increases in cerebral length, occipital cortex weight, and the cholinesterase/acetyl-cholinesterase ratio in occipital cortex than in rats exposed to the usual enriched conditions of the Berkeley studies.

Our version of the superenrichment apparatus (see Fig. 2) was simply fashioned out of three standard wire mesh gang cages (Wahmann LC-27). Each of four interconnecting tunnels contained a centered gate which could be positioned for one- or two-way

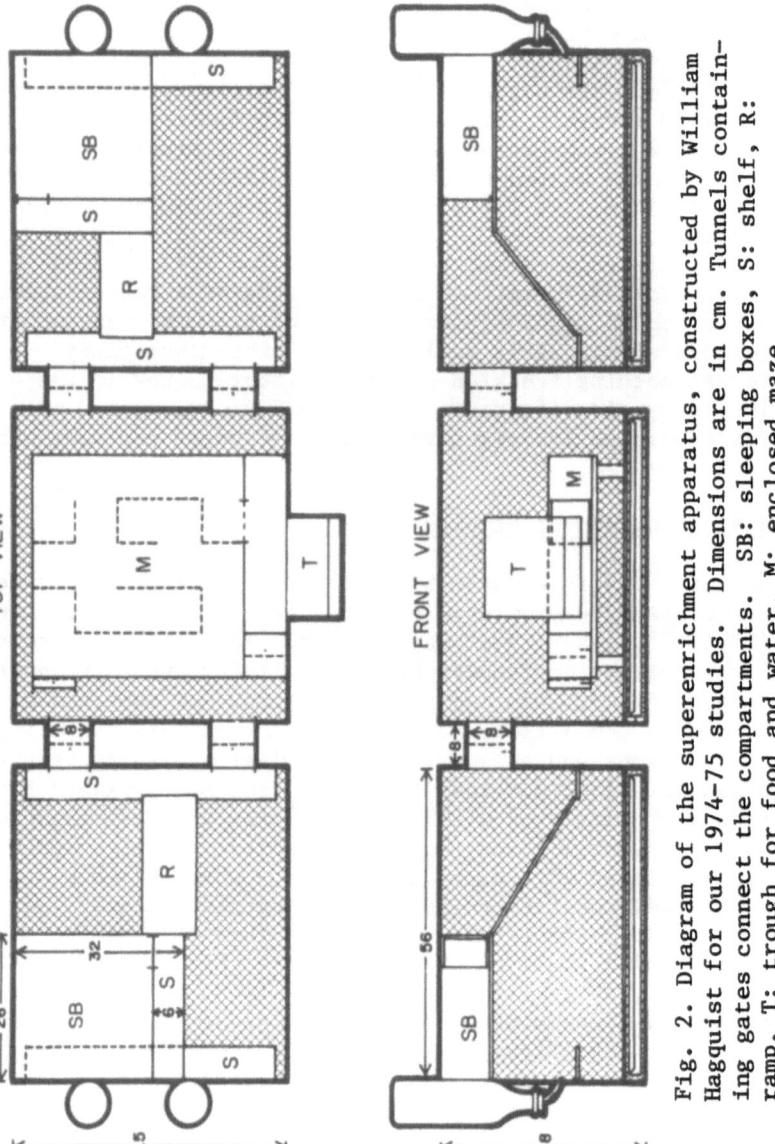

Fig. 2. Diagram of the superenrichment apparatus, constructed by William Hagquist for our 1974–75 studies. Dimensions are in cm. Tunnels containing gates connect the compartments. SB: sleeping boxes, S: shelf, R: ramp, T: trough for food and water, M: enclosed maze.

swing. The colors of the gates (white on one side, brown on the other) cued the direction of swing on certain days and were uncorrelated with the direction on other days. The compartments contained objects (those used in our previous studies) and other features indicated in Fig. 2. The maze, located in the center compartment during a portion of the exposure period, differed from the symmetrical maze in being much smaller, completely enclosed so as to have a dark interior, and usually occupied by several rats, since it seemed to be a favorite sleeping location. One end of the maze was aligned with a food (or water) trough which was mounted on the outside of the center compartment's front door; one-way entrance and exit gates like those in the tunnels were located at the ends of one side of the maze.

With 45 rats in this apparatus simultaneously, the level of activity was often strikingly high, during both light (0500-1900 hr) and dark (1900-0500 hr) portions of the daily cycle. We followed Kuenzle and Knüsel's practice of requiring the rats to learn various ways to obtain food or water by changing apparatus features approximately every third day during a 34-day period, except that we substituted some simple changes (e.g. reversing the food and water locations) for their most difficult tasks of rope-climbing and jumping for food in order to minimize the risk of subjecting our hypothyroid rats to severe food or water deprivation.

Preweaning conditions in our 1974-75 studies were similar to those in our first enrichment experiments except that exposure to 0.2% thiouracil was reduced to a period from gestation Day 17 to postnatal Day 10, some additional mothers and litters were exposed to propylthiouracil (PTU) in varying doses, and weaning was delayed until Day 36 because of the immaturity of the PTU-treated pups. The thiouracil-treated offspring and their controls constituted the main experiment, in which 45 rats (21 T, 24C) occupied the superenrichment apparatus from Day 36 to Day 70 and an extensive battery of behavioral tests was administered. The PTU rats were used for a supplemental study with a different design which we will describe later.

The main experiment had eight treatment combinations generated by the thyroid, environment, and sex variables in a 2 x 2 x 2 factorial design. Except for discarding some surplus females in the E subgroups which were pregnant at the beginning of maze testing, the selection of six rats for each of the eight subgroups was made randomly from a larger pool of 90 rats. At least four different litters were represented in each subgroup, and for each of the four combinations of the thyroid and sex variables comparisons could be made in littermates. (No systematic litter effects appeared in the behavioral data, however.)

Although none of the E rats appeared to have difficulty in
getting to food and water in the superenrichment apparatus, mean
body weights of males were lower for E than for I rats in both the
hypothyroids (TE:302 g, TI: 331 g, p< .10) and the controls (CE:
346 g, CI: 388 g, p< .01) on Day 70. This weight difference has
been a frequent finding in studies of rearing environments (Rosenzweig et al 1972). During a 5-day period in which all rats were
individually housed with unlimited access to food and water, the
weights of the E and I groups showed no convergence. (Later we
found these weight differences in the males to persist through
Day 240). On Day 75 we instituted the food deprivation schedule
(85% target weights adjusted for normal growth of a given treat-
ment-combination).

The chronology of the behavioral testing is provided in Table
I.   In the symmetrical maze on Days 80-132 the rats received problems P-1, P-2, P-3, and T-2 (in place of the usual P-4) for practice and T-6, T-9, T-10, and T-11 (in place of the usual T-12) for
regular test problems. The test problems were run to the usual
criterion in a single session and after problem T-9 a four-trial
retention test was given at least 2 days after each problem's
acquisition session before proceeding to the next problem:
retention intervals varied from 2 to 4 days for individual rats
on a given problem, but this variation did not correlate with
retention error scores. We gave additional tests in passive
avoidance, barpressing, and running-wheel activity situations
for reasons we will clarify later. After these tests, the males
were set aside for neuroanatomical studies and the females were
returned to the symmetrical maze for two final problems at
200-210 days of age.

TABLE 1
1974-75 Thiouracil Experiment: Chronology of Testing Procedures

Procedure	Age in Days
Enriched and isolated environments	36 - 70
Body weight test, ad libituum feeding,	70 - 75
Maze pretraining and practice problems	77 - 98
Maze problems T-6 through T-11	99 - 132
Passive avoidance testing	148 - 152
Barpressing acquisition	157 - 162
Barpressing extinction	164 - 166
Barpressing reacquisition and VI shcedule	167 - 183
Activity: 20-min sessions	172 - 182
Activity: 5-day periods (females only)	185 - 195
Maze problems T-7 and T-8 (females only)	200 - 210

1. <u>Maze learning results</u>. The initial symmetrical maze acquisition results, summarized in Fig. 3, were clear: the learning deficit shown by the superenriched hypothyroid rats was sharply reduced
in comparison to that displayed by the isolated hypothyroids. We
found, in fact, an overall 62% reduction in terms of the ratio of
group mean error differences as calculated previously (TI-TE/TI-
CI). For females the reduction averaged 77%, for males 47% (this
was not a statistically significant sex difference, however). Thus
the enriched thiouracil rats generally performed more like the two
groups of normal rats, which again showed no effect of the environmental conditions, than like the isolated thiouracils. These findings were consistent over the four maze problems (see Fig. 4) and
results for the trials-to-criterion measure were highly similar to
the error data.

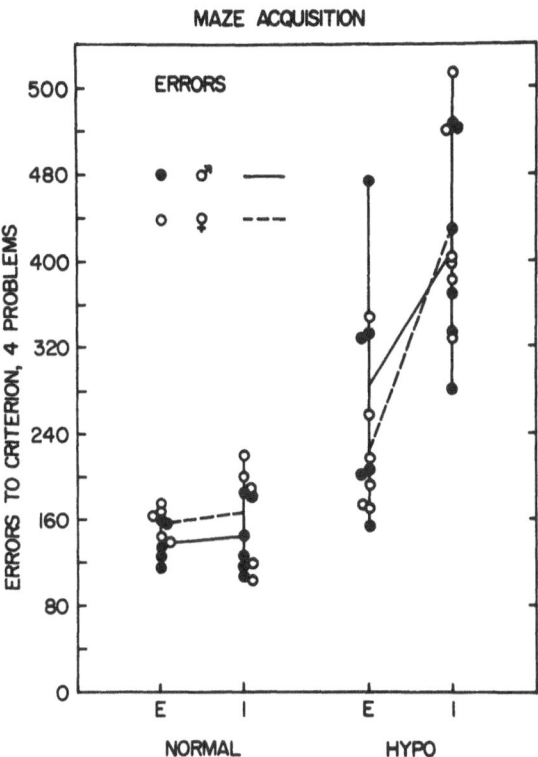

Fig. 3. Acquisition errors, totaled over four symmetrical maze
problems, made by superenriched (E) and isolated (I) normal and
hypothyroid rats tested at 99-132 days of age in our 1974-75
thiouracil study. The filled (male) and unfilled (female) circles
represent individual scores. Subgroup means are indicated by the
connecting lines.

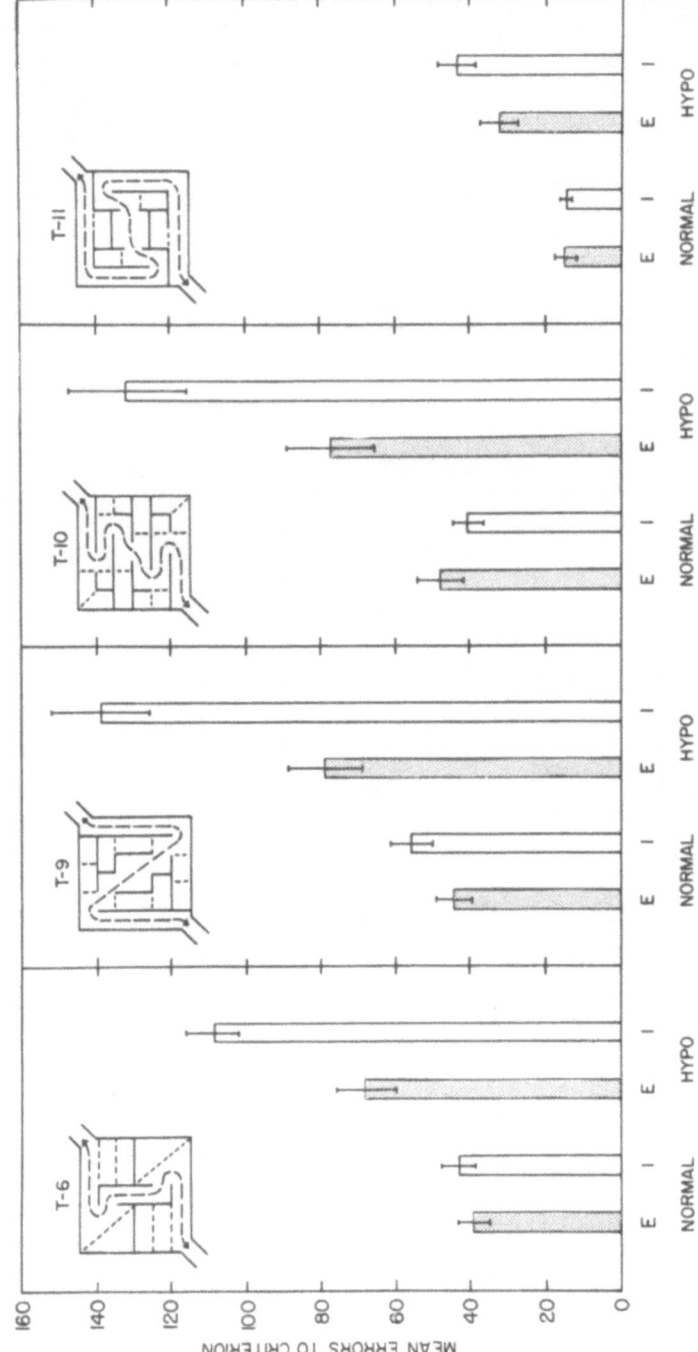

Fig. 4. Means and standard errors of acquisition error scores on each of the initial four symmetrical maze problems, for superenriched (E, shaded bars) and isolated (I, open bars) normal and hypothyroid rats in our 1974-75 thiouracil study.

In an overall analysis of variance of the error scores, the interaction between the environment and thyroid factors was significant ($\underline{F}$ = 12.61; $\underline{df}$ = 1, 37; $\underline{p}$ < .005), as was the difference between the TE and TI groups ($\underline{t}$ = 4.30, $\underline{p}$ < .001). The TE group's error scores still represented a significant ($\underline{p}$ < 01) deficit in comparison to the two control groups, but it is worth noting that seven of the 12 rats in this group fell within the range of the controls' error scores (Fig. 3) whereas none of the 12 TI rats did.

2. <u>Maze retention results</u>. The four-trial retention tests on maze problems T-9, T-10, and T-11 (Fig. 5) revealed our first clear evidence of longterm memory deficit in early-hypothyroid rats. More importantly for our present purposes, they also showed more dramatic evidence of deficit-reduction by enrichment than the original learning scores on these problems did. Calculated as before, the overall reduction of retention errors in the TE group was 97%.

Analysis of the retention error scores showed that the thyroid ($\underline{F}$ = 8.60) and environmental ($\underline{F}$ = 8.01) main effects were significant ($\underline{df}$ = 1, 37; $\underline{p}$ <.01 for each). The interaction between these factors

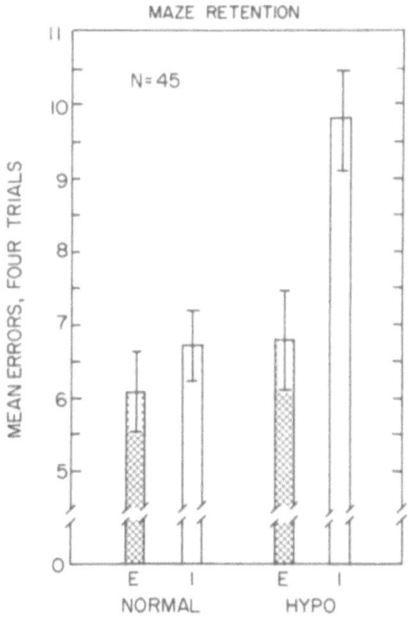

Fig. 5. Longterm memory in the maze: means and standard errors of symmetrical maze retention error scores, averaged over problems T-9, T-10 and T-11, for superenriched (E) and isolated (I) normal and hypothyroid rats in our 1974-75 thiouracil study. These data were obtained two to four days after each problem was run to criterion in a single acquisition session.

only approached significance (p <10), reflecting the fact that an unreliable environmental effect in the controls was in the same direction as the highly reliable (t = 3.13, p < .01) effect in the hypothyroids. Again sex differences were nonsignificant.

3. <u>Durability of environmental effects on the maze</u>. The final two problems in the maze, which we administered to the female subgroups at 200 days of age, provided some impressive evidence that postweaning superenrichment can be a durable form of "therapy" (Fig. 6). In acquisition errors the deficit-reduction (calculated as before) was 54.3%, and in errors on the first two retention trials (46–48 hr after acquisition for each rat) it was 87.4%. These percentages represent relatively small declines from the corresponding reductions of 77% and 100% which the thiouracil females displayed in their initial maze testing nearly 3 months earlier.

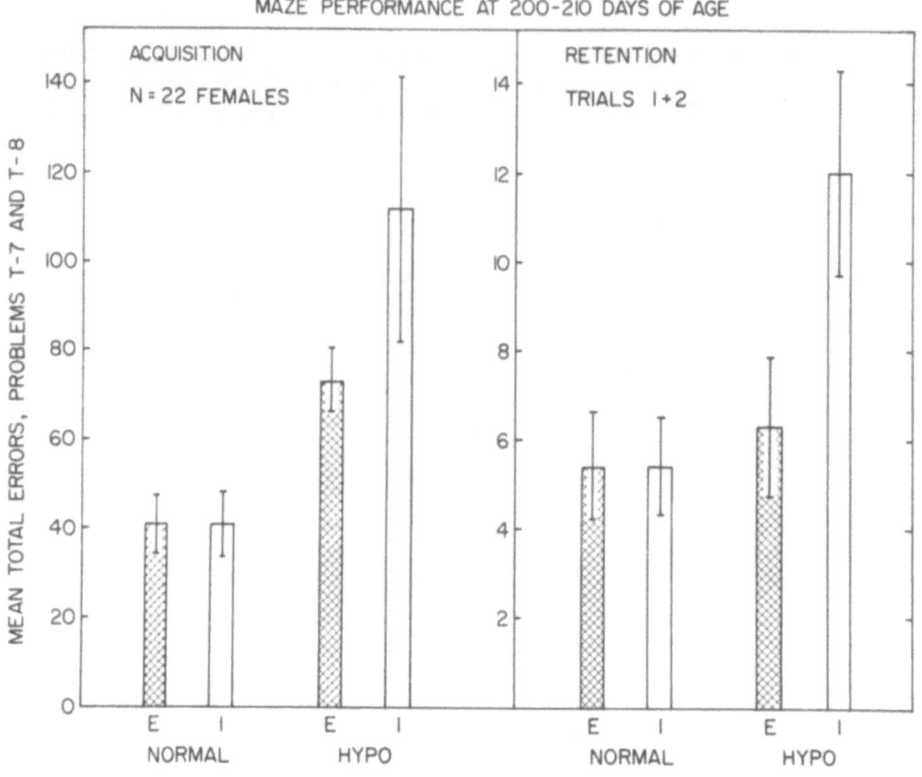

Fig. 6. Results in the final tests of symmetrical maze acquisition (left panel) and retention (right panel), administered to the female subgroups of the 1974-75 thiouracil study 130-140 days after the end of the superenrichment (E) and isolation (I) treatments. Means and standard errors of error scores, averaged over problems T-7 and T-8, are depicted.

4. Severity of maze learning deficit. Some further evidence
of environment-facilitated maze learning came from   supplemental
study with propylthiouracil (PTU) treated rats. This was a small-
scale study with 18 offspring of eight mothers which were exposed
to mash diets containing PTU in doses ranging from 0.01 to 0.2%
from gestation Day 7 or 17 to postnatal Day 10. At all doses of
PTU we found a surprisingly high incidence of teratogenic effects
(fetal resorption, reduced litter size, stillbirths), and the
surviving offspring showed no more severe retardation of physical
growth than the thiouracil-treated pups of the main experiment
which were reared concurrently. They also displayed, at 65 days
of age, the most severely deficient maze performance we have observed in our six years of experience with the symmetrical maze.
On problem T-6, which was given after the standard pretraining
and practice problems, only five of the 18 rats reached criterion
within 48 trials.

From weaning until the completion of this problem, all of the
PTU-treated rats had been housed individually in standard rack
cages. After the problem they were assigned to E and I groups
(five males, four females in each) which were equated for errors
on problem T-6 and average PTU dose. The E group was placed in
the superenrichment apparatus from 71 to 103 days of age, while
the I group remained in the individual cages. Four days after
the end of the E treatment and the reinstitution of food deprivation, maze testing resumed with problem T-9 administered in a 6
trials/day procedure.

On the first day the E males made only half as many errors
as the I males (means of 41.6 and 81.8, no overlap of the score
distributions, $p < 01$). One extremely high error score by an E
rat prevented a similar trend in the females from attaining statistical significance. No environmental effects appeared in retention tests on later days. Because of time restrictions and
the absence of control groups, we did not test the PTU rats
further. Although only a scrap of evidence, the T-9 acquisition
results seem to be an important indication that even severely
deficient rats can be benefited in their learning performance by
an enriched environment and that the stimulation from such an
environment need not be restricted to the immediate postweaning
period in order to exert this effect.

5. Passive avoidance. The maze retention results shown by the
thiouracil-treated rats in the main experiment prompted us to
examine performance in a quite different paradigm single-trial
passive avoidance -- which is popular among researchers in memory
consolidation. For this task we used a step-down apparatus that
was fashioned from two Gerbrands operant conditioning chambers
(with rear walls removed) placed back-to-back. The grid floor

of one chamber was covered with clear Plexiglas. Step-down latencies from the Plexiglas floor to the exposed grid floor were recorded on three (nonshock) adaptation trials and a single acquisition trial (0.5 ma shock, duration determined by the rat's escape
by returning to the Plexiglas floor) on Day 1 and on two (nonshock)
test trials 72 hr later on Day 2. Trials were spaced about 1 hr
apart on each day. This testing was conducted during a temporary
period of ad libitum feeding from Day 133 to 153.

As Fig. 7 shows, we found an expected deficit in thiouracil
rats' passive avoidance, but no reliable effect of the environment
variable, in contrast to the previous maze results. Analysis of
step-down speeds (reciprocalized latencies) on the first test trial
showed a significant thyroid effect ($\underline{F}$ = 10.73; $\underline{df}$ = 1, 37; $\underline{p}$<.005)
and no other significant effect or interaction. A suggestion of lower
speeds in the TE than TI rats appeared on the second test trial, but
this was also far short of significance.

6. <u>Barpressing extinction</u>. We administered the free-operant
barpressing tasks in four identical Gerbrands chambers which we
equipped with retractable levers. The 45 rats received five 10-min
acquisition sessions in which barpressing was continuously reinforced
(CRF) with 45-mg food pellets, three 20-min extinction sessions, two
10-min CRF reacquisition sessions, and ten 10-min sessions on a
variable-interval (VI 30 sec) schedule of reinforcement. Some interesting group differences emerged on the first day of acquisition and
in the VI sessions which we prefer to present later as motivational

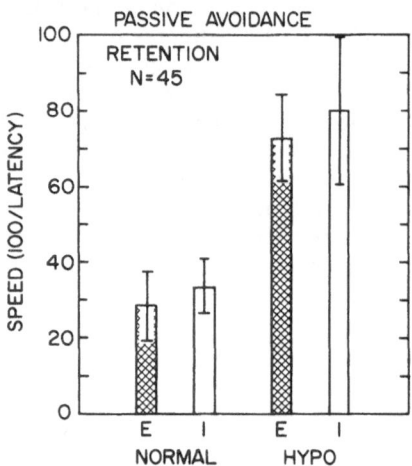

Fig. 7. Passive avoidance retention: means and standard errors of
step-down speeds on Trial 5, given 72 hr after the single shock
trial, for the same superenriched (E) and isolated (I) rats as in
Figs. 3-5.

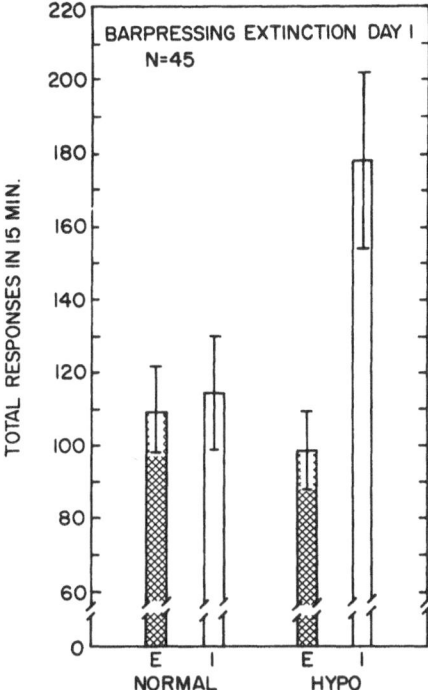

Fig. 8. Resistance to extinction of barpressing: means and standard errors of total presses in the first extinction session for the same superenriched (E) and isolated (I) rats as in Figs. 3, 4, 5, and 7.

effects. The groups performed almost identically on the later days of acquisition, but in extinction we found a normal-hypothyroid difference in the I condition which may be classed as a learning (or response-inhibition) deficit and another striking effect of the superenrichment treatment (Fig. 8).

In line with some nonsignificant trends which we have observed previously (Davenport and Dorcey, 1972; Davenport, et. al 1976), the thiouracil isolates of both sexes were more resistant to extinction than their corresponding controls. On the other hand, the enriched thiouracils extinguished rapidly, much like controls, thus showing an effect of the superenrichment experience that resembled the reductions of acquisition and retention deficits in the maze. Analysis of barpressing totals on Day 1 of extinction showed a significant environmental effect ($\underline{F}$ = 6.04; $\underline{df}$ = 1, 37. $\underline{p}$ <.025) and a significant interaction between the environment and thyroid variables ($\underline{F}$ = 4.62; $\underline{df}$ = 1, 37; $\underline{p}.$ <.05). By subsequent $\underline{t}$ tests, both the deficit in the isolates (TI vs. CI, p<.05) and the enrichment reduction of the deficit (TI vs. TE, p<.01) proved to be reliable effects. Findings were similar for the 3-day extinction period.

We also examined spontaneous recovery in terms of changes in barpressing rates from the last 5 min of one extinction session to the first 5 min of the next. In contrast to Davenport and Hennies' (1976) finding of significantly greater spontaneous recovery of barpressing in thiouracil-treated female rats, no reliable group differences appeared in transitions from extinction Day 1 to Day 2 or from Day 2 to Day 3 in the present data.

7. <u>Motivational tasks.</u> Simple conditioning tasks such as acquisition of barpressing or runway locomotion do not usually bring out abnormalities in early-hypothyroid rats which can be categorized as learning deficits. They can, however, reveal emotional or motivational differences which sometimes may result in paradoxically "better" performance by hypothyroid than normal rats. Recently, for example, we have found more rapid acquisition of bar-touching and barpressing tasks in thiouracil-treated than in normal female rats (Davenport and Hennies, 1976). We intrepreted this to reflect reduced fearfulness in thiouracil females, since these animals showed somewhat unusual tameness in handling and in adapting to other apparatuses, in line with some early observations of neonatally thyroidectomized rats by Eayrs and Lishman (1955). We have also found elevated VI barpressing, running-wheel activity, food and water intake, and oxygen consumption in early hypothyroid rats (Davenport and Hennies, 1976), which may suggest a persistent hypermetabolic state, although the VI barpressing and activity elevations could reflect a generalized "disinhibition syndrome."

We gave our superenriched and isolated rats some of these tasks to see whether hypothyroid rats' motivational aberrations could be normalized by the E conditions. The first task, barpressing, acquisition, was negative on this point, but showed some interesting environmental and sex differences in normal rats. On the first day of acquisition (see Fig. 9), we replicated the Davenport and Hennies result for females -- faster acquisition by isolated thiouracils than by isolated normals -- and confirmed that the same effect is much smaller or nonexistent in males. Viewed another way, normal females, but not males, seem to be disadvantaged in this simple task by their natural fearfulness (possibly enhanced by prior shock experience in the similar avoidance chamber). The effect of the superenrichment condition was (again) to reduce the disadvantage, rendering the normal E females about equal to thiouracil (E or I) females and all four male subgroups. In separate analyses of the Day-1 barpressing scores, the females showed a significant ($p<.05$ interaction between the environment and thyroid factors, while the males showed no reliable effects; a subsequent t test verified that the female CI subgroup was significantly ($p<.05$) below the other three females subgroups.

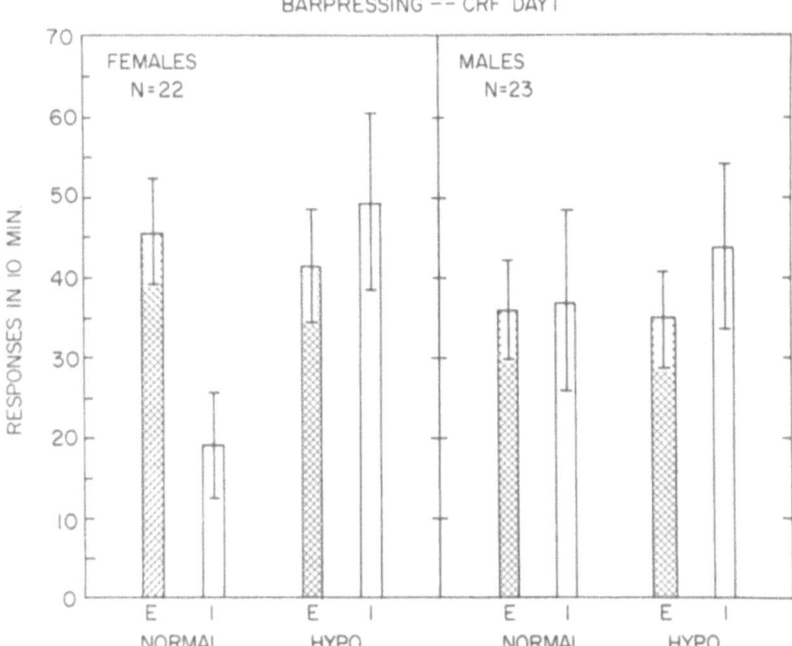

Fig. 9. Adaptation to the barpressing situation: means and standard errors of total presses on the first day of CRF barpressing
acquisition for each of the eight subgroups in the 1974-75 thiouracil study. Because of the rats' prior familiarity with
pellet feeders in the maze, magazine training was not given in
the barpressing apparatus before acquisition. E: superenriched,
I: isolated.

Trends were similar in the rats' initial exposure to the maze
(practice problem P-1), the avoidance apparatus (first adaptation
trial of Day 1), and the running wheels (first session). In each
case, the CI females were the slowest female group to adapt in
terms of quantitative measures, significantly so on the first two
trials of maze problem P-1 ($p < .01$) and the first trial in the
avoidance chamber ($p < .02$). Interestingly, the only deviation in
these other tasks from the pattern shown by all eight subgroups
on Day 1 of barpressing acquisition (Fig. 9) was another significant effect of the E-1 conditions in the males --faster trial times
by the TE males than by the other three male subgroups ($p \leqslant 05$)--
on maze practice problem P-1, which was the first task encountered
by the rats after the enrichment experience. Thus we have some
fairly extensive evidence that this experience reduces a rather
persistent fearfulness in normal female rats and a more transient
fearfulness in thiouracil-treated male rats.

On the VI 30 sec barpressing schedule, TI females responded
excessively relative to CI females, confirming Davenport and
Hennies (1976). TE females did not show this elevation (Fig. 10).
Because of high variability, the overall TI-TE difference in the
female was not statistically reliable. Taken with Davenport and
Hennies' result, the TE reduction suggests a normalization effect
of the environment paralleling the extinction results (Fig. 8).
Males, in contrast, performed identically at rates significantly
($\underline{p} < .05$) below the females'.

Following each of the first nine VI sessions, the rats were
given a 20-min activity session in standard Wahmann running wheels.
No conclusive results were found in these activity tests other than
significantly ($\underline{p} < .001$) higher activity levels in females than
males.

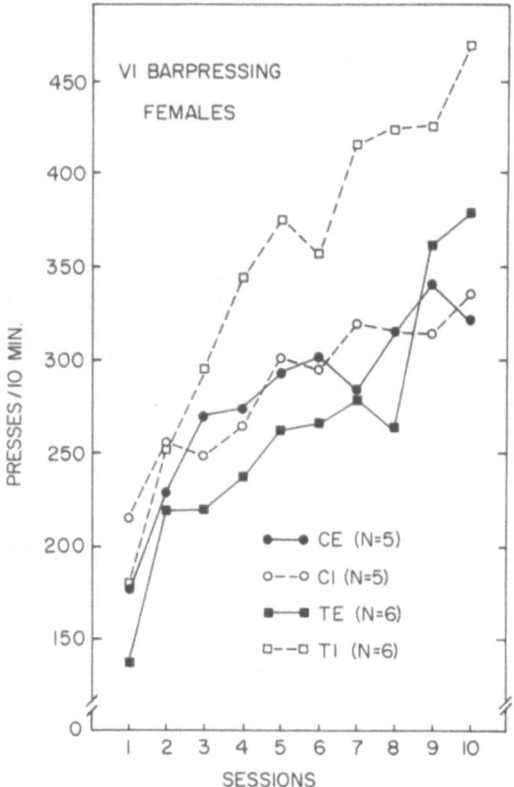

Fig. 10. Mean response rates over ten VI 30-sec barpressing sessions
for the normal-superenriched (CE), normal-isolated (CI), hypothyroid-
superenriched (TE), and hypothyroid-isolated (TI) female subgroups
of the 1974-75 thiouracil study.

C. Summary and Interpretations

We will begin a discussion of our findings with the following summary:

1. In terms of learning-memory tasks, superenrichment reduced hypothyroid rats' deficits very substantially in maze acquisition and almost totally in maze retention and barpressing extinction, but not at all in passive avoidance performance.

2. Lasting benefits of the experience were found in the extinction task over 3 months after completion of the environmental manipulation and in final tests of maze learning and retention nearly 5 months after these treatments.

3. Maze learning deficits were also partially alleviated by postweaning enriched conditions like those of the Berkeley studies in thiouracil-treated rats (our 1972 finding which did not replicate) and by superenriched conditions administered during early adulthood to more severely-deficient PTU-treated rats (1974-75 supplemental study).

4. In terms of motivational tasks, we found some fairly clear indications that excessive VI barpressing in female hypothryoid rats was normalized by superenrichment and that this treatment improved adaptation to novel apparatus settings in normal females.

5. Environmental effects in our studies were differential for hypothyroid and normal rats; in all four tasks which revealed normalization of behavior in hypothyroid rats, no significant effect of environmental stimulation appeared in normal rats.

The enrichment-facilitated learning by our hypothyroid rats could be interpreted in terms of one or more of the following: (a) positive transfer of specific associations from the enriched environment to the later test situations; (b) differences between the E and I rats in exploratory tendencies, gross activity levels, emotionality, or other motivational functions; (c) "developmental acquisition of competence" (cf., Hunt, this volume) in the E rats or, conversely, "learned helplessness" (cf.,Seligman, 1975) in the I rats; or (d) improved learning capacities of a more general nature. In this section and the next, we will argue that the last of these alternatives best fits our overall results and is also consistent with the behavioral and neuroanatomical effects of environmental stimulation which have been reported in studies with normal animals.

The main point to be raised against the first three interpretations is that, with one minor exception, differential rearing experience did not significantly affect our normal rats. In task after task, these control groups failed to show any influence of

specific transfer or differences along a competence-helplessness
contimuum and the only clear suggestion of superiority in adapt-
ting to various apparatuses. Other data (e.g. Davenport et al.,
1970; Davenport and Dorcey, 1972) indicate that our typically
small differences between E and I normal groups in symmetrical
maze learning were probably not due to floor effects, and we have
additional data showing that this task is abundantly sensitive
to manipulations of hunger (Davenport and Gonzalez., 1973) and
amount of reward (unpublished data, 1973) in normal rats. The
very familiar barpressing extinction task seems similarly untaint-
ed by floor effects or lack of sensitivity.

The nearly-equivalent performances by our control groups do not
completely negate the potential roles of transfer or motivational
mediation in the hypothyroid rats; possibly the latter were
somehow more subject to these influences than the normal rats.
Particularly in the case of the maze acquisition data in our 1974-
75 studies, we would not contend that there was no facilitative
transfer of specific learnings from the tunneling and enclosed-
maze experiences in our superenrichment apparatus. It is also
conceivable that at least a small part of the E-I difference in
the hypothyroids' maze learning could stem from differences in
learned competence or helplessness.

Notice, however, that it is more difficult to deal with our
maze retention and barpressing extinction results in these
terms. Here, in both cases, performance was measured after all
eight subgroups had been trained to comparable levels of mastery
(i.e. to the common criterion of learning in each maze problem
and to virtually identical asymptotic levels in barpressing acquisition). In terms of effects on longterm memory or resistance
to extinction, the influence of specific associations from the
superenrichment setting would seemingly be quite overshadowed by
the equated learnings in the acquisition phases of these tasks.
So also would the more general form of transfer represented by the
concepts of learned competence or helplessness; in Seligman's (19-
75) terms, these mastery experiences ought to have provided enough
"immunization" to render the groups fairly equal on the competence-
helplessness continuum. Finally, if enriched environments can
retroactively interfere with retention (Parsons and Spear, 1972),
proactive interference cannot be completely ignored as a factor
which might have given the impoverished animals an advantage in
retention or rate of extinction.

Motivational mediation fares even less well as an explanation
of the facilitations in our hypothyroid rats. Generally, there was
very little evidence, in our activity or open-field tests, in other
auxiliary measures (e.g performance in maze practice problems), or
in casual observations, that E and I hypothyroids (or normals)
differed in arousal levels or exploratory tendencies, and the sig-

nificant group differences which we found in apparent fearfulness did not correlate with group differences on the maze or extinction tasks. A similar lack of correlation held for some non-significant differences in exploration which we observed in the latter practice problems of the maze in our 1974-75 thiouracil study. After reviewing over a dozen studies reporting E-I differences in exploration in normal rodents (see discussions by Rosenzweig, 1972; Smith, 1972: and Walsh and Cummins, in press), we are highly skeptical that learning, memory and extinction effects can be attributed to such differences.

The surviving interpretation is that environmental stimulation improved certain learning capacities in our hypothyroid rats. "Learning capacities" cannot be defined precisely at this time, but may be taken to include abilities to form, store, and retrieve associations, to acquire spatial orientation, and to inhibit maladaptive responding. All things considered, we feel that it is easier to account for the data in our studies in terms of impairment of such abilities by early hypothyroidism and remediation of these impaired abilities by environmental stimulation. As one would expect with changes in learning abilities, both of these effects seem to be durable. Noting that the persisting behavioral impairments from early thyroid deficiency are correlated (in a general fashion, at least) with apparently enduring central nervous system abnormalities (Eayrs, 1971), we favor an expansion of the "capacity" interpretation to include the notion that the remediation effect probably reflects enhanced neural growth of the types revealed in enrichment studies (e.g. Greenough, 1975). In particular, the remediation of maze retention deficit (Fig. 5) and the durability of this effect evidenced by our final maze tests (Fig. 6) carry the implication that retentive capacity was improved in our impoverished hypothyroid rats through relatively permament "wiring changes" in the brain. This broader view also suits our findings of facilitated maze acquisition and barpressing extinction in the hypothyroids. Perhaps it also accounts for the normalization of their elevated VI barpressing.

If relatively general and durable learning capacities are enhanced by the enriched rearing conditions, individual hypothyroid rats showing therapeutic successes on one learning task ought to show similar remediation on other learning tasks which reliably detect normal-hypothyroid differences, and therapeutic failures should show consistently poor performance across the same tasks. These expectations were confirmed in our main study. The five rats in the enriched hypothyroid (TE) group which were relatively "unremediated" in comparison to seven "normalized" rats in this group whose maze acquisition error scores fell within the total score range of the 21 normal rats (see Fig. 3) were also among the poorest performance in the maze retention and barpressing extinction tasks in nearly every instance. Thanks also to the con-

TABLE 2

Listing of Studies on Effects of Differential
Experience on Learning in Normal Rats,
Since Hebb (1949)

Reference	Treatment Age	Task
A. Findings of Enhanced Learning in Enriched Rats		
Hymovitch (1952)	30 - 75	Hebb-Williams maze
Forgays & Forgays (1952)	29 - 90	Hebb-Williams maze
Bingham & Griffiths (1952)	21 - 51	Warner-Warden, incli-ned-plane mazes
Forgus (1954)	24 - 84	Multiple-T maze
Cooper & Zubek (1958)	25 - 65	Hebb-Williams maze
Woods (1959)	23 - 154[a]	Hebb-Williams maze
Woods et al (1960)	21 - 90	Hebb-Williams maze
Woods et al (1961)	25 - 155	Hebb-Williams maze (low drive)
Forgays & Read (1962)	0 - 109[b]	Hebb-Williams maze
Krech et al (1962)	25 - 55	Visual discrimination reversal
Schwartz (1964)	30 - 95	Hebb-Williams maze
Schweikert & Collins (1966)	25 - 75	Hebb-Williams maze
Nyman (1967)	30 - 80[c]	Alternation & Hebb-Williams mazes
Brown (1968)	20 - 100[d]	Hebb-Williams maze
Denenberg et al (1968)	0-21,21 - 50	Hebb-Williams maze
Edwards et al (1969)	25 - 85	Brightness discrimina-tion
Ray & Hochauser (1969)	21 - 85	Lashley III maze, ac-tive avoidance
Bennett et al (1970)	25 - 185[e]	Visual reversal dis-crimination, and Dash-iell, Lashley, & H.W. mazes
Brown & King (1971)	25 - 105	Visual discrimination
Sturgeon & Reid (1971)	21 - 81	Hebb-Williams maze
Bernstein (1972)	21 - 66	Brightness discrimina-tion
Doty (1972)	300 - 660	Discrimination, active avoidance reversal, passive avoidance
Freeman & Ray (1972)	25-55, 28 - 88	Lashley maze, passive avoidance
Greenough et al (1972a)	23 - 53	Lashley III maze, runway speed
Ough et al (1972)	21 - 70	DRL 20-sec barpressing
Smith (1972)	21 - 55	Hebb-Williams maze
Tanabe (1972)	26 - 60	Hebb-Williams maze
Wells et al (1972)	21 - 100	Hebb-Williams maze
West & Greenough (1972)	23 - 53	Lashley III maze

TABLE 2 (Cont'd)

Bernstein (1973)	21 - 84	Brightness disc., Lashley III maze
Cummins et al (1973)	21 - 530	Hebb-Williams maze
Greenough et al (1973)	23 - 53	Lashley III maze, brightness disc.

B. Findings of No Significant Enhancement of Learning in Enriched rats.

Hymovitch (1952)	27 - 78	Multiple T-maze
Bingham & Griffiths (1952)	21 - 51	Visual discrimination
Woods et al (1960)	21 - 215	Visual discrimination
Woods et al (1961)	25-60, 25 - 155	Hebb-Williams maze (high drive)
Krech et al (1962)	25 - 55	Visual discrimination (acq.)
Hughes (1965)	33 - 66	Hebb-Williams maze
Gill et al (1966)	21 - 81	Visual discrimination
Reid et al (1968)	21 - 81	Hebb-Williams maze
Bennett et al (1970)	25 - 120[e]	Visual reversal discrimination
Doty (1972)	300 - 600	Active avoidance acquisition
Freeman & Ray (1972)	28 - 55	Active avoidance, Y-maze
Ough et al (1972)	21 - 70	CRF barpressing acquisition
Gonzalez & Davenport (1972)	30 - 60	Symmetrical maze acquisition
Davenport (1974-75)	36 - 70	Symmetrical maze acquisition & retention, passive avoidance, barpressing extinction & VI

---

[a]Three different treatment ages: 23-63, 23-154, and 66-154.

[b]Five different treatment ages: 0-21, 22-43, 44-65, 66-87, and 88-109.

[c]Three different treatment ages: 30-40, 50-60, and 70-80.

[d]Three different treatment ages: 20-60, 60-100, and 20-100.

[e]Positive" findings by Bennett et al (1970) or Rosenzweig (1971) at 25-55, 25-85, and 25-185 in visual reversal discrimination and at 25-55 and 60-90 in Lashley III maze learning. Their Dashiell and Hebb-Williams results, also positive, were not published. "Negative" findings at 60-90 and 90-120 in visual reversal discrimination.

sistency of the seven normalized rats over the three tasks, maze acquisition correlated positively with maze retention (r = .69, p <.02) and with barpressing extinction (r = .55, p <.06) in the TE group as a whole; corresponding correlations were .28 (p<.20) and .52 (p <.10) in the TI group and much lower in the control groups.

The absence of an environmental effect in the hypothyroids' passive avoidance performance contrasted sharply with our results in other tasks. At the time we inserted this task into our test battery, we considered it an interesting way to compare two very different memory paradigms -- maze retention vs. passive avoidance retention -- with respect to thyroid and environmental effects. More recently, however, we have become convinced that our normal-hypothyroid difference in passive avoidance (Fig. 7) represents a combination of motivational abnormalities rather than a memory deficit. This conviction stems from having noticed, literally hundreds of times, how much less capable of "sitting still" in a confined space thiouracil-treated rats are in comparison to normals during weighing and other handling. We now prefer the interpretation that the poor inhibition on passive avoidance test trials by hypothyroids reflects such "fidgetiness," and other motivational aberrations (e.g. reduced fearfulness and more general hyperactivity) which we have quantified in these animals (Davenport and Hennies, 1976).

Such motivational attributes seem unlikely to be normalized by environmental stimulation, and we speculate that a considerable range of behavioral capacities will prove to be unalterable by enrichment of experience, perhaps including early-maturing vegetative functions, homeostatic drives, fixed-action patterns, and the ability to acquire simple conditioned responses. This leaves many other capacities having greater intellectual and social significance, however, which may turn out to be very fortunate from a therapeutic standpoint.

III. Other Behavioral Studies of Differential Experience

A. Normal Animal Populations

Our consistent failure to obtain significant environmental effects in normal rats has led us to take a more detailed look at the behavioral literature in this area. Several reviews (e.g. Bennett et al 1970; Gluck and Harlow, 1971; Rosenzweig, 1971: Rosenzweig et al 1972) have emphasized the inconsistency of the effect of enriched rearing in normal animals' learning performance. Has this picture changed recently?

Table 2 suggests that it has. In this table we have listed chronologically all of the studies we have been able to find on learning in enriched and more-impoverished (isolated or social-

control) normal rats. In most of these studies the features of the
enriched environments were similar to those in the Berkeley studies--
group housing in a large cage with objects -- but the age at which
the rats were exposed to the E condition (given in the center column of the table) varied considerably.

The number of positive demonstrations of enrichment-facilitated
learning in normal rats has now grown to almost three dozen studies,
and over four dozen enriched treatment groups, not counting some
studies (e.g., Bennett et al 1970;Morgan, 1973) showing better learning in social-control than isolated rats, or studies showing E-
facilitation in mice (Greenough et al   1972[b]; Henderson, 1970).
We have also found about one dozen negative findings, including
an anomalous result showing poorer performance by enriched rats
(the 60-90 group in Bennett et al 1970). In nine of the negative
reports, the same authors presented positive findings in other learning tasks, usually in the same groups of rats. Even allowing for
an unknown number of negative results which never got into print,
this quantitative summary amounts to impressive evidence of facilitated learning by environmental stimulation. Although most of the
pre-1970 studies relied on the Hebb-Williams maze, and some of these
probably obtained facilitation that resulted from specific transfer (see Gluck and Harlow, 1971), the more recent studies from
Greenough's laboratory and the positive results in the simpler tasks
used by Freeman and Ray (1972), Doty (1972), and Ough et al (1972)
provide sufficient diversity to warrant a tentative conclusion that
a fairly general learning capacity is increased by enrichment relative to impoverished rearing conditions.

Regarding other species, about a half-dozen studies of E-I
effects have been conducted with dogs (reviewed by Bennett et al
1970, and Gluck and Harlow,1971) and one (Wilson et al 1965) in
cats. It seems fair to count most of these as positive findings,
although to a greater extent than in rats the studies in dogs,
particularly Lessac and Solomon's (1969), have emphasized the deleterious emotional and cognitive consequences of isolated rearing
conditions. Gluck et al (1973) have presented the first compelling
evidence of enrichment-facilitated learning in rhesus monkeys.
After earlier studies in their laboratory had failed to find such
an effect in object discrimination, learning set, delayed response,
and avoidance conditioning (see Harlow et al 1971)these researchers
found that monkeys reared in enriched "nuclear family" environments
performed significantly better than partial isolates in oddity
learning set, under conditions in which this effect could not readily be attributed to specific transfer in the enriched monkeys or
poor adaptation in the isolates. Their results have since been
confirmed in a comparison of enriched and social-control (mother-
and peer-reared) monkeys in oddity learning set (S. Suomi, personal communication). Another recent study by R.K. Davenport et al

(1973), found that eight wild-born chimpanzees scored higher than
six chimpanzees reared for the first two years of life in restricted laboratory environments in object discrimination transfer
index testing, after both groups had lived under similar laboratory
conditions for long periods prior to this adult testing. An earlier
study from the Yerkes group (Davenport and Rogers, 1970) had shown
better discrimination, delayed-response, and oddity performance in
feral-reared than deprived chimpanzees. The positive trends in the
rodent and primate studies over the past five years suggest that environmental stimulation increases learning capacities in essentially
all subhuman mammalian species. (See also Hunt, this volume).

        Our negative results in normal rats, then, are exceptional,
particularly considering the similarity of our symmetrical maze
apparatus to the Hebb-Williams maze. The absence of E-I effects in
our control groups provides a distinct advantage in ruling out transfer and motivational factors as responsible for the reduction of
deficits in hypothyroid rats, but we are understandably concerned
about reconciling our control-group results with the many positive
findings. Some studies (e.g., Woods et al, 1960, 1961; Reid et al,
1968) have suggested that E-I effects in normal rats tend to disappear under high motivation and after extended pretraining. Since
our food deprivation conditions were moderately severe and our rats
were well-adapted even in the first of their tasks, these factors
might account for the discrepancy. We are currently studying the
interaction of hunger levels, pretraining conditions, and differential postweaning experience in the symmetrical maze to clarify
matters. In any event, we do not take the close similarities in
performance by our control groups to represent equivalence in underlying learning capacities. Rather, we assume from the evidence in
Table 2 that at least a small difference in favor of superior capacities in our enriched controls was induced by environmental stimulation, but that the capacities of the impoverished controls were
sufficient for performance that was nearly as proficient as the enriched controls, under our particular testing conditions.

        Only a few of the studies showing enhanced learning in enriched
normal rats have pursued the important question of the durability of
this effect. Denenberg et al (1968) demonstrated facilitation by enrichment in Hebb-Williams maze performance over 300 days after the
end of their E and SC conditions; this durable effect surprisingly
resulted from pre- as well as postweaning enrichment. Earlier studies by Forgays and Forgays (1952) and Forgays and Read (1962) also
showed facilitations in the Hebb-Williams task over intervals of four
weeks to 90 days. Rosenweig (1971), however, has reported rapid
diminutions of postweaning E-I effects in this task, in visual
discrimination, and in the Lashley III maze. The only other information on this question in the normal-rat literature seems to be in
Sturgeon and Reid's (1971) work, in which rats exposed to E cond-

itions for 60 days immediately after weaning clearly outperformed isolates in their first series of Hebb-Williams problems starting at Day 110 but performed only slightly better on a second testing at Day 190. This study emphasizes the durability of our E-I effects in hypothyroid rats, since their maze tests were given at ages comparable to our first and final symmetrical maze tests. (Interestingly, Sturgeon and Reid also employed a procedure which involved a greater range and variety of stimulation than the usual Berkeley procedure). Since these investigators merely retested their rats on the same Hebb-Williams problems in their Day-190 testing, however, their groups may have converged because of a floor effect, such that durability did not get a fair test in their study.

In any event, our finding of lasting but slightly declining benefits in the more difficult symmetrical maze fits quite well with work from Berkeley (Bennett et al 1974) showing persistence of brain weight and enzyme changes from the standard E condition for over six weeks after the rats are transferred from E to I conditions (see also Walsh and Cummins, this volume). This report by Bennett et al also contains evidence of somewhat larger cerebral effects from still another kind of superenriched environment (one devised by Ferchmin et al 1970) than from the standard E treatment, in agreement with Kuenzle and Knüsel (1974) and paralleling Sturgeon and Reid's (1971) finding that their superenriched rats made fewer errors than their standard-E-reared rats in the initial maze testing. Similarly, Brown and King's (1971) study indicated that increments in variety of stimulation (but not increases in amount, or formal training in discrimination) contribute significantly to differences between social-control and various enrichment conditions in cholinergic enzyme activities and in visual discrimination performance. These recent findings point to the likelihood that both cerebral and behavioral changes may become larger and more durable as the variety of stimulation is increased in the rearing environment. The "capacity" interpretation of enrichment effects has gained credence from these latest studies.

B. Other Disadvantaged Populations

Our literature searches have yielded only a few studies of environmental effects on learning in other disadvantaged animal populations. We have netted two malnutrition studies (Wells et al 1972; Tanabe, 1972), two brain-lesion studies (Schwartz, 1964; Hughes, 1965), and some generic studies (Cooper and Zubek, 1958; Bennett et al 1970, Henderson, 1970, 1972), all except Henderson's using rats.

We have summarized the main results of most of these in Table 3, for comparison with our findings in hypothyroid rats. Henderson's work is discussed separately, and we have added an interesting study of prenatal growth hormone-treated rats by Ray and Hochhauser (1969) that fits into this framework.

Table 3 is arranged for comparisons of how groups of normal rats
(first and second columns, designated CE and CI as in our studies)
and disadvantaged experimental groups (third and fourth columns,
designated XE and XI) were differentially affected by enriched (E)
and more-impoverished (I) conditions within each study. Note, however, that in Ray and Hochhauser's case the("gifted") growth hormone
groups are placed on the left and their normally poorer-performing
controls, being relatively disadvantaged (as in earlier prenatal
growth hormone studies by Clendinnen and Eayrs, 1961, and Block and
Esssman, 1965), are to the right; similarly, Cooper and Zubek's
"maze-bright" and "maze-dull" strains are located on the left and
right, respectively. The raw-score difference between E and I subgroups within each study is expressed, separately for C and X populations, as a percentage reduction from the corresponding I-con-
dition score. The fifth column expresses the reductions of deficit
in the disadvantaged rats (XI-XE) in terms of how far along the
score dimension enrichment has moved the XE subgroups toward normal-
enriched (CE) performance levels -- a "percentage normalization"
measure. Note that this measure is 100 x (XI - XE/ (XI-CE), i.e.,
"normal" is defined in terms of the most favorable control (CE)
condition, unlike our previous index of deficit-reduction with which
we summarized Figs. 3-6 in terms of an XI-CI divisor.

Some remarkable facts are disclosed by Table 3:

1. In the disadvantaged groups, all 11 E-1 differences favored
E rats.

2. These E-I differences were larger, percentagewise, than in
C groups in all comparisons except for Cooper and Zubek's bright
and dull strains.

3. In contrast to our measures, in which E-I differences in
normals were negligible, the other six studies show less-differential
effects, i.e., the effects tended to be superimposed in parallel upon
C and X groups alike.

4. Across all studies and nearly all measures, percentage
normalization was high!

The reduction of deficits was consistent across these studies
despite considerable variation in the E conditions. Wells et al
exposed their E rats to a variety of apparatuses (runway, T-maze,
running wheel, activity chamber, and open field, for exploration
rather than reinforced training) on Days 76-100 in addition to more
standard E conditions on Days 21-100. Tanabe gave his singly-housed
E rats daily 5-hr placements in a fairly typical group-with-objects
environment on Days 26-60. Schwartz's rats lived continuously in

TABLE 3

Summary of Scores and Deficit-Reductions in Various
Studies of Environmental Effects in Disadvantaged
Rat Populations

	Controls		Disadvantaged		Percentage Normalization*
	CE	CI	XE	XI	
Wells et al (1972): X = Malnourished; Hebb-Williams Maze Errors					
Mean	135	182	166	263	
% Diff.		25.8		36.9	75.8
Tanabe (1972): X= Malnourished; Hebb-Williams Maze Errors					
Mean	119	147	137	183	
% Diff.		19.0		25.1	71.9
Schwartz (1962): X = Early Cortisol-Lesioned; Hebb-Williams Maze Errors					
Mean	65	125	95	205	
% Diff.		48.0		53.7	78.6
Hughes(1965): X = Hippocampal-Lesioned; Hebb-Williams Maze Errors					
Mean	109	118	154	223	
% Diff.		7.6		30.9	60.5
Cooper and Zubek(1958): C = Bright, X= Dull: Hebb-Williams Maze Errors					
Mean	111	170	120	170	
% Diff.		34.7		29.4	84.7
Ray and Hochhauser(1969);C = Growth Hormone, X = Normal; Lashley Maze Errors.					
Mean	18.5	23.0	19.5	27.0	
% Diff.		19.6		27.8	88.2
Gonzalez and Davenport (1972)X = Hypothyroid: Symmetrical Maze Errors					
Mean	160	160	473	629	
% Diff.		0.0		24.8	33.3
Davenport (1974-75): X = Hypothyroid; Symmetrical Maze Acquisition Errors					
Mean	148	154	256	422	
% Diff.		3.9		39.3	60.6
Davenport (1974-75): X = Hypothyroid; Symmetrical Maze Retention Errors					
Mean	6.08	6.79	6.72	9.79	
% Diff.		10.5		21.1	57.3
Davenport (1974-75): X = Hypothyroid; Barpressing Extinction Responses					
Mean	109	114	98	178	
% Diff.		4.4		44.9	115.9
Davenport (1974-75): X = Hypothyroid females; VI Responses on Days 1 - 10					
Mean	280	286	269	354	
% Diff.		21.		24.0	114.9

* Percentage normalization = 100 (XI-XE)/(XI-CE)

the typical environment from Day 30 to Days 94 or 96, as did Hughes'
rats on Days 33-66, and Cooper and Zubek's rats on Days 25-65. Ray
and Hochhauser had their standard-type E cages located in a busy
corridor of the laboratory for extra stimulation. Our conditions
were standard (Gonzalez and Davenport, 1972) and superenriched
(1974-75 study), as described earlier, on Days 30-60 and 36-70, respectively. What we have called I treatments were individual-housing
isolation conditons in all cases except for the social-control conditions used by Schwartz (two to six rats/cage), Cooper and Zubek
(9 or 13/cage), and Ray and Hochhauser (two/cage). The study by
Hughes had, in addition to enriched and isolated groups, social controls (group-housed without objects) whose performance scores were
indistinguishable from his isolated sham-operated and lesioned
rats' scores given in Table 3.

There is a tantalizing suggestion in these studies of a correlation between the experimental variations and the extent to which
disadvantaged animals were selectively influenced by the E and I
conditions. Omitting the growth hormone study, we can roughly rank
-order the remaining seven studies in terms of how much their
E and I environments differed, the maximal contrast probably being
our (1974-75) superenriched- vs. - isolated conditions, followed by
Wells et al Hughes, Gonzalez and Davenport, Schwartz, Tanabe, and
Cooper and Zubek. This order does not correlate with percentage
normalization but it does tend to relate to the difference between
$XI - XE$ and $CI - CE$ percentages (in the same order, 35.4 for our
1974-75 maze acquisition task, 11.1, 23.3, 24.8, 5.7, 6.1, and
-5.3). The best-controlled comparison on this point is between
our 1972 and 1974-75 figures (24.8 with standard environment vs.
35.4 with superenrichment, and corresponding percentage normaliza-
tions of 33.3 and 60.6), where type and degree of disadvantage as
well as the task were the same. One implication is that increments
of stimulation added to already-enriched environments may selectively benefit learning by disadvantaged subjects, including many types
not yet studied, to a proportionately greater extent than learning
by normal subjects.

Some caution should be exercised in interpreting the surprisingly high percentage-normalization figures in Table 3. None of the
deficits in the malnutrition, brain-lesion, or genetic studies
listed, except perhaps in Hughes' hippocampal-lesioned rats, appear
large in relation to the variability of the scores (i.e., XI and
CI distributions probably overlapped considerably), whereas in both
of our hypothyroidism studies the deficits were severe (no overlap
in maze acquisition -- see Fig. 3). Under these latter conditions
a 50-to-60% normalization by enrichment may represent a more impressive effect than an 80% normalization of a disadvantaged group that is
already closer to normal. This reasoning seems particularly applicable when the lower percentage represents an E-I effect which is

selective for disadvantaged subjects.

In the other genetic studies involving learning measures, things are more complicated. Bennett et al (1970) have compared E, social control (SC), and I conditions in rats of the Berkeley S_1 strain (descendents of Tryon's "maze-bright" rats) and in S_3 ("maze-dull") rats, concluding that enrichment did not improve visual reversal discrimination performance in comparison to the social-control treatment in the S_1 strain (both E and SC rats were superior to the I rats), but that it did in the S_3 strain (SC and I rats did not differ). They also concluded that this pattern of results was in essential agreement with Cooper and Zubek's (1958) three-condition comparisons of McGill bright and dull strains in the Hebb-Williams maze. However, the S_1 and S_3 strains were not compared within the same experiment. In addition, Bennett et al note that S_3 rats paradoxically perform better than S_1 rats on the visual reversal discrimination task, which obviously clouds the analogy to the McGill strains and raises other questions. To make matters worse, Cooper and Zubek's E and SC groups (the latter are designated CI and XI in Table 3, and were reared in 9 or 13 rats/cage settings) were evidently reared and tested concurrently within the same experiment, but what they call "control groups" were reared and tested in a different experiment (Hughes and Zubek, 1956), probably a year or two earlier. The only specification of the rearing conditions for these "controls" given by Cooper and Zubek is that they were "raised in a 'normal' laboratory environment," and it is apparent that they represented a different generation of the McGill bright and dull lines. In comparing their results to Cooper and Zubek's Bennett et al seem to have mistaken these groups for SC-treated rats and the 9 or 13/cage "restricted" groups for isolates. About all that can be salvaged from this, by simply dismissing Copper and Zubek's dubious "controls" and the Bennett et al SC groups from consideration, is a conclusion that the former study found significant E-SC differences in both McGill strains (shown in Table 3) and the latter study found significant E-I differences in both Berkeley strains (performance measures not given by Bennett et al). Apparently, in neither case was the enhancement of learning by E conditions differential for "brights" and "dulls."

Henderson (1970) studied environmental influences in 384 mice from six well-known Jackson Laboratory strains and their 30 F_1 crosses. In all 36 offspring groups, the mice were reared from birth to six weeks of age (weaning was at three weeks) in enriched or social-control litter cages. The enriched cages were larger and contained a hollow log, small maze, steel tube, rocks, and wood and wire-mesh ramps. In the seventh week an unusual food-seeking task was administered in which each mouse, 24-hr deprived, was given up to 60 min in one trial to reach food in a complicated apparatus probably involving elements of both learning and exploration.

Henderson's enriched mice performed better on this task, by our count, in 25 of the 36 groups, but in at least four of the genetic combinations performance was distinctly worse in the E than the SC mice (the other seven combinations showed no appreciable difference). The six inbred strains were generally inferior to the 30 hybrid crosses, but the magnitude of the enrichment effect averaged about the same for both. Considering just the 30 crosses in Henderson's table of mean times to reach food, however, we found that the hybrids which performed worst tended to be most benefited by E rearing and those which had the shortest times were least benefited or worsened by enrichment. We calculated a Pearson correlation coefficient of +.68 (p < .001) between mean times under SC conditions and percentage reduction (plus or minus) of these times under E conditions. For all 36 pairs of groups the correlation was +.59 (p < .001). The same calculation for the 25 (21 hybrids and 4 inbreds) improved-by-enrichment pairs was, of course, lower (+.40) but still significant (p < .05), and none of these correlations seems to be an artifactual result of ceiling or floor effects. So here again the "more room for improvement" principle emerges. Difficulties remain, however, in that we do not know what was improved, because of the nature of the task and its resemblance to the enriched environment: exploration, specific transfer, or some more meaningful kind of learning capacity?

In Henderson's (1972) second study, involving 768 mice and again 36 genetic combinations, no effects appeared in T-maze spatial discrimination, T-maze reversal, or in black-white and vertical - horizontal visual discriminations. As Table 2 indicates, such discrimination tasks have been inconsistent at best in revealing E-I effects in rats, and by using aversive (escape from shock or water) rather than appetitive reinforcers in all of them, Henderson may have further reduced their sensitivity. A derived measure based on performance differences in the two visual problems did show significantly greater improvement in the enriched hybrid crosses (but not in inbred strains), however.

We will consider a final study dealing with motivational effects of rearing environment in early-malnourished rats. Levitsky and Barnes (1972) reared normal and low-protein male rats in three different environments from birth to seven weeks of age, which was also the duration of the undernutrition treatment. Their environments were an enriched (E) condition, which involved daily handling of the pups during the 3-week nursing period, and 4 subsequent weeks of individual housing plus 1-hr placements in a Berkeley-type enrichment cage 5 times per week; an isolated (I) condition, consisting of individual housing and once-weekly handling during the postweaning period and an unusual (for rats) "super-isolation" (SI) condition, in which the weanlings were housed individually in wire cages enclosed within lightproof, sound-attenuating chambers and not handled. Ten weeks after these conditions the rats were tested in open-field locomotion, in exploration of a small chamber which could be entered from the open field, and in social behavior (following and fighting behaviors by two rats at a time in the open field).

The experimental effects were large and differential for malnourished and normal rats in all four measures. In malnourished groups, abnormally high locomotion scores in the SI condition became normalized in the E condition and partially so in the I condition. A comparison of the SI and E conditions only in exploration showed a similar effect, in that the SI-malnourished rats displayed much lower exploration scores than the E-malnourished, SI-normal, and E-normal groups, whose scores were closely similar. In the six groups' social tests, abnormally low following behavior in the malnourished rats was also monotonically normalized as stimulation increased, and fighting was monotonically elevated from a normal level under SI conditions to supernormal levels under E conditions in these rats; the three normal groups were virtually indistinguishable on the social measures. Levitsky and Barnes indicate that their results (excepting fighting) can be viewed in terms of "therapeutic" normalization of behavior, possibly by direct reversal of known brain dysfunction in isolated malnourished rats (e,g,, decreased brain size, DNA content, cortical dendritic growth, and cholinesterase content). Alternatively, the findings can be viewed in terms of exaggeration of the abnormal behavioral consequences of malnutrition by extreme impoverishment of the rearing environment, or from the standpoint that certain of these consequences (e.g., apathy, excessive food-orientation) restrict the organism's interactions with its environment, resulting in inadequate motivational and cognitive development unless these constrains are overcome by increasing the stimulation in the environment. Presumably the best-fitting of these alternative interpretations will be revealed by further work at the level of neural tissue and closer examination at the behavioral level of how much self-imposed impoverishment of the rearing environment actually occurs during and after malnutrition (see chapters by Levine and Richardson this volume).

Levitsky and Barnes' study is also interesting in that their large effects showed impressive durability, occurring over 10 weeks after the end of differential rearing. Secondly, although only motivational effects were assessed, its agreement with the effects shown by Wells et al (1972) and Tanabe (1970) in malnourished rats suggest that the therapeutic implications of rodent studies using such measures as open-field activity may often be no less than those employing explicit learning measures. Levitsky and Barnes' findings rather nicely provide a rounding-out of this cluster of studies with disadvantaged animals, which presents a generally consistent, and most encouraging picture.

IV. Current and Future Work in This Area

In our hypothyroidism research we have concluded that the
large and durable reductions of deficits by increased environmental
stimulation which we found primarily represent enhanced behavioral
capacities. Our findings, however, do not yet permit the conclusion
that cerebral changes from enrichment were responsible for the reduction of the behavioral deficits. Recognition of this has dictated
a shift to collaborative neuroanatomical studies in our work
with hypothryoid rats. This work should profit from the abundant
suggestions in both the thyroid and enrichment literatures regarding appropriate measures, brain sites, and techniques.

In addition to studying the relatively gross anatomical measures (e.g., cortical weight and thickness) which have so consistently revealed environmental effects in the Berkeley studies,
we hope to show how superenriched, social-control, and isolated
hypothyroid rats differ from their controls in branching and spine
densities of basal and apical dendrites in the cerebral cortex,
using the rapid-Golgi staining methods employed by Globus et al.,
(1973) and Greenough (1975) and focusing on the same cortical
laminae which these investigators and Eayrs (1971 , in hypothyroid
rat brains) have studied. Ultrastructural analysis of the same
regions for measurements of synaptic size (West and Greenough, 1972;
Møllgaard et al 1971) and thickness of dendritic spine stalks (Van
Harreveld and Fifkova, 1975) also seems likely to be fruitful. In
addition, we think similar attention should be directed to the hippocampal region, in view of the environmental effects shown by Walsh
et al (1969) in that region, because of resemblances in the dis-
inhibited behaviors of early-hypothyroid and hippocampal-or sep-
tal-lesioned rats (Altman et al 1973), and because the hippocampus is considered by many to be importantly involved in the memory
and response-inhibition functions on which our superenriched and
isolated hypothyroids differed.

In further behavioral work, we are currently studying environmental influences in neonatal-hyperthyroid rats. Whether the learning deficits which have so consistently appeared in these rats (Eayrs,
1964; Schapiro, 1968; Davenport and Gonzalez, 1973; Davenport et al
1975; Stone and Greenough, 1975) can be reduced by postweaning stimulation is particularly interesting because of how they differ neuro-
histologically and neurochemically from thyroid-deficient rats.
While synaptogenesis is reduced in both hyper- and hypothyroid rats,
in the former this appears to be due to premature termination of
neural proliferation (Nicholson and Altman, 1972a, b), resulting in
reduced cell numbers as indexed by DNA content (Balasz et al 1971),
and not due to underdeveloped dendritic arborization, which in fact
may be overstimulated in early-hyperthyroids. Conceivably, with
neural processes already elaborately differentiated and fewer cells

to work with in the first place, the early-hyperthyroid rat will
display less plasticity in response to environmental stimulation
than the early-hypothyroid rat.

Some recent unpublished evidence (Sjöden and Söderberg, at
Uppsala), however, indicates that preweaning enrichment durably
normalizes the tendency for neonatal-hyperthyroid rats to be hyperactive in open-field tests during adolescence and adulthood.
In our latest work we have extended this result, finding that a
month of postweaning experience in the superenrichment apparatus
substantially reduces the hyperactivity shown by neonatal-hyperthyroid rats in a quadrant activity chamber at around 60 days of
age. Thus there may be hope for this type of disadvantaged rat
despite our gloomier expectations.

We wonder, of course, whether enrichment-facilitated performance will be found in other animal populations in which enduring
behavior disorders have been experimentally induced, such as oxy-
gen-deprived, phenylketonuric, lead-poisoned, or microcephalic rats,
and thyroid-altered, brain-lesioned, or phenylketonuric rhesus
monkeys. Presumably there are limits somewhere, since we can
readily visualize brain dysfunctions (e.g., anomalous congenital
malformations, massive brain lesions) in which enriched experience
would probably be of little benefit despite plenty of "room for
improvement."

Other chapters in this book provide ample evidence that the
study of environmental stimulation effects in human intellectual
functioning has begun in earnest. From what we have seen with
normal and disadvantaged animals in this chapter, the efforts of
these investigators at the human level are clearly warranted. By
now it is a foregone conclusion, we feel, that animal studies will
provide some valuable guidance to them as to the types and timing
of effective environmental therapies and the specific kinds of
behavioral impairment in normal (e.g., aged) and early-disadvantag-
ed human beings which will most likely be remediated by those therapies.

Acknowledgments

* Publication No. 15-025 of the Wisconsin Regional Primate Research
Center. The editorial-sounding "we" throughout this chapter refers
in part to the students and staff of the Center's Learning Unit,
whose contributions to this work were enormous. Louis M. Gonzalez
initiated our research on environmental effects in hypothyroidism,
and conducted the first study in 1972. Major roles in the program
were played by John C. Carey in literature reviews, Steven B.
Bishop in conducting the 1974-75 experiments, and William W. Hagquist in apparatus design. In addition, skilled assistance was
provided by Bruce M. Preslan, Steven E. Shelton, Richard S. Hennies,
and Robert DeRubeis in the testing, Susan L. Engelke in the data
analyses, and Mary Iwen in the preparation of the manuscript. This
work was supported by Grant GB-31992 from the National Science Foundation and Grants HD-06060 and FR-00167 from the National Institutes
of Health.

REFERENCES

Altman, J., Brunner, R.L., and Bayer, S.A. 1973. The hippocampus and behavioral maturation. Behav. Biol. 8:557-596.

Balasz, R. 1971. Biochemical effects of thyroid hormones in the developing brain. UCLA Forum in Medical Sciences, No. 14, pp. 273-320.

Balasz, R., Cocks, W.A., Eayrs, J.T., and Kovacs, S. 1971. Biochemical effects of thyroid hormones on the developing brain , pp. 357-379. In M. Hanburgh and E.J.W. Barrington (Eds.), Hormones in Development. Appleton-Century-Crofts, New York.

Bennett, E.L., Rosenzweig, M.R., and Diamond, M.C. 1970. Time courses of effects of differential experience on brain measures and behavior of rats, Pp. 55-88. In W.L. Byrne (Ed.). Molecular Approaches to Learning and Memory. Academic Press, New York.

Bennett, E.L., Rosenzweig, M.R., Diamond, M. C., Morimoto, H., and Herbert, M. 1974. Effects of successive environments on brain measures. Physiol. Behav. 12:621-631.

Bernstein, L. 1972. The reversability of learning deficits in early environmentally restricted rats as a function of amount of experience in later life. J. Psychosom. Res. 16:71-73.

Bernstein, L. 1973. A study of some enriching variables in a free-environment for rats. J. Psychosom. Res. 17:85-88.

Bingham, W.E., and Griffiths, W.J. 1952. The effect of differential environments during infancy on adult behavior in the rat. J. Comp. Physiol. Psychol. 45:307-312.

Block, J.R., and Essman, W.B. 1965. Growth hormone administration during pregnancy: A behavioral difference in offspring rats. Nature 205:1136-1137.

Brown, C.P., and King, M.G. 1971. Developmental environment : Variables important for later learning and changes in cholinergic activity. Develop. Psychobiol. 4:275-286.

Brown, R.T. 1968. Early experience and problem solving ability. J. Comp. Physiol. Psychol. 65:433-440.

Clendinnen, B.G., and Eayrs, J.T. 1961. The anatomical and physiological effects of prenatally administered somatotrophin on cerebral development in rats. J. Endocrinol. 22:183-193.

Cooper, R.M., and Zubek, J.P. 1958. Effects of enriched and restricted early environments on the learning ability of bright and dull rats. Canad. J. Psychol. 12:159-164.

Cummins, R.A., Walsh, R.N., Budtz-Olsen, O.E., Konstantinos, T., and Horsfall, C.R. 1973. Environmentally-induced changes in the brains of elderly rats. Nature 243:516-518.

Davenport, J.W. 1970. Cretinism in rats: Enduring behavioral deficit induced by tricyanoaminopropene. Science 167: 1007-1009.

Davenport, J.W., and Dorcey, T.P. 1972. Hypothyroidism: Learning deficit induced in rats by early exposure to thiouracil. Hormon. Behav. 3:97-112.

Davenport, J.W., and Gonzalez, L.M. 1973. Neonatal thyroxine stim-
    ulation in rats: Accelerated behavioral maturation and subse-
    quent learning deficit. J. Comp. Physiol. Psychol. 85:397-408.
Davenport, J.W., and Hennies, R.S. 1976. Perinatal hypothyroidism
    in rats: Persistent motivational and metabolic effects. Develop.
    Psychobiol., in press.
Davenport, J.W., Hagquist, W.W., and Rankin, G.R. 1970. The sym-
    metrical maze: An automated closed-field test series for rats.
    Behav. Res. Meth. Instrum. 2:112-118.
Davenport, J.W., Gonzalez, L.M., Hennies, R.S., and Hagquist, W.W.
    1976. Severity and timing of early thyroid deficiency as fact-
    ors in the induction of learning disorders in rats. Hormon. Behav.,
    in press.
Davenport, J.W., Hagquist, W.W., and Hennies, R.S. 1975. Neonatal
    hyperthyroidism: Maturational acceleration and learning deficit
    in triiodothyronine-stimulated rats. Physiol. Psychol. 3:231-
    236.
Davenport, R.K., and Rogers, C.M. 1970. Differential rearing of
    the chimpanzee. Chimpanzee 3:337-360.
Davenport, R.K., Rogers, C.M., and Rumbaugh, D.M. 1973. Long-term
    cognitive deficits in chimpanzees associated with early impov-
    erished rearing. Develop. Psychol. 9:343-347.
Denenberg, V.H., Woodcock, J.M., and Rosenberg, K.M. 1968. Long-
    term effects of preweaning and postweaning free-environment
    experience on rats' problem-solving behavior. J. Comp. Physiol.
    Psychol. 66:533-535.
Doty, B.A., 1972. The effects of cage environment upon avoidance
    responding of aged rats. J. Gerontol. 27: 358-360.
Eayrs, J.T. 1961. Age as a factor determining the severity and
    reversibility of the effects of thyroid deprivation in the rat.
    J. Endocrinol. 22:409-419.
Eayrs, J.T. 1964. Effect of neonatal hyperthyroidism on maturation
    and learning in the rat. Anim. Behav. 12:195-199.
Eayrs, J.T. 1968. Developmental relationships between brain and
    thyroid, Pp. 239-255. In R.P. Michael (Ed.), Endocrinology and
    Human Behavior,Oxford University Press, London.
Eayrs, J.T. 1971. Thyroid and developing brain: Anatomical and
    behavioral effects, Pp. 345-355. In M. Hamburgh and E.J.W.
    Barrington (Eds.), Hormones in Development. Appleton-Century-
    Crofts, New York.
Eayrs, J.T., and Goodhead, B. 1959. Postnatal development of the
    cerebral cortex in the rat. J. Anat. 93:385-401.
Eayrs, J.T., and Lishman, W.A. 1955. The maturation of behavior in
    hypothyroidism and starvation. Brit. J. Anim. Behav. 3:17-24.
Edwards, H.P., Barry, W.Y., and Wyspianski, J.O. 1969. Effect of
    differential rearing on photic evoked potentials and brightness
    discrimination in the albino rat. Develop. Psychobiol. 2:133-
    138.
Ferchmin, P.A., Eterovic, V.A., and Caputto, R. 1970. Studies of
    brain weight and RNA content after short periods of exposure to
    environmental complexity. Brain Res. 20:49-57.

Forgays, D.G., and Forgays, J.W. 1952. The nature of the effect of free-environmental experience in the rat. J. Comp. Physiol. Psychol. 45:322-328.

Forgays, D.G., and Read, J.M. 1962. Crucial periods for free-environmental experience in the rat. J. Comp. Physiol. Psychol. 55: 816-818.

Forgus, R.H. 1954. The effect of early perceptual learning on the behavioral organization of adult rats. J. Comp. Physiol. Psychol. 47: 331-336.

Freeman, B.J., and Ray, O.S. 1972. Strain, sex, and environmental effects on appetitively and aversively motivated learning tasks. Develop. Psychobiol. 5:101-109.

Gill, J.H., Reid, L.D., and Porter, P.B. 1966. Effects of restricted rearing on Lashley stand performance. Psychol. Rep. 19:239-242.

Globus, A., Rosenzweig, M.R., Bennett, E.L., and Diamond, L.C. 1973. Effects of differential experience on dendritic spine counts in rat cerebral cortex. J. Comp. Physiol. Psychol. 82:175-181.

Gluck, J.P., and Harlow, H.F. 1971. The effects of deprived and enriched rearing conditions on later learning: A review. pp. 103-119. In L.E. Jarrard (Ed.), Cognitive Processes of Nonhuman Primates. Academic Press, New York.

Gluck, J.P., Harlow, H.F., and Schiltz, K.A. 1973. Differential effect of early enrichment and deprivation on learning in the rhesus monkey (Macaca mulatta). J. Comp. Physiol. Psychol. 84:598-604.

Gonzalez, L.M., and Davenport, J.W. 1972. Partial alleviation of learning deficit in hypothyroid rats by environmental enrichment. Unpublished manuscript.

Greenough, W.T. 1975. Experimental modification of the developing brain. Amer. Sci. 63:37-46.

Greenough, W.T., Madden, T.C., and Fleischmann, T.B. 1972a. Effects of isolation, daily handling, and enriched rearing on maze learning. Psychon. Sci. 27:279-280.

Greenough, W.T., Wood, W.E., and Madden, T.C. 1972b. Possible memory storage differences among mice reared in environments varying in complexity. Behav. Biol. 7:717-722.

Greenough, W.T., Yuwiler, A., and Dollinger, M. 1973. Effects of posttrial eserine administration on learning in "enriched"- and "impoverished"-reared rats. Behav. Biol. 8:261-272.

Harlow, H.F., Dodsworth, R.O., and Harlow, M.K. 1965. Total social isolation in monkeys. Proc. Nat. Acad. Sci. 54:90-97.

Harlow, H.F., Schiltz, K.A., Harlow, M.K., and Mohr, D.J. 1971. The effects of early adverse and enriched environments on the learning ability of rhesus monkeys, Pp. 121-148. In L.E. Jarrard (Ed.), Cognitive Processes of Nonhuman Primates, Academic Press, New York.

Hebb, D.O. 1949. The Organization of Behavior, Wiley, New York.

Hebb, D.O., and Williams, K.A. 1946. A method of rating animal intelligence. J. Gen. Psychol. 34:59-65.

Henderson, N.D. 1970. Genetic influences on the behavior of mice can be obscured by laboratory rearing. J. Comp. Physiol. Psychol. 73:505-511.

Henderson, N.D. 1972. Relative effects of early rearing environ-ment and genotype on discrimination learning in house mice. J. Comp. Physiol. Psychol. 79:243-253.

Hughes, A.M. 1944. Cretinism in rats induced by thiouracil. End-ocrinol. 34:69-76.

Hughes, K.R. 1965. Dorsal and ventral hippocampus lesions and maze learning: Influence of preoperative environment. Canad. J. Psychol. 19:325-332.

Hughes, K.R., and Zubek, J.P. 1956. Effect of glutamic acid on the learning ability of bright and dull rats: I. Administration during infancy. Canad. J. Psychol. 10:132-138.

Hymovitch, B. 1952. The effects of experimental variations on pro-blem solving in the rat. J. Comp. Physiol. Psychol. 45:313-321.

Krech, D., Rosenzweig, M.R., and Bennett, E.L. 1962. Relations between brain chemistry and problem solving among rats raised in enriched and impoverished environments. J. Comp. Physiol. Psychol. 55:801-807.

Kuenzle, C.C., and Knüsel, A. 1974. Mass training of rats in a superenriched environment. Physiol. Behav. 13:205-210.

Lessac, M.S., and Solomon, R.L. 1969. Effects of early isolation on the later behavior of beagles: A methodological demonstra-tion. Develop. Psychol. 1:14-25.

Levitsky, D.A., and Barnes, R.H. 1972. Nutritional and environ-mental interactions in the behavioral development of the rat: Long-term effects. Science 176:68-71.

Møllgaard, K., Diamond, M.C., Bennett, E.L., Rosenzweig, M.R., and Lindner, B. 1971. Qualitative synaptic changes with differen-tial experience in rat brain. Internat. J. Neurosci. 2:113-128.

Morgan, M.J. 1973. Effects of post-weaning environment on learn-ing in the rat. Anim. Behav. 21:429-442.

Nicholson, J.L., and Altman, J. 1972a. The effects of early hypo-and hyperthyroidism on the development of the rat cerebellar cortex: I. Cell proliferation and differentiation. Brain Res. 44:13-23.

Nicholson, J.L., and Altman, J. 1972b. The effects of early hypo-and hyperthyroidism on the development of the rat cerebellar cortex: II. Synaptogenesis in the molecular layer. Brain Res. 44:25-36.

Nyman, A.J. 1967. Problem solving in rats as a function of exper-ience at different ages. J. Genet. Psychol. 110:31-39.

Ough, B.R., Beatty, W.W., and Khalili, J. 1972. Effects of isola-ted and enriched rearing on response inhibition. Psychon. Sci. 27:293-294.

Parsons, P.J., and Spear, N.E. 1972. Long-term retention of avoidance learning by immature and adult rats as a function of environmental enrichment. J. Comp. Physiol. Psychol.80:297-303.

Ray, O.S., and Hochhauser, S. 1969. Growth hormone and environmental complexity effects on behavior in the rat. Develop. Psychol.
1:311-317.

Reid, L.D., Gill, J.H., and Porter, P.B. 1968. Isolated rearing
and Hebb-Williams maze performance. Psychol. Rep. 22:1073-1077.

Rosenzweig, M.R. 1971. Effects of environment on development of
brain and behavior, Pp. 303-342. In E. Tobach, L.R. Aronson,
and E. Shaw (Eds.), The Biopsychology of Development. Academic
Press, New York.

Rosenzweig, M.R. 1972. Environmental enrichment, brain plasticity,
and behavior. Paper delivered at AAAS meeting, December, 1972,
Washington, D.C.

Rosenzweig, M.R., Bennett, E.L., and Diamond, M.C. 1972. Brain
changes in response to experience. Sci. Amer. 226:22-29.

Schapiro, S. 1968. Some psychological, biochemical, and behavioral consequences of neonatal hormone administration: Cort-
isol and thyroxine. Gen. Comp.Endocrinol. 10:214-228.

Schwartz, S. 1964. Effect of neonatal cortical lesions and early
environmental factors on adult rat behavior. J. Comp. Physiol.
Psychol. 57:72-77.

Schweikert, G.E., and Collins, G. 1966. The effects of differential postweaning environments on later behavior in the rat.
J. Genet. Psychol. 109:255-263.

Seligman, M.E.P. 1975. Helplessness: On Depression, Development, and
Death. Freeman and Co., San Francisco.

Smith, H.V. 1972. Effects of environmental enrichment on open-
field activity and Hebb-Williams problem solving in rats. J.
Comp. Physiol. Psychol.80:163-168.

Stone, J.M., and Greenough, W.T. 1975. Excess neonatal thyroxine:
Effects on learning in infant and adolescent rats. Develop.
Psychobiol., 8:479-488.

Sturgeon, R.D., and Reid, L.D. 1971. Rearing variations and Hebb-
Williams maze performance. Psychol. Rep. 29:571-580.

Tanabe, G. 1972. Remediating maze deficiencies by the use of
environmental enrichment. Develop. Psychol. 7:224.

Van Harreveld, A., and Fifova, E. 1975. A mechanism for potentiation and short-term memory. Proceedings, Konikl. Nederl.
Akademie Van Wetenschappen--Amsterdam, Series C, 78, No. 1
pp. 21-24.

Volkmar, F.R., and Greenough, W.T. 1972. Rearing complexity
affects branching of dendrites in the visual cortex of the
rat. Science 176: 1445-1447.

Wallock, D., and Davenport, J.W. 1970. Early motor development
and adult learning deficits in neonatally thyroidectomized
rats. Unpublished data.

Walsh, R.N., and Cummins, R.A. 1976. The open field test: A
critical review. Psychol. Bull, in press.

Walsh, R.N., Budtz-Olsen, O.E., Penny, J.E., and Cummins, R.A.
1969. The effects of environmental complexity on the histology of the rat hippocampus. J. Comp. Neurol. 137:361-366.

Wells, A.M., Geist, C.R., and Zimmermann, R.R. 1972.   Influence of
    environmental and nutritional factors on problem solving in the
    rat. Percept. Mot. Skills 35:235-244.
West, R.W., and Greenough, W.T. 1972.   Effect of environmental com-
    plexity on cortical synapses of rats: Preliminary results.
    Behav. Biol. 7:279-283.
Wilkins, L. 1965.   The Diagnosis and Treatment of Endocrine Dis-
    orders in Childhood and Adolescence, 3rd Ed. Charles C. Thomas,
    Springfield, Ill.
Wilson, M., Warren, J.M., and Abbott, L. 1965.   Infantile stimula-
    tion, activity and learning by cats. Child. Devel. 36:843-853.
Woods, P.J. 1959.   The effects of free and restricted environment-
    al experience on problem-solving behavior in the rat. J. Comp.
    Physiol. Psychol. 52:399-402.
Woods, P.J., Ruckelshaus, S.I., and Bowling, D.M. 1960.   Some
    effects of "free" and "restricted" environmental rearing con-
    ditions upon adult behavior in the rat. Psychol. Rep. 6:191-
    200.
Woods, P.J., Fiske, A.S., and Ruckelshaus, S.I. 1961.   The effects
    of drives conflicting with exploration on the problem-solving
    behavior of rats reared in free and restricted environments. J.
    Comp. Physiol. Psychol. 54:167-169.

THE EFFECTS OF TOTAL SOCIAL ISOLATION REARING ON

BEHAVIOR OF RHESUS AND PIGTAIL MACAQUES*

Gene P. Sackett, Richard A. Holm, Gerald C.
Ruppenthal and Carol E. Farhrenbruch

University of Washington, Psychology Department
Regional Primate Research Center
Child Development and Mental Retardation Center

I. INTRODUCTION

Rhesus monkeys (M. mulatta) raised in social isolation exhibit
a variety of post-rearing abnormalities which are so consistent that
they have been termed "The Isolation Syndrome" (Sackett and Ruppenthal, 1973). This syndrome includes deviant personal behavior
such as body rocking, self-clutching, peculiar postures, stereotyped locomotion, self-directed aggression, and a type of "waxy
flexibility" in which an arm or a leg floats upward uncoordinated
with other ongoing behavior. Isolates are also low in exploratory
behavior, have almost no positive social interaction, and are
abnormal as adults in sexual and maternal behavior. The only major
type of behavior not showing pronounced abnormality is learning.
Compared with socialized controls including wild-born monkeys,
rhesus isolates are not deficient in discrimination, delayed
response, or learning set performance (Gluck and Harlow, 1971;
Harlow, et al., 1968).

The extent of rhesus isolation deficits depends on the type
of isolation environment, duration of isolation from birth, and
sex (Sackett, 1972a). Infants totally isolated exhibit profound
abnormalities, especially in personal behavior while infants
reared in partial isolation, with visual, auditory, and olfactory
stimulation from other monkeys but no physical contact show less
severe effect. Rhesus infants may recover from 3 months of total
isolation, but isolation for 6 months or more appears to yield
lasting abnornmalities. One exception to this generalization was
reported by Suomi and Harlow (1972), who socialized 6-month total
isolates with less mature, 3-month-old infants immediately after
emergence from isolation. This therapy commenced immediately

115

after emergency from isolation, eliminated many components of the
isolation syndrome.

Sex differences in rhesus responses to total and partial isolation appear in both social and exploratory behavior (Sackett,
1972b; Sackett, et al., 1975). Female total isolates are more
willing to expose themselves to novel stimulation than males.
This difference is pronounced in partial isolates, where males
show large deficits but females do not differ in response to
novelty from socialized controls. During social playroom tests,
female total isolates are less deviant in personal behavior and
respond more to the inanimate environment than males, although
neither female nor male total isolates show positive social interactions. Partial isolate females are also less personally deviant
and more exploratory than partial isolate males, and partial isolate females interact socially to a much greater degree than males.
Although the sources of such sex differences in vulnerability to
environmental deprivation are not understood, female rhesus seem
to be better able to withstand impoverished rearing than males.

The effects of isolation rearing in rhesus monkeys have been
viewed as a model for studying etiology and therapy of human
abnormal behavior (e.g. Sackett, 1968; Harlow, et al., 1972). Aspects of the isolation syndrome resemble many motor behaviors seen
in autistic, schizophrenic, and mentally retarded children, and in
depressed human children and adults. Chimpanzees raised in total
isolation also perform many of the abnormal behaviors seen in
rhesus monkeys, although chimpanzee isolates engage in more social
interaction than rhesus (Menzel, 1964; Davenport and Menzel, 1963).
Thus, on face value, it seems that rhesus isolate behavior has good
concordance with the behavior of at least one other nonhuman primate
species and with some human behaviors.

In 1970, we moved our laboratory from the University of Wisconsin to the University of Washington Regional Primate Research
Center. The Washington Primate Center specializes in pigtail
monkeys (M. nemestrina), with 600 breeders in the colony. Pigtail
and rhesus Macaques are closely related taxanomically, share similar
anatomy, size, and physiology (although pigtails have a larger
brain/body weight ratio), and appear similar in free-ranging social
organization. They did evolve in different areas, however -- rhesus
in India, pigtails in tropical areas of Malaysia and Indonesia.

Our move brought about a change in species of infant subjects,
but little change in equipment, techniques, or personnel. The new
laboratory contained the same rearing and testing apparatus, and
many of the same people that had been used in studying rhesus isolates during the previous 8 years.

Our first major experiments at Washington involved rearing pigtail newborns in total social isolation. One purpose was to assess the degree of similarity in response to isolation between rhesus and pigtail monkeys prior to initiating studies of genetic and prenatal factors in sex differences between total isolates. Unfortunately, we failed to find very close similarity between the two species. The purpose of this article is to report our comparisons between rhesus and pigtail monkeys reared under identical conditions of total social isolation.

II. SUBJECTS AND REARING CONDITIONS

Ninety-two newborns were studied over a 10-year period in four experiments. Sample sizes for Wisconsin rhesus and Washington pigtail subjects are given in Table I. All newborns were normal in health and birth weight.

TABLE I. Sample sizes and age (months) at start of social playroom testing for pigtail and rhesus subjects

Species	Rearing Conditions	Males	Sex Females	Age
M. nemestrina	Total Social Isolates	20	5	7-9
	Socialized	15	16	7-10
M. mulatta	Total Social Isolates	8	8	8-9
	Socialized	10	10	10-12

Rhesus subjects were involved in two studies. The first (Sackett, 1966; Pratt, 1969) raised total social isolates ($\underline{n}$=12) from birth through 8 months in cages totally enclosed by Masonite walls. Some subjects received colored slides and motion pictures during rearing, while others received no stimulation added to the isolation environment. These groups did not differ in post-rearing behavior (Pratt, 1969). Socialized controls ($\underline{n}$=8) in this experiment were reared without mothers, but with two or more agemates in standard laboratory wire cages. In the second experiment (Sackett, et al., 1972), total isolates ($\underline{n}$=4) were raised from birth through 7 months in enclosed, sound-attenuating chambers. Socialized controls were raised either in (i) pens with their mother and other mother and other mother-infant pairs ($\underline{n}$=4), (ii) agemate pairs without mothers in standard laboratory wire cages ($\underline{n}$=4), or (iii) agemate pairs in enclosed, sound-attenuating, isolation chambers ($\underline{n}$=4).

Analysis of post-rearing behavior revealed no important differences
between these socialized groups or between these groups and the
socialized controls in the first experiment. Therefore, all rhesus
socialized groups were combined. Only minor differences appeared
in the post-rearing behavior of total isolates from the two studies,
so all isolate data were combined.

Pigtail infants also served in two experiments. Experiment
1 (Sackett, et al., 1975) raised newborns from birth through 7 months
in cages enclosed by Masonite walls (n=9). Socalized controls
(n=15)were reared with their mothers in groups containing other
mother-infant pairs and nonmaternal adults. In Experiment 2 (Holm,
1975) newborns were raised in enclosed, sound-attenuating, chambers
(n=16). Half of these isolated infants received added input from
telemetered electrical brain stimulation, but postrearing behavior
did not differ between stimulated and unstimulated animals. Socialized controls (n=16) in this experiment were reared identically to
those of pigtail Experiment 1. Statistical comparisons between the
total isolates and between the socialized controls in these two
studies revealed no important differences, so data within each
rearing group were combined.

The sound-attenuating isolation chambers measured $1.81-m^3$,
and contained a .71x.71x91-m inner living cage. Solid and liquid
food were dispensed into the living cage through ports in one wall.
A diurnal cycle of 16 hr light on and 8 hr off was maintained. Behavior was viewed through a 1-way glass in the rear wall. Masonite-
walled cages were .71x.81x.81-m, and also contained provision for
feeding without opening the cage door. Behavior was viewed through
1-way windows constructed from circuit boards with very small
holes. A 16-8 diurnal light cycle was also imposed on these
cages.

During the first weeks of life, isolates were bottle fed a
similac formula by human caregivers. This was accomplished with
minimal handling and other physical contact. When isolates attained self-feeding at 1-3 weeks of age, their cages were opened
only for cleaning and health checks. The only other temporally
varied stimulation available to sound-chamber isolates was from
their own movements and from visually scanning the cage interior.
Masonite cage isolates did receive auditory input from laboratory
sounds. Socialized subjects raised without mothers in agemate
groups also received hand-feeding during weeks 1-3. Subsequently,
they lived together in wire cages approximately the same size as
those used to house total isolates. We emphasize that the sound
chambers, their associated living cages, and the Masonite cages
housing rhesus and pigtail isolates were the same units, transported from Wisconsin to Washington. Also, the feeding and
maintenance procedures used with the two species were identical.

III. TEST CONDITIONS AND MEASUREMENT PROCEDURES

Two types of test situations were studied. The first involved observation of total isolates in their home cages during the isolation period. The second involved social grouping in a playroom situation, which presented the first extensive opportunity for social interaction by total isolates.

A. Isolation Cage Tests

Observations in isolation cages were made 3-5 days per week throughout rearing. In this article, we report on behaviors during the last month in isolation. Observation occurred for 5 min periods during times of relatively high behavioral activity. During these home cage tests, isolates received no input from pictures or brain stimulation, and the laboratory was relatively quiet. Pigtail data was collected at 6-7 months of age, rhesus data at 7-8 months.

B. Playroom Tests

Post-rearing tests at Wisconsin and Washington were conducted in approximately equal size playrooms (2.44-m wide, 1.98-m high, 3.05-m deep), containing similar shelves, ladders, toys, and a large 2-way observation window. (All sessions were 30 min long, with each subject scored for two 5-min periods. Two observers scored each subject once per session.) As shown in Table I, testing began at 7-12 months of age in different experiments. Duration of testing varied from 2-3 months, with both pigtail and rhesus subjects receiving each duration. Sessions occurred 3-5 times per week.

Isolates and socialized controls were tested in between-group pairs, or in groups of four consisting of two monkeys from each rearing condition. Approximately equal numbers of pigtails and rhesus were tested under each group size. Subjects received individual playroom adaptation prior to the start of formal social testing. No reliable rearing differences were found between two and four monkey groupings, although socialized animals played during four-animal tests but had little play in two-animal pairs. This test group size variable was, therefore, excluded from analysis.

C. Observation Methods

Human observers employed a standard coding system for isolation cage and playroom tests (Sackett et al., 1973). Although coding instruments differed between some experiments (a digital electronic system in all pigtail experiments and in rhesus Experiment 2, a clock-counter and pencil-paper system in rhesus Experiment 1), coding categories were identical for all studies. High intra-observer reliability ($r \geq 0.85$) was obtained for all categories in

all studies, and one of the observers collected data in all four
experiments.

For analysis purposes, specific isolation cage behaviors were
combined into four categories which accounted for 99% of responding
during the total test time. These categories were (i) Sleep-
Passive, behaviors in which no active responses occurred, except
perhaps slow visual scanning; (ii) Abnormal, the personal and locomotor behaviors described above which define the isolation syndrome;
(iii) Exploration, behaviors involving manual and/or oral manipulation of the environment, locomotion, and normal self-manipulation
such as grooming; and (iv) Play, highly active behavior involving
chasing, wall-bouncing, and other locomotion-manipulation actions
classified as play during actual social interactive behavior. The
dependent variables reported for isolation cage tests were derived
from the total number of seconds spent in each behavior. Time per
category was divided by the 300 sec total test time, and these percentage scores were averaged over all 5 min observations during the
last month in total isolation.

Specific behaviors scored during playroom tests were also combined for analysis purposes. Three pooled nonsocial and three
pooled social categories accounted for 99% of playroom activities.
The pooled nonsocial categories were (i) Sleep-Passive, no active
responses except perhaps slow visual scanning; (ii) Play-Explore-
Sex, behaviors involving manual and/or oral manipulation of the inanimate environment and normal self-manipulation; and (iii) Abnormal,
those behaviors involving self-directed clutching, body rocking,
stereotyped locomotion, and withdrawal which define the isolation
syndrome. The pooled social categories were (iv) Play-Explore-Sex,
behaviors involving normal social interaction, sexual activity, and
grooming; (v) Aggression, threat and physical attack; and (vi)
socially-elicited Fear-Withdrawal-Disturbance.

On playroom tests during rhesus Experiment 1, frequence of
occurrence, but not duration, was scored. In all other experiments
both frequency and duration measures were obtained. Coding categories on all playroom tests were mutually exclusive and exhaustive,
thereby yielding a measure of total number of behavior changes. The
dependent variable reported for playroom tests is probability of occurrence (frequency per category divided by total behavior changes)
per 5 min of testing for each of the six pooled categories. These
probabilities were averaged over all 5 min observations for each
subject.

D. Data Analyses

Results were evaluated using the harmonic mean, unequal $\underline{n}$,
ANOVA technique (Winer, 1971). Separate ANOVAs were performed for

each isolation cage and playroom category. The 2x2x2 independent groups design used to assess isolation cage behavior tested effects of Species, Type-of-Isolation (sound chamber versus Masonite cage), and Sex. The 2x2x2 independent groups design used to study playroom behavior tested effects of Species, Rearing Condition (isolates versus socialized), and Sex. Where required, simple interaction effects were assessed by $\underline{t}$ tests.

IV. SPECIES DIFFERENCES IN BEHAVIOR DURING ISOLATION

Table II presents the percentage of test time spent in each behavior. Sex differences and interactions with sex were not statistically reliable (all $\underline{p} > 0.05$). The results can be described as follows.

(i) Sleep-Passive. A significant Species X Type-of-Isolation interaction ($\underline{p} < 0.01$) revealed that pigtails reared in Masonite cages had lower inactivity scores than any of the other groups. The two rhesus groups did not differ from each other or from pigtails reared in sound chambers (all $\underline{p} > 0.05$). This suggests that the auditory input available in Masonite cages facilitated responsivity of pigtail isolates, but not of rhesus isolates.

(ii) Isolate Syndrome Behaviors. A significant Species effect occurred ($\underline{p} < 0.001$), with no reliable main effect of Type-of-Isolation or interaction. Although rhesus developed a high amount of isolate syndrome behavior while in isolation, pigtails did not.

(iii) Exploration. A significant Species effect was found ($\underline{p} < 0.001$), with no Type-of-Isolation main effect but a reliable interaction ($\underline{p} < 0.05$). Pigtail isolates explored 4 times more than rhesus. Rhesus did not differ by caging type, but Masonite-caged pigtails explored more than sound chamber pigtails ($\underline{p} < 0.05$). This again suggests that the auditory input available in Masonite cages facilitated responsiveness for pigtails, but not for rhesus.

(iv) Play. No reliable main effects were found, but the Species X Type-of-Isolation interaction was significant ($\underline{p} < 0.05$). The two rhesus groups did not differ from Masonite-caged pigtails in play, while sound chamber pigtails were lower than the other groups. (all $\underline{p} < 0.05$). This suggests that total lack of stimulation depresses highly active behavior in pigtail isolates, but does not do so for rhesus.

These results show two remarkably different patterns of behavioral development under isolation. Pigtail monkeys spent a large portion of their time in environment and self-directed normal exploratory and manipulatory activity. Pigtails failed to develop the "typical" isolate syndrome to any marked degree. Rhesus, on

TABLE II. Percentage of total test time during isolation cage
           5 min trials for pigtail and rhesus total social iso-
           lates living in sound-attenuating chambers or enclosed
           Masonite cages

Behavior Category	Pigtails		Rhesus	
	Sound Chamber	Enclosed Cage	Sound Chamber	Enclosed Cage
Sleep-Passive	33.9	7.2	29.0	25.5
Isolate Syndrome	1.5	7.0	51.0	47.3
Exploration	62.8	78.4	16.0	21.2
Play	1.8	7.0	4.0	6.0
Sample Size	16	9	4	12

the other hand, had greatly reduced exploratory behavior, and
showed their typically high level of isolate syndrome behavior.

V. PLAYROOM TESTS: SPECIES AND REARING CONDITION DIFFERENCES

     Table III presents results of ANOVAs for each of the six play-
room behaviors. Figure 1 presents behavioral probability profiles
for each species and rearing group. Sex differences did appear and
will be discussed below. However, almost all main effects and interactions involving Species and Rearing effects were reliable irrespec-
tive of sex differences. The results can be summarized as follows.

     (i) Passive. A Species main effect occurred, with no reliable
Rearing main effect or interaction. This was due to greater passive
behavior by pigtails ($\bar{X}$ probability = 0.39) than by rhesus ($\bar{X}$ = 0.28).

     (ii) Nonsocial Play-Explore-Sex. Both main effects and the
interaction were significant. As shown in Figure 1, pigtail isolates had a higher probability of responding to the inanimate environment than rhesus isolates. However, socialized rhesus had a
much higher probability of these normal nonsocial behaviors than
socialized pigtails. It is also clear that isolation rearing depressed environment-directed behaviors for both species, but did so
much more for rhesus than for pigtail isolates.

     (iii) Isolation Syndrome Behavior. Both main effects and the
interaction were significant. Rhesus isolates had a mean probability of 0.55 for isolate syndrome behavior, while pigtail isolates

TABLE III. Analyses of variance for species differences by male and female socialized and total isolate 1-year old monkeys. Results are given for each of the six pooled behavior categories measured during playroom tests. All effects were tested with $\underline{df}$ = 1/84.

Variance Source	MS	F	MS	F	MS	F
			Nonsocial Behaviors			
	Passive		Play-Explore		Abnormal	
Species (SP)	.244	42.36‡	.395	86.44‡	.344	63.53‡
Rearing (R)	.021	3.66	1.642	359.69‡	2.999	554.60‡
Sex	.017	3.00	.029	6.35*	.004	.78
SP x Sex	.001	.04	.766	167.90‡	.437	80.85‡
SP x R	.001	.06	.047	10.35*	.026	4.88*
R x Sex	.033	5.78*	.030	6.57*	.001	.17
SP x R x Sex	.011	1.95	.004	.79	.022	4.07*
Error	.006		.005		.005	
			Social Behaviors			
	Play-Explore		Aggression		Fear-Disturbance	
Species (SP)	.281	55.51‡	.003	15.75†	.038	17.16‡
Rearing (R)	.682	134.75‡	.003	14.10†	.284	127.61‡
Sex	.009	1.71	.002	10.32†	.001	.59
SP x R	.159	31.50‡	.003	13.79†	.043	19.16†
SP x Sex	.021	4.10*	.002	9.33‡	.008	3.47
R x Sex	.001	.20	.001	5.99*	.004	1.82
SP x R x Sex	.002	.46	.002	7.26†	.004	1.90
Error	.005		.0002		.002	

$^{*}\underline{p}$ < 0.05 $^{\dagger}\underline{p}$ < 0.01 $^{\ddagger}\underline{p}$ < 0.001

had half that value ($\bar{X}$ = 0.27). Socialized subjects of both species had almost no isolate syndrome responses.

(iv) <u>Social Play-Explore-Sex</u>. Both main effects and the inter-

action were reliable. As shown in Figure 1, socialized pigtails
had a three times higher probability of normal social interaction
than socialized rhesus. Isolates of both species had low social
interaction probabilities. However, the fact that pigtail isolates did engage in more positive social interaction was revealed
by a chi square analysis. Twenty-one of the 25 pigtail isolates
had social interaction probabilities greater than zero, but only
3 of the 16 rhesus isolates had non-zero interaction probabilities
(p < 0.001). Thus, as a species, pigtails engaged in more positive
social interaction, and these behaviors did appear, although at reduced levels, in pigtail isolates.

(v) <u>Aggression</u>. Although threat and attack behavior was
generally low, significant main effects and interaction did occur.
This was due to a 0.03 aggression probability by socialized rhesus.
Rhesus isolates and pigtail monkeys of both rearing conditions did
not exceed probabilities of 0.003. Thus, isolation depressed aggression toward agemates in rhesus, but did not affect aggression
in pigtails.

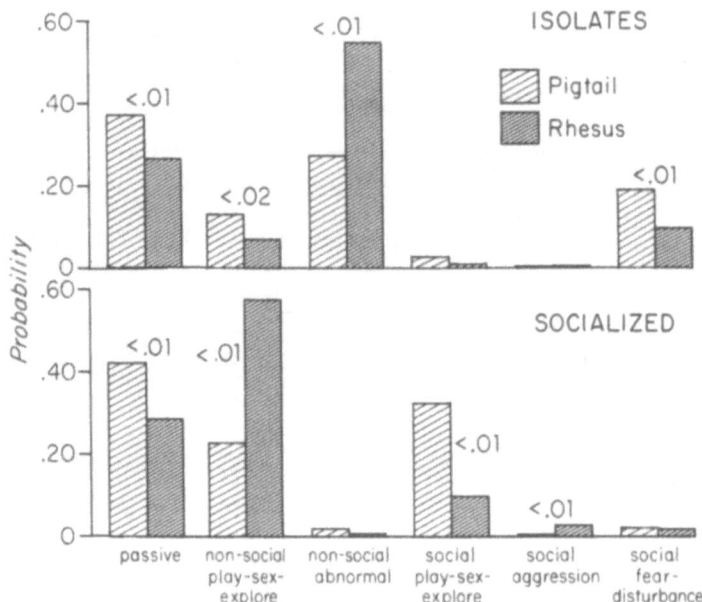

FIG. 1. Behavioral profiles for pigtail (<u>M. nemestrina</u>) and rhesus
(<u>M. mulatta</u>) 1-year-old monkeys showing probability of occurrence of
three nonsocial and three social behavior categories during playroom
social behavior tests. Upper graph compares monkeys raised in total
social isolation from birth through 7-9 months. Lower graph compares
socialized controls reared during infancy with mothers and/or peers.

(vi) <u>Social Fear</u>. Both main effects and the interaction were significant. The probability of pigtail isolates exhibiting socially-elicited fear was twice that of rhesus isolates, while the socialized groups did not differ. Although higher social fear could be viewed as a negative reaction to isolation, our opinion is that greater social fear reflected greater social awareness by pigtail isolates. Also, the fact that pigtail isolates engaged in some positive social interaction increased their opportunity for exhibiting socially-evoked fear.

Like the isolation cage results presented above, the social playroom data also reveal overall species differences and important differences in behavior following isolation rearing. Regardless of rearing condition, pigtails were more passive, less aggressive, and more socially responsive than rhesus of the same age. Socialized pigtails were, however, less exploratory than their rhesus counterparts.

Differences between the socialized groups could be due to differences in the quality of socialization available during infancy. However, the fact that isolation-reared pigtails showed a similar behavior profile to socialized pigtails that differed from the rhesus profiles on the same behavior categories suggests that quality of socialization will not account for overall species effects. Rather, these differences appear to reveal a basic genetic effect, appearing independently of the rearing environment.

Species comparisons between isolates reveal that the isolation syndrome does occur for both species, but is much more extensive in rhesus monkeys. Thus, pigtail isolates responded more to the non-social environment, had less abnormal behavior, showed some positive social interaction, and seemed to exhibit greater social awareness. These results suggest that basic genetic differences between pigtail and rhesus monkeys interact with deprived rearing conditions in determining whether the monkey will, or will not, be susceptible to developing extensive abnormal behavior.

Follow up studies of rhesus isolates reveal failure to develop normal behavior even after years of post-rearing socialization (e.g., Sackett, 1968, 1972a). The only rhesus isolates not showing the isolation syndrome were those who received extensive therapy in interactions with <u>much younger</u> infants immediately after emergence from isolation (Suomi and Harlow, 1972). On the other hand, pigtail isolates show less severe isolation effects upon emergence from isolation. Follow up studies still in progress suggest that post-rearing social experience with <u>same-age</u> partners has a normalizing effect on pigtail isolate social behavior.

VI. PLAYROOM TESTS: EFFECTS OF SEX

Table III shows a number of significant Sex main effects and interactions with the Species and Rearing variables. These playroom test results are summarized as follows.

(i) Sleep-Passive. The Rearing x Sex interaction was significant. This was due to male isolates ($\bar{X}$ probability = 0.28), who showed less inactive behavior than female isolates ($\bar{X}$ = 0.36) or male ($\bar{X}$ = 0.36) or female ($\bar{X}$ = 0.35) socialized monkeys.

(ii) Nonsocial Play-Explore-Sex. A reliable Sex main effect occurred, with females ($\bar{X}$ = 0.27) exhibiting a slightly higher probability of responding to the inanimate environment than males ($\bar{X}$ = 0.23). Significant Rearing x Sex and Species x Sex interactions are presented in Table IV. Although socialized animals of either sex responded to the environment with higher probabilities than isolates, socialized females exhibited more normal nonsocial behavior than socialized males. The Species x Sex interaction shows that, although rhesus females explored more than rhesus males (independent of rearing condition), no sex difference in exploration appeared among pigtails. These complicated species effects probably deserve further study and no more comment at this time.

(iii) Isolate Syndrome Behavior. The Species x Sex and Species x Rearing x Sex interactions were significant. The 3-way interaction is presented in Table V. Among pigtails, male isolates had slightly more abnormal behavior than females, but this was not significant. Among rhesus isolates, males had a 10% higher probability of isolate syndrome behavior than females (p < 0.01). Socialized animals had very low levels of abnormal behavior, with no reliable sex differences appearing in either species. These findings suggest a need for further research concerning the interaction of genetic predispositions with deprivation rearing.

TABLE IV. Rearing x Sex and Species x Sex interactions in average probability of nonsocial Play-Explore-Sex during playroom social behavior tests

	Rearing x Sex		Species x Sex	
	Isolates	Socialized	Pigtails	Rhesus
Males	.103	.356	.183	.276
Females	.103	.434	.172	.365

TABLE V. Species x Rearing Condition x Sex interaction in average probability of abnormal, isolate syndrome, behaviors during social playroom tests

	Pigtails		Rhesus	
	Isolates	Socialized	Isolates	Socialized
Males	.282	.026	.597	.012
Females	.253	.021	.505	.001

(iv) Social Play-Explore-Sex. The only reliable effect was the Species x Sex interaction. Pigtail males ($\bar{X}$ probability = 0.20) played reliably more ($p < 0.05$) than pigtail females ($\bar{X}$ = 0.14), while no significant difference appeared between rhesus males ($\bar{X}$ = 0.05) and females ($\bar{X}$ = 0.06).

(v) Aggression. All sex effects were significant. Table VI clearly shows the source of these effects. Pigtails of either sex or rearing condition had almost no threat or attack behavior. Among rhesus, socialized animals were more aggressive than isolates ($p < 0.001$). Thus, as a species, rhesus were more aggressive than pigtails, rhesus males being particularly so. Male rhesus isolates did not have reliably more aggression than female rhesus isolates, and the male isolate probability was much lower than that for socialized male rhesus. Isolation rearing thus appeared to suppress the species-typical high aggression level of rhesus males toward agemates, while for pigtails, isolation had neither an enhancing nor a depressing effect on aggression in either sex.

These sex differences and interactions generally agree with those reported elsewhere (e.g., Sackett et al., 1975). As found previously, the magnitude of sex effects were generally greater on

TABLE VI. Species x Rearing Condition x Sex interaction in average probability of threat and aggression behavior during social playroom tests

	Pigtails		Rhesus	
	Isolates	Socialized	Isolates	Socialized
Males	.003	.002	.005	.047
Females	.002	.003	.001	.010

nonsocial than social behaviors. However, the addition of the species variable in this experiment throws a new complication on an old problem. Although the direction of sex differences between isolates was generally the same, the magnitude of differences was much greater for rhesus monkey isolates. This may reflect counteracting genetic variables.

Rhesus monkeys, as a species, appear to be more susceptible to isolation rearing effects than pigtails. On the other hand, a wealth of data attests to the idea that males are more vulnerable than females to postnatal insult. Thus, the relative insensitivity of pigtails to isolation rearing effects may decrease the magnitude of measurable sex differences in pigtail isolates. The relative susceptibility of rhesus to isolation effects may, conversely, serve to magnify sex differences in rhesus isolates. Although complex, this interaction of genetic variables with impoverished rearing conditions may yet prove to be an excellent experimental model for the study of individual differences in abnormal behavior.

VII. CONCLUSION

Studies of various species, reviewed extensively in this volume, reveal deficits in behavior and central nervous system anomalies following environmental deprivation. Some studies also suggest that environmental enrichment can produce both a behaviorally more competent and a neurally more developed individual. Previous work on rhesus monkey social isolates leads one to suspect that nonhuman primates in general should respond to deprivation rearing in the same manner as their human and nonprimate relatives. Behaviorally, this is the case for rhesus monkeys. Unfortunately, few well-controlled studies of brain anatomy and/or biochemistry have been performed to compare rhesus CNS abnormalities with those of other species.

The results of the present experiment, however, suggest a word of caution concerning generalization of behavioral, and probably also CNS, effects of isolation rearing across species. Sex differences suggest that environmental restriction has attentuated effects on rhesus females. Anatomical and chemical CNS studies by Rosenzweig (1974, personal communication) suggest that the same type of sex difference occurs among rats subjected to environmental deprivation. Thus, even within a species, there appear to be genetic factors involved in vulnerability to, or relative buffering against, abnormalizing effects of deprivation.

Our species difference results only serve to underscore this problem. These results show that the generality of rearing condition effects, even across very closely related nonhuman primate species, must be experimentally tested--not simply assumed. This seems especially true when dealing with models of important human problems such as are involved in the area of "Environments as Therapy for Brain Dysfunction."

Rosenblum and Kaufman's (1967) studies of infant pigtail and bonnet monkey reactions to separation from their mothers further illustrates the basic problem. Pigtail infants become depressed when separated from their mother, while bonnet infants do not. When cross-fostering was studied, pigtails reared by bonnet mothers failed to show their typical depression on separation. Surprisingly, bonnet infants reared by pigtail mothers also did not become depressed on separation. Thus, pigtail infants were highly influenced by their rearing experiences, while bonnet infants were genetically or prenatally buffered against showing separation effects regardless of their rearing environment. Like Rosenblum and Kaufman's pioneering effects in studying species differences among primates in effects of environments on social development, the present study has also revealed a major species difference between Macaques in response to the powerful variable of social isolation in infancy.

ACKNOWLEDGMENTS

A brief summary of the material presented in Figure 1 of this article has been submitted to Science magazine as a brief report. Portions of the pigtail isolation work are included in R. Holm's doctoral dissertation and were supported by NSF Grant GB-31149 to G. Sackett. NIH grants supporting this work over a 10-yr period were RR-0167 to the Wisconsin Regional Primate Research Center, MH-11894 to the Wisconsin Primate Laboratory, RR-00166 to the Washington Regional Primate Research Center, and HD-02274 to the Washington Child Development and Mental Retardation Center.

REFERENCES

Davenport, R. K., Jr., and Menzel, E. W., Jr. 1963. Stereotyped Behavior of the Infant Chimpanzee. Arch. Gen. Psychiat. 8: 99-104.

Gluck, J. P., and Harlow, H. F. 1971. The Effects of Deprived and Enriched Rearing Conditions on Later Learning: A Review, pp. 105-120. In L. E. Jarrard (ed.). Cognitive Processes of Nonhuman Primates. Academic Press, New York.

Harlow, H. F., Gluck, J. P., and Suomi, S. J. 1972. Generalization of Behavioral data between nonhuman and human animals. Amer. Psychol. 27:709-716.

Harlow, H. F., Schiltz, K. A., and Harlow, M. K. 1968. Effects of Social Isolation on the Learning Performance of Rhesus Monkeys, pp. 178-185. In C. R. Carpenter (ed.). Proc. II International Congress of Primatology, Vol. 1. Karger, New York.

Holm, R. A. 1975. The Effects of Isolation Rearing on the Pigtail Monkey (M. nemestrina): With and Without Electrical Brain Stimulation. Doctoral Dissertation, University of Washington.

Menzel, E. W., Jr. 1964. Patterns of Responsiveness in Chimpanzees Reared Through Infancy Under Conditions of Environmental Restriction. Psychol. Forsch. 27:337-365.

Pratt, C. L. 1969. The Developmental Consequences of Variation in Early Social Stimulation. Doctoral Dissertation, University of Wisconsin.

Rosenblum, L. A., and Kaufman, I. C. 1967. Laboratory Observations of Early Mother-Infant Relations in Pigtail and Bonnet Macaques, pp. 33-41. In S. A. Altmann (ed.). Social Communication Among Primates. University of Chicago Press, Chicago.

Sackett, G. P. 1966. Monkeys Reared in Visual Isolation with Pictures as visual stimulation: Evidence for an Innate Releasing Mechanism. Science 154:1468-1472.

Sackett, G. P. 1968. The Persistence of Abnormal Behavior Following Isolation Rearing, pp. 3-37. In The Role of Learning in Psychotherapy. CIBA Foundation, London.

Sackett, G. P. 1972a. Is-lation Rearing in Monkeys: Diffuse and Specific Effects on Behavior, pp. 61-110. In R. Chauvin (ed.). Ethology and Human Behavior. Colloques Inter. du. C. N. R. S., Paris, France.

Sackett, G. P. 1972b. Exploratory Behavior of Rhesus Monkeys as a Function of Rearing Experiences and Sex. Develop. Psychol. 6: 260-270.

Sackett, G. P., and Ruppenthal, G. C. 1973. Development of Monkeys After Varied Experiences During Infancy, pp. 52-87. In S. A. Barnett (ed.). Ethology and Development. Lippincott, Philadelphia.

Sackett, G. P., Tripp, R., and Grady, S. A. 1972. Monkeys Reared in Isolation with Added Social, Nonsocial, and Electrical Brain Stimulation: A Preliminary Study. Paper presented Ann. Meet. Amer. Psychol. Assoc., Margaret Harlow Memorial Symposium, Hawaii.

Sackett, G. P., Stephenson, E., and Ruppenthal, G. C. 1973. Digital Data Acquisition Systems for Observing Behavior in Laboratory and Field Settings. Behav. Res. Meth. Instrum. 4:344-348.

Sackett, G. P., Holm, R. A., and Landesman-Dwyer, S. 1975. Vulnerability for Abnormal Development: Pregnancy Outcomes and Sex Differences in Macaque Monkeys, pp. 59-76. In N. R. Ellis (ed.). Aberrant Development in Infancy. Erlbaum Associates, New Jersey.

Sackett, G. P., Ruppenthal, G. C., and Fahrenbruch, C. E. 1975. Effects of Prior Mothering on the Response of Pigtail Monkeys to Social Isolation Rearing. In preparation.

Suomi, S. J., and Harlow, H. F. 1972. Social Rehabilitation of Isolate-Reared Monkeys. Develop. Psychol. 6:487-496.

Winer, B. J. 1971. Statistical Principles in Experimental Design, (2d ed.), pp. 599-603. McGraw-Hill, New York.

ENVIRONMENTS OF DYSFUNCTION: THE RELEVANCE

OF PRIMATE ANIMAL MODELS[1]

Helen L. Morrison and William T. McKinney, Jr.

Department of Psychiatry
University of Wisconsin Medical School
Madison, Wisconsin 43706

I.   INTRODUCTION

It has long been known that the environment plays a role in
both the production and alleviation of patterns of aberrant behavior. The way in which organisms adapt to their milieux and the
processes by which this occurs are concerns shared by most scientists. Developmental psychology, behavioral genetics, psychiatry,
ethology, neurophysiology, and systems theory are among the many
specialties that contribute to our understanding of the genesis
and maintenance of behavior. All have recognized that combinations
of environmental stimuli or excesses or deficits of stimuli have
behavioral consequences. This adjustment of the animal to internal
and external pressures inherent in the demands of survival is reflected in its behavior. Comprehensive understanding of behavior
will require both behavioral observation and studies of basic mechanisms involved in the behavior.

In terms of the title of this volume, one can experimentally
produce "brain dysfunction" and know whether social, surgical, or
pharmacologic variables were responsible for the dysfunction. The
same is true for the therapies used in reversing this dysfunction.
However, the multiplicity and interaction of variables present in
most forms of human psychopathology prevent the study in humans of

1 The writing of this chapter was supported by Research Grant
MH-21892 and by Research Scientist Development Award MH-47353
(WTM), both from the National Institute of Mental Health, and
by the Wisconsin Psychiatric Research Institute.

these variables in isolation from each other. It also prevents the isolation of a given variable and its contribution to the condition. In animals, manipulation of one variable at a time is often possible and permits the direct observation of the consequences of that manipulation.

The ideal situation is to study the results of these experimental conditions in the species in which they are most frequently observed or in which the particular problem being studied is most appropriate. Many experiments with human subjects which could add to our knowledge of behavior are prohibited by both practical and ethical considerations. Federal regulations that led to needed formation of Human Subjects Committees also have led to more restrictive and occasionally overly rigid standards for human experimentation. As such, the use of model systems in humans is both less advantageous and available. Thus, animal models using mice, rats, cats, dogs, birds, and multiple primate species have been utilized in many situations (Wildt and Dukelow, 1974; Meldrum et al., 1975; Newberne, 1975; Rall, 1969). The determination of the kind of animal for the model all too frequently is based on nonexistent criteria. This can be translated to mean the unfamiliarity of the investigator in working with all but one species.

This chapter will discuss the current status of experimental psychopathology and will concentrate on animal models. The advantages and disadvantages and the criteria for the development and assessment of animal models will be discussed. The various social and biologic environmental induction techniques and concomitant rehabilitative techniques of a biologic and social nature will then be presented. Included are correlative studies of biologic systems affected by these techniques. We have not included sections on ethology or on the history of comparative psychology or of the production of psychopathology. The reader is referred to many excellent and detailed writings on these topics (Waters et al., 1960; Hinde, 1974; White, 1974).

II. ANIMAL MODELS: RELEVANCE AND CRITERIA FOR EVALUATION

Acceptance of an animal model does not imply equality with the "real" observed syndrome in its "natural" species. Too frequently models are expected to provide more than they can. Specific limitations exist, depending on the syndrome being studied, and not all conditions are amenable to the concept of animal modeling. Marked difficulties also exist in the acceptance of phenomena which are observed in nonhuman animals as equivalent to their analogous phenomena in the human (Broadhurst, 1953; Birch, 1961; Mason, 1968a; Levy, 1952; Lorenz, 1971). The popularization of animal behavior research has led some to ignore a major ethological maxim, that similarity of

behaviors in different species does not imply similarity of mechanisms or meanings of those behaviors. Publications which commit
this major fallacy in that they attempt to equate humans to our
relatives in the animal kingdom have seemed to proliferate unchecked
in recent years. None of this "popular" work is representative of
scientific work in the field of animal models.

Skepticism regarding the relevance of psychopathological models
in animals to human disorders has been voiced by many workers in
several disciplines. For Kubie (1939), a psychiatrist and leading
spokesman against acceptance of animal models, behavior was only the
"sign language" of underlying symbolic disorder, the real core of
psychopathology. And for others concerned with the inability to
generalize from studies done in the early period of this discipline,
little relevance existed beyond the situation in which the behavior
was produced. In many cases, methodologic flaws hampered the utility
of early animal models in both generating and testing hypotheses.

The definition of the abnormality of animal behavior and subsequent assessment of its relevance are both necessary aspects in
the evaluation of models. Both aspects can be accomplished through
the rigorous definition of criteria of behavior considered applicable
to animals. Hebb (1947; Hebb and Thompson, 1954) was one of the first
authors to select criteria and he began by defining neurosis of the
human in non-verbal, behavioral terms. This permitted the use of the
definition at the level of animals. In 1966, Senay put forth the
concept of human depression reflected in an animal model. This
followed his observation that depressive symptomatology occurred in
puppies when separated from the investigator. Upon reunion with the
investigator, the symptoms abated. As the literature continued to
report the effects of loss and disruption of previous affectional
bonds, the need for systematic experimentation and evaluation became
critical.

This need, where the interactional and social variables can be
manipulated in an organized, logical manner was described by McKinney
and Bunney (1969). Their five criteria and requirements for an animal model of depression were: (1) the behaviors of the depression
so induced should be reasonably analogous to those seen in human
depression; (2) there should be observable behavioral changes which
can be evaluated objectively; (3) independent observers should agree
on objective criteria for drawing conclusions about the subjective
state; (4) the treatment modalities effective in reversing depression in humans should reverse the changes seen in animals, and (5)
the system should be reproducible by other investigators. Adherence
to this system, noted to be "no easy task," permits further elucida-
tion of the variables and also allows for greater diversity in behavioral and biochemical studies.

It is important for the reader to be aware of several points before we proceed to the remainder of our discussion. We are talking about observable behavioral changes, leaving the subjective dimension to workers who have subjects other than monkeys. Definitions of behavioral scoring categories will not be presented in detail but include a wide range of self- and other-directed social behaviors, activity measures and multiple environmental categories. The objectivity of the scoring system permits almost no subjective bias and distortion. We also must emphasize that although behavioral similarities are observable between our animals and various clinical syndromes in man, no similarities are implied in either etiology or in the significance of these observable behaviors. Many labels have been applied to the behavioral manifestations of these monkeys, and inadequate behavioral description has too frequently accompanied them. Labels such as phobia, autism, experimental neurasthenia, and anxiety are meaningless terms in defining the study of animal models without substantially more documentation than has been done.

III. THE ENVIRONMENT OF INDUCTION

The specific description of various induction techniques used in the production of abnormal behaviors in primates, will be discussed later in this section. Our focus will turn initially to those general concepts felt to be necessary for the reader to more clearly comprehend the detailed studies presented below. A brief history of the study of the environment with its contribution to the induction of psychopathology is followed by more recent findings which describe basic developmental characteristics in primates. These discoveries provided the background work which allowed the investigation of the formation of maladaptive behavior patterns to be systematically described.

In any discussion of the effects of early experience upon the later development and behavior of an organism, stimuli from the physical environment play a considerable role. At birth, the organism begins a process of adaptation to a particular environment with successful development requiring physiologic, morphologic, and behavioral adaptation within the circumscribed conditions of that environment. The clinical literature notes that deprivation, or reduced or simplified stimulation, has consequences in both intellectual and emotional spheres (Goldfarb, 1955; O'Connor, 1968; Yarrow et al., 1972). Some workers, following the publication of Hebb's Organization of Behavior (1949), have studied the effects of restriction in early life on later functioning of the organism. The lack of environmental stimulation in dogs and rats has been noted to lead to deficits in perception (Riesen, 1950), emotionality, social behavior, activity level and motor coordination (Thompson and Solomon, 1954; Reiss, 1954) and intelligence (Forgays and Forgays, 1952). Tinkelpaugh (1929) and

Foley (1934, 1935) described the effects of rearing rhesus monkeys
in wire-cage isolation from other monkeys and subsequent abnormal
behaviors of self-mutilation, toe and thumb sucking and aberrant
sexual behavior. An infant chimpanzee, isolated during early development also showed disturbed affective responses (McCulloch and
Haslerud, 1939).

Attachment in animals had been recognized since Lorenz (1935)
described innate mechanisms, both auditory and visual, that were
involved in a process known as imprinting, defined as responses of
following behaviors in fish and infant birds. Several authors then
systematically investigated variables which were thought to contribute to the maintenance and development of imprinting (Hinde et al.,
1956; Jaynes, 1958; Hess, 1959; Fabricius, 1962). The observations
of affectional attachments in monkey and chimpanzee infants has been
noted by many authors (Yerkes, 1913; Zuckerman, 1932; Carpenter,
1942) with considerable controversy concerning the development and
underlying mechanisms of attachment. Of the postulated theories,
the most dominant posited drive reduction as a basis of learning by
which affection became a derived, self-supporting drive (Dollard and
Miller, 1950; Mussen and Conger, 1956). The importance of innate
needs such as clinging to mother, needs relating to movement, temperature and contact and the need to orally suck a breast have been
stressed by psychoanalytic writings (Bowlby, 1958; Ribble, 1943;
Winnicott, 1948). Attempts to integrate theories and experimental
evidence were limited because of the paucity of data which would
have permitted the cirtical evaluations of proposed theories. De-
ductions and intuitions did not yield data which would permit an
analysis of the many variables attendant in the theories of affectional development.

It was not until 1958, when Harlow first spoke of the attachment behaviors in primates from his work on surrogates, that systematic study of the importance of these bonds could be attempted
(Harlow, 1958; Harlow and Zimmerman, 1959; Harlow and Suomi, 1970b).
Two surrogate types were used initially by the Wisconsin researchers.
The cloth surrogate had a wood base, was covered with sponge rubber
and terrycloth fabric in a tan color. Heat radiated from a light
bulb placed at the height where the infant would normally encounter
a breast. The wire surrogate, made of a wire mesh, was adequate to
provide nursing and support functions, and also had radiant heat.
The two surrogates had as their only difference the quality of contact comfort available to them. The initial condition, the dual
mother surrogates described above, was designed to test the variables
of contact comfort and nursing comfort and these variables were rated
as to their relative importance. Lactation was found to be of almost
negligible importance while contact comfort was overwhelmingly important.

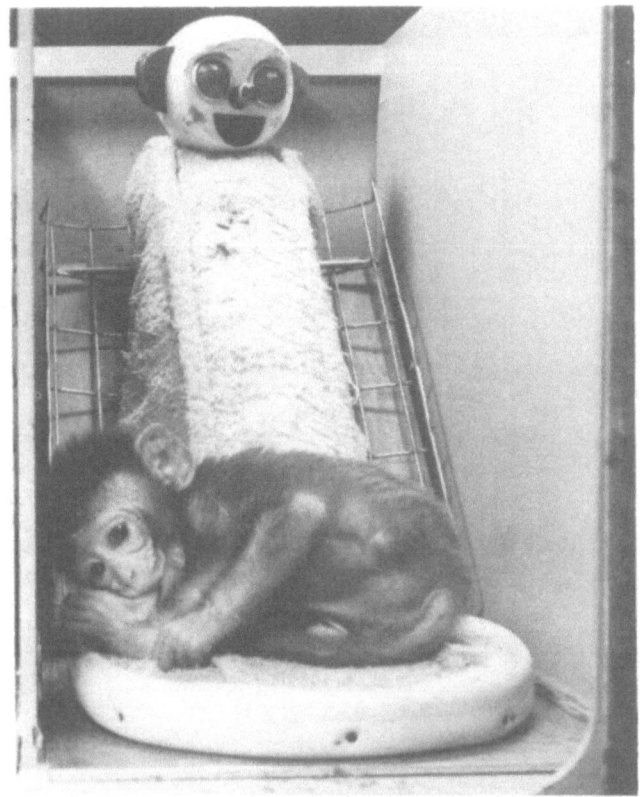

Fig. 1. Cloth-mother surrogate.

The infants over an increasing period of time also showed de-
creasing preferences for the lactating wire mother and increased
preference for the non-lactating cloth mother which did not support
the then dominant view that the attachment was a derived drive where
the infant was conditioned to the figure of mother because of thirst-
hunger reduction.

Another paradigm used was fear-producing stimuli to measure
the strength of the affectional bonds. A typical fear response to
a threatening stimulus was that of clinging tightly to the mother,
again with consistent preference shown for the cloth mother. This
seems to parallel the fearful human child who clings to its mother
when the situation becomes more dangerous or fearful.

The human child, at certain developmental stages, will react
to the strangeness of a previously unexperienced environment by
seeking security from the mother. In the primate, this situation
of unfamiliarity was tested in an "open field" environment. When

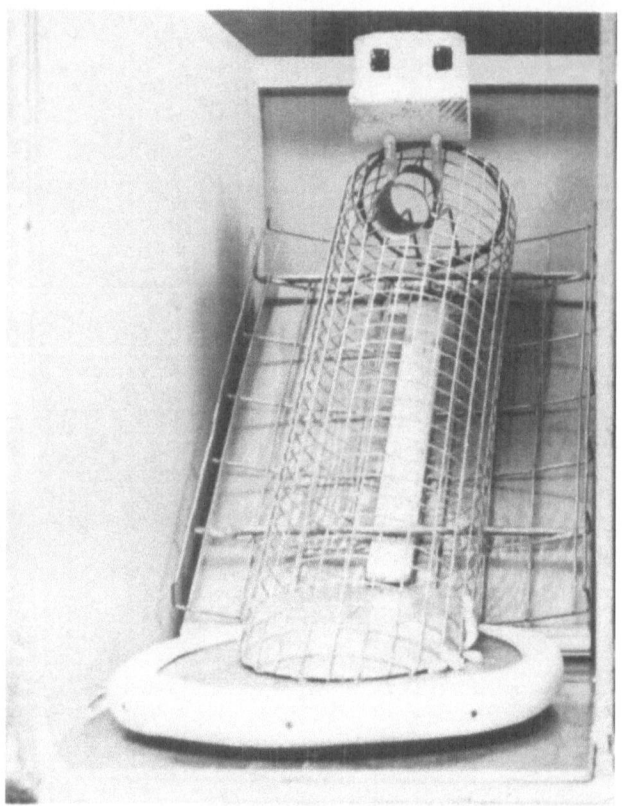

Fig. 2.   Wire-mother surrogate.

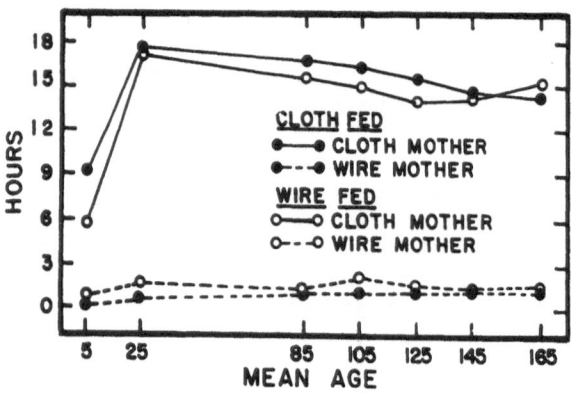

Fig. 3.   Preference of cloth-mother over wire-mother regardless of presence or absence of lactation.

the cloth mother was present, the infants would explore their environment and return to the mother before continuing the exploration.
If the mother was absent, the infants would scream and cry while
clutching their bodies or cloth diapers which, it would appear, did
not satisfy them. These behaviors were not different from those observed in the presence of the wire mother.

Several other variables appeared to be important in the formulation of the nature of the bond between infant and mother. When
contact comfort was equated in surrogate mothers, the lactating surrogate was preferred by the infant. Facial expression was important
but only in the sense that the infant exhibited a fear response if
the face was changed. Infants also showed a preference for cloth
surrogates if given a choice among vinyl, rayon or rough grade sand-
paper. Proprioceptive stimulation or a rocking motion has been
noted to be important in the mother-infant bond, in the human and
subhuman literature (Mason, 1968b). Monkeys prior to 140 or 150
days of age were found to prefer rocking mothers but this preference
disappeared after that age. Temperature variables were also implicated in attachment bond formation. Infants raised with a surrogate
that was heated by coils and then cooled showed attachment behaviors

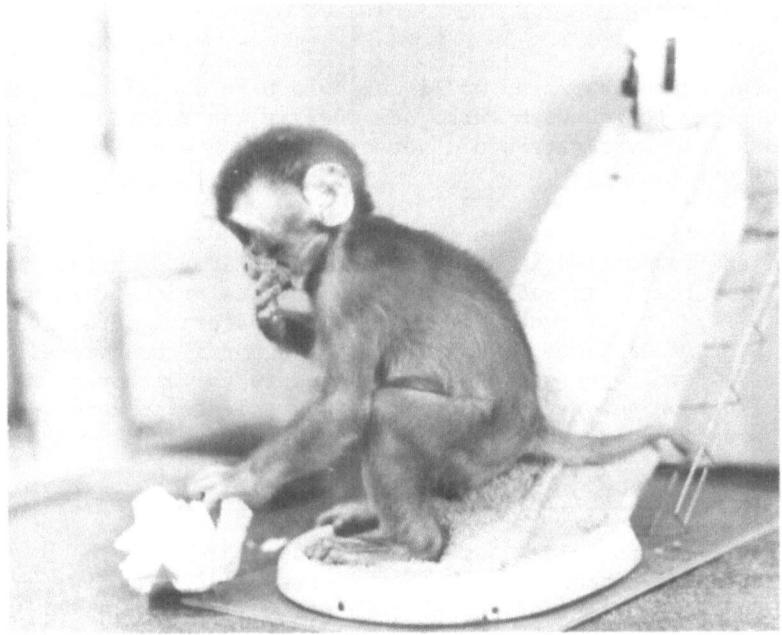

Fig. 4. Environmental exploration in "open field" testing by infant in presence of cloth surrogate.

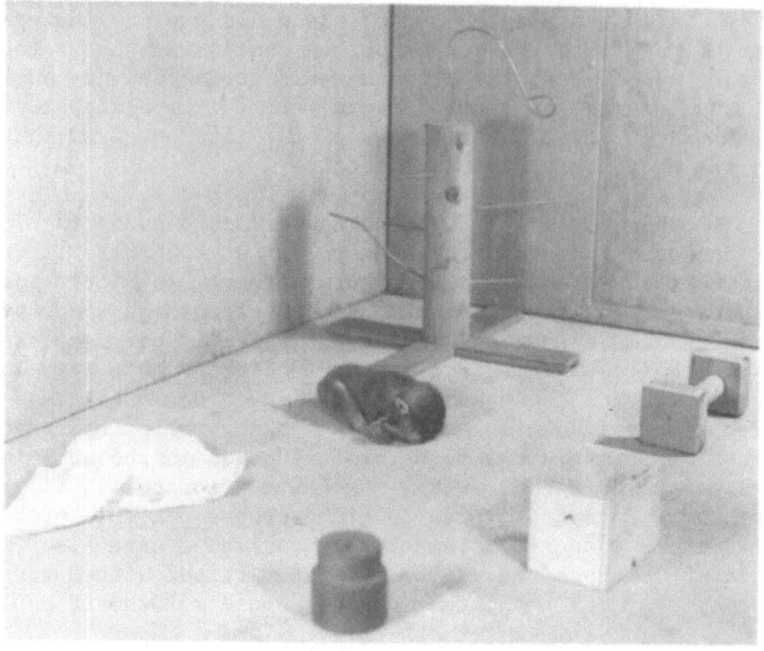

Fig. 5. Infant response to lack of mother surrogate in "open
field" testing.

when the surrogate was warm, would not attach to a cold surrogate,
but would cling to the warm surrogate when it was returned. Infants
raised on a cold surrogate would not attach, even when a warm surrogate was offered.

     Several attachment stages or "affectional systems" have been
described and documented in the developing primate organism. These
include: (1) the infant-mother, (2) the mother-infant, (3) the
peer-peer, (4) the heterosexual, and (5) the paternal affectional
systems (Harlow and Suomi, 1970a). Both the normal behavioral
characteristics of each stage and the sequence in which they matured
needed definition before there could be any scientific understanding
of the disruptions in or failure of their development.

A. Induction: The Physical and Social Environment

     The question formulated by the work reported above led to a
series of studies concerned with the effects of early social environments on the development of social competency (McKinney, 1974a).
Major social rearing conditions in use at the Wisconsin Primate

Laboratory include:

1. <u>Feral Monkeys</u>. Born and reared in the wild, these monkeys are then captured and brought to the laboratory.

2. <u>Nursery Rearing</u>. The newborns are removed from the mother at birth and housed in a closely supervised nursery situation. They are fed initially every 2 hours and, through the feeding process, are in intimate physical contact with humans. Self-feeding occurs around 15 to 20 days of age after being trained to drink from a bottle in a wire rack from ten days of age.

3. <u>Surrogate-Only Rearing</u>. This condition occurs following the 30-day nursery situation and has been discussed previously.

4. <u>Peer-Only Rearing</u>. Following the 30-day nursery period, the infants are placed in groups of two, four or six animals. Social stimulation is provided by exclusive placement with peers the same age. Delayed maturation of social behaviors has been noted following this living condition (Harlow and Harlow, 1971).

5. <u>Mother-Peer Rearing</u>. One of the most complex of laboratory rearing environments in which the animal lives with his mother in a "playpen" situation with basic living occurring in one of the four corner units and access to a central play area. Infants can play with each other and mothers are not able to interfere in the play activity but can observe their infants.

6. <u>Mother-Only Rearing</u>. These infants are reared with their biological mothers but have no physical interaction with peers or adults. The resultant social behavior deficits are primarily reflected in their avoiding play interactions, a tendency toward hyperaggressiveness when in contact with peers, and contact shyness. The longer they are denied the opportunity to interact with peers, the more severe are their social deficits (Alexander, 1966; Novak, 1974).

7. <u>Nuclear Family</u>. Four families live in one of four compartments bordering three sides of a play area equipped with objects to stimulate motor and social play. Mothers, fathers, other adults of both sexes, siblings and peers provide interfamily contacts, as well as intrafamily interaction. The infants are provided continued access to their mothers and fathers but have limited access to other adults and peers (Harlow, 1971). More sophisticated patterns of social behavior were noted to develop in this condition (Ruppenthal et al., 1974). Higher levels of activity and dominance behaviors and lower measures of passive and submissive behaviors are seen than occur in mother-peer reared animals (Suomi, 1974).

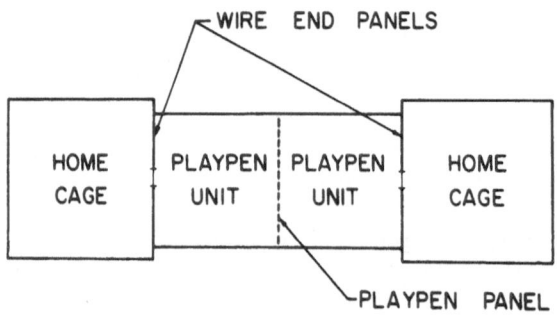

Fig. 6. Playpen situation in the mother-peer rearing environment.

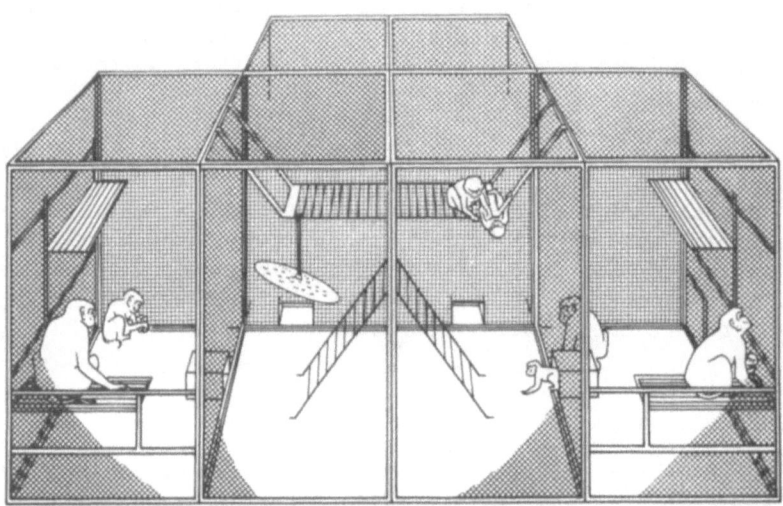

Fig. 7. Apparatus of nuclear family. Central play area surrounded
by four outer living cages (behind and on each side of the apparatus) with one adult male-female pair in each living cage.

There is no doubt that the most devastating impairment of social functioning results from the rearing condition of social isolation, with more severe effects a result of total isolation as compared to the condition of partial isolation. <u>Partial social isolation</u> involves placing an animal from birth in bare wire-mesh cages which prohibit it from physical interaction or contact with other animals but allow visual and auditory contact. This condition is the environment most commonly used for housing in primate laboratories. Studies of monkeys housed alone from birth or within the first six weeks of life for a duration of 1 to 10 years of age show that aberrant behaviors increase in frequency and severity as the duration of the partial isolation increases (Cross and Harlow, 1965). They typically show excessive self-orality, self-clasping and stereotyped patterns of rocking. There is a general withdrawal from social initiations with other animals and they lack the frequency and sophis-

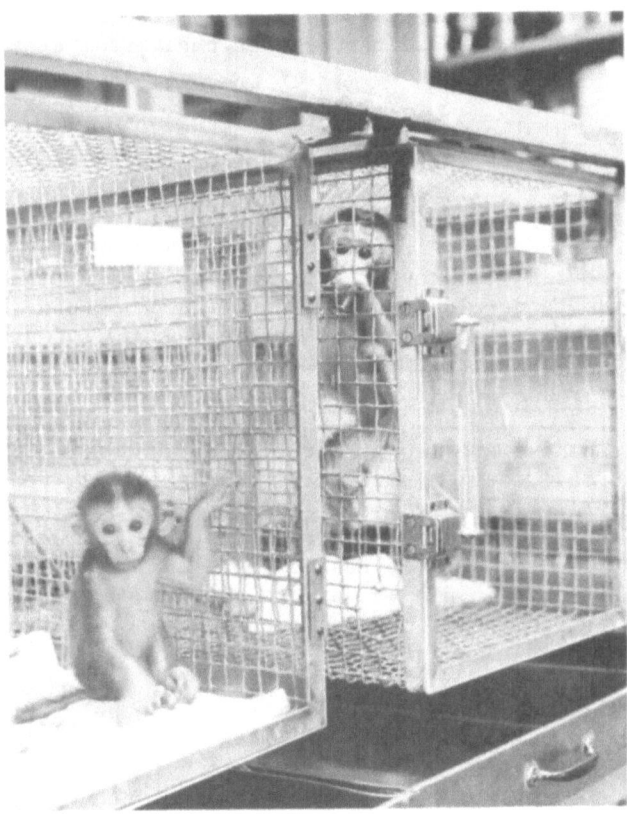

Fig. 8. Individual rhesus infants housed in the environment of partial social isolation.

tication of play or grooming activities of competent age-mates.
Aggressive behavior is inappropriate and sexual behavior is less
than adequate. Maternal behavior is most often characterized by
infifference without the brutality usually seen in "motherless-
mother" monkeys. These partial isolates do eventually show rudiments
of play behavior if repeated interactions are permitted with age
mates.

In the above rearing conditions we have seen that complex social
environments result in larger repertoires of complex social behaviors.
This is in stark contrast to the condition known as total social
isolation. The isolation syndrome has also been studied in dogs, in
cats, and in chimpanzees and although the specific techniques of both
isolation and measurement of behaviors vary, persistent patterns of
abnormal behavior have been found (Berkson et al., 1963; Nissen et
al., 1951; Thompson and Melzack, 1956; Fuller, 1967; Konrad and
Bagshaw, 1970). Nevertheless, species variability may be critical
in determination of the effects of the social isolation syndrome.
For example, Sackett in his study of pigtail macaques reared in
social isolation has not found the adverse behavioral effects noted
above (Sackett et al., this volume).

In total social isolation studies monkeys are placed in chambers,
metal encased enclosures which deny visual or tactual contact with
any social agents or environments (Rowland, 1964; Harlow et al.,
1964). Food, water and milk preparations are delivered to the monkeys within the chamber itself (Blomquist and Harlow, 1961) and diffuse light is provided to prevent optic nerve degeneration (Riesen,
1965). The "primate deprivation syndrome" (Mason, 1968b) shows the
symptoms of abnormal movements and posturing, excessive arousal or
fearfulness, lack of integration of motor patterns and communication
difficulties.

If rhesus monkeys are isolated for three months of life, severe
behavioral abnormalities may necessitate force feeding for survival
because of the animal's refusal to eat or drink. Upon removal from
the isolation chamber there are decreases in oral and manual exploration of the environment with increases in self-directed orality.
Although they improved in play behaviors and showed few long-term
learning deficits, the three month isolates did not become behaviorally normal (Boelkins, 1963).

Total social isolation for the first six months of life produces
sequelae differing not only in degree but also in persistence of
deficits as compared to three month isolates. Upon removal from
isolation into a social environment the abnormal behaviors are maintained at levels often higher than that seen in the isolation chamber.
The repertoire of behaviors in itself is not unusual in that, as in
humans, behavioral abnormalities reflect variations of the norm.

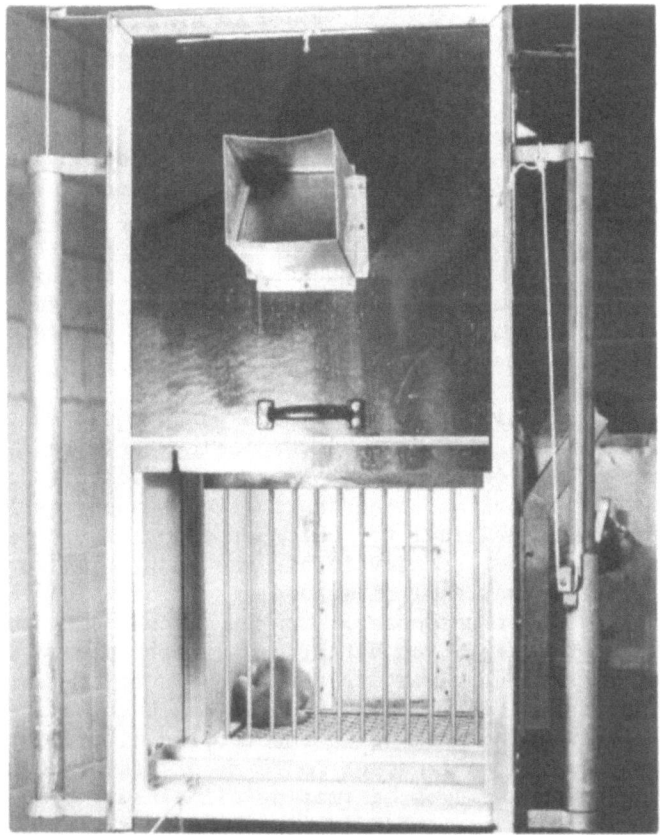

Fig. 9. Total social isolation chambers which deny visual or
tactual contact with the environment with front panel open.

The sucking reflex, if a surrogate is not present, is turned to a
pattern of self-orality which is abnormal only in its excessiveness.
Denial of a clinging reflex leads to self-clasping, and the lack of
kinesthetic stimulation, also denied the isolate, seems to be substituted by stereotypic rocking behaviors. Placement into social
environments with age-mate peers reveals an absence of appropriate
social interactions. Aggressive activity is inappropriate. Attack
on the self, on a dominant adult male or on a neonate -- all inappropriate aggressive activities are rare occurrences in normally
socialized monkeys, is the rule rather than the exception for these
isolates (Mitchell et al., 1966; Arling et al., 1969; Boelkins and
Heiser, 1970). Sexual behavior is usually characterized by infantile
heterosexual behavior or none at all (Mason, 1965) with maternal be-

havior towards offspring (conceived through insemination or forced
breeding) frequently characterized by physical attack and occasional
fatal injury to the newborn.

Varying the timing of placement in isolation tends to result in
less behavioral deviation. With six months of isolation beginning
at six months of age, neither the intensity or range of abnormal behaviors is seen as noted above. Isolation initiated at three months
of age reveals primary abnormalities in the sphere of aggression with
hyperaggressiveness the most noted change (Clark, 1968; Mitchell and
Clark, 1968). Feral born animals are said to be unaffected by social
isolation if this occurs during the second or later years of life.
However, extensive data are not available.

1. _Proposed Mechanisms_. We still lack substantive data which
would clarify the interactions of neurobiologic, social and rearing
conditions. Sackett (1968) discusses learning deficits, postulated
to be caused by early environmental deprivation, which may lead to
failure of experiences critical to basic perceptual-motor development. This is felt to permanently impair the adaptation to change.
Physiologic substrates may fail to mature resulting in an inability
to process information or responses. Sensory mechanisms, which are
known to mature soon after or at birth, may atrophy due to deprivation. Finally, emergence trauma, or the reaction to removal from
an environment deficient in stimuli to one rich in stimuli, could
produce uneven functioning from which recovery is difficult if not
impossible. Defining an environment in terms of its homogeneity of
factors rather than in terms of maximizing all sensory processing
modes is beginning to be explored for its contribution to the concept of "normal" development (Riesen, 1975).

Mirsky (1968) and Miller et al. (1967) have concluded that the
difficulty in social interaction is based on inability to integrate
response or communication rather than a lack in the components of
behavior. Failure of an infant to develop the potential for later
functioning because of atrophy or "missing" of the critical period
is not supported by the work in rehabilitation of the isolation
syndrome which is discussed extensively below.

2. _Neurophysiologic Effects_. Neurophysiologic substrates attendant in the isolation paradigm are less available for evaluation.
In regard to effects of isolation on the endocrine system, several
authors report increased plasma corticosterone levels (Sackett, 1972)
and increased urinary 17-hydroxycorticosteroid levels in monkeys and
humans when environmental stimulation was increased (Mason and Brady,
1965). However, these changes could well reflect the stress the
animal was experiencing. Metabolic changes of hyperphagia and poly-
dipsia without apparent neuroendocrine dysfunction have also been
reported (Miller et al., 1971). Electroencephalographic abnormali-

ties from sensory relay nuclei, limbic system structures and cerebellum are discussed by Heath (1972). Decreased alpha frequency in
humans subjected to isolation was noted by Zubeck et al. (1969,
1971).

Early environmental deprivation and its effects on developing
behavior can also be tested by means of the vertical chamber apparatus described in detail elsewhere (Suomi and Harlow, 1969; Harlow
et al., 1970). The use of the apparatus showed that infants confined for six weeks beginning at six weeks of age exhibit abnormal
social behaviors on removal (Harlow and Suomi, 1970). Rocking,
huddling, self-clasping, and social withdrawal were seen most frequently. Rhesus monkeys at age three years also showed behavioral
deficits after confinement in the vertical chamber. Clinging behaviors and decreased locomotion were the primary effects (McKinney
et al., 1972). As previously noted, the variable of age may have
altered the nature of the effect.

3. _Clinical Observations_. Studies of the mother-infant relationship in primates have focused on the infant's response to
separation as the major evidence for bond formation. Separation
induced depression in humans was first described by Spitz (1946) in
terms of the syndrome of anaclitic depression. Stages of responses
were defined with a "protest" stage, characterized by attempts to
return to mother and increased agitation, a "despair" stage, with
decreased activity and crying, and a "detachment" phase, a final
withdrawal from the environment and rejection of the mother's initial
attempts to reestablish the dyad on her return (Robertson and Bowlby,

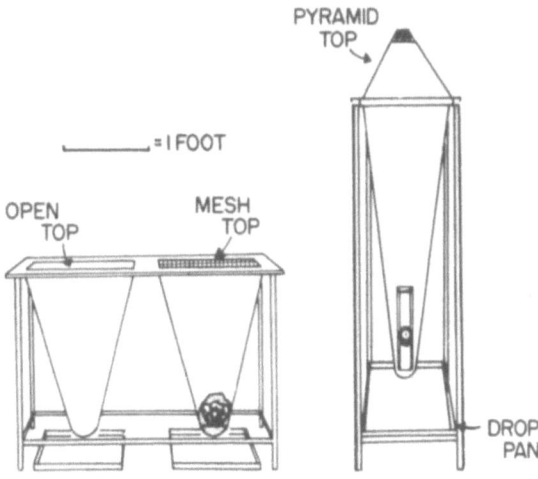

Fig. 10. Vertical chamber apparatus; two versions.

1952). The disruption of attachment bonds, or separation, is thought
to be of major import in the development of depression as well as
other psychopathology in humans. Many investigations of separation
in various species have stemmed from these clinical observations
(Hinde and Spencer-Booth, 1971; Hofer, 1975; Kaufman and Rosenblum,
1967a; McKinney et al., 1973; Seay et al., 1962; Seitz, 1959; Senay,
1966).

Separation from mother is not the only factor which can precipitate a depressive-like syndrome in many species. Some evidence
to support this contention can be illustrated in the Agapornis parrot ("love bird"). If an individual member of this species is unable
to have normal social interaction in the presence of an observable
bond formation, it will die. This most frequently occurs if three
African parrots are placed in a cage, and two form a pair; the non-
paired bird loses its plumage and within six months is dead. Of
interest is that one love bird left alone and not in the presence of
an observable pair will survive well (Dilger, 1960).

Before discussing the paradigms of separation studies and their
effects on the behavior of the infant, a clear understanding of the
definitions of "object loss" and "separation" is required. These
terms are so frequently overused in their application to a range of
responses and resultant behavioral characteristics that we lose sight
of their basic meaning. The implication that the event of loss and
separation leads to depression so frequently denies the multifactoral
dimension of the events involved (McKinney, 1975; McKinney et al.,
1971; Akiskal and McKinney, 1973; Akiskal and McKinney, 1975).
Systematic integration of genetic, environmental and neurobiological
components is a primary focus of the experimental psychopathology
research approach in the Wisconsin Primate Laboratory (Morrison and
McKinney, 1976). Variables involved in the response of an organism
are also being explored from the viewpoint of the influence of the
organism on its environment in the production of the abnormal behaviors (Lewis and Rosenblum, 1974; Hofer, 1975; see Beckwith, this
volume). It has been in the question of underlying mechanisms of
the response to separation that animal models have been especially
useful (McKinney, 1974a,b).

4. _Primate Separation._ Studies of mother-infant separation in
monkeys have reported Bowlby's protest and despair stages for rhesus
(Spencer-Booth and Hinde, 1967) and pigtail monkeys (Rosenblum and
Kaufman, 1968) while marked intraspecies differences have been noted
in both severity and duration of symptoms (Seay and Harlow, 1965).
Generally, separation from mother after living together for the
first three to six months of life leads to a biphasic response of
the infant. Within 36 hours following separation, the infant's behavior is characterized by increased activity and vocalizations and
attempts to return to mother, the "protest stage." Following this

is the "despair" stage of inactivity, huddling and withdrawal. In some animals, a gradual spontaneous recovery occurs over a six-week period. Not only have species differences been noted in response to separation but a great deal of variability has been observed in the infant's behavior (Lewis and McKinney, 1975). The comparisons among five studies of mother-infant separation with 20 rhesus monkeys did not provide support for a singular concept of the protest-despair response. Changes in the infant's behavior were neither stable nor predictable enough to use this as an induction method for the production of animal models for the purpose of neurobiological or rehabilitative studies.

Exploratory work on the effect of separating monkeys who had been raised from birth without mothers but with peers led to the conclusion that peer separation was a possible model for depression (Bowden and McKinney, 1972). Repetitive peer separations where animals are separated for two-week periods (McKinney et al., 1972b; Suomi et al., 1970) provide methodologic advantages in the study of depression. It also provides a greater potential for crossover designs and repeated treatments. Both of these factors are of utmost importance for the study of antianxiety and antidepressant medications.

Age and developmental stages have been noted to be factors requiring consideration in determining the reaction of peers to separation. Infants tend to exhibit the biphasic response described above while adolescent age monkeys show no evidence of the despair stage. Early experience, most notably that of previous separation, is another variable in the production of depression in peer separation (McKinney et al., 1973a; Young et al., 1973). In peer separation subjects confined in a vertical chamber apparatus showed high levels of self-directed activities and lower levels of socially-directed activities than counterparts separated in wire cages (Suomi, 1973). Total and partial isolates may differ on the basis of sex in their responses to isolation in terms of exploratory and social behaviors with males being more severely affected (Sackett et al., 1975).

Adult monkeys reared in the nuclear family develop and maintain social attachments, described by Ruppenthal et al. (1974). In a study designed to evaluate the response to separation from the nuclear family in semi-adult monkeys, Suomi et al (in press) noted that group housed subjects revealed little reaction to removal from the family units but those housed individually showed reactions similar to those of infants with anaclitic depression.

Seligman et al. (1968) has introduced the term "learned help-lessness." The concept is concerned with subjects learning that the electric shock they are experiencing is uncontrollable and ceasing

.

to respond to escape it. This model lends itself to social and
biological rehabilitation studies and provides study for one aspect
of human depression. Another social technique is that of alteration
of dominance patterns described by Price (1967).

Biologic effects of maternal and peer separation studies are
currently underway. Animals in the protest stage show increases in
serotonin in the hypothalamus and elevation of the catecholamine-
synthesizing enzymes in the adrenal gland but no noted changes in
norepinephrine, dopamine or serotonin levels (Breese et al., 1973).
The focus of current research is on turnover rates of biogenic amines
and effects on the neuroendocrine system following these social and
environmental manipulations.

B.   Induction: The Biologic Environment

Syndromes of psychopathology induced through biochemical techniques have facilitated our exploration and understanding of the
relationships between abnormal behaviors and neurotransmitter
functioning. This technique is relatively new and involves alteration and selective depletion of neurotransmitters while observing
resultant alteration in behavior. Subsequent work deals with the
consequent biological effects of social environment manipulations
previously discussed in this chapter. Another aspect is that of
biologic rehabilitation after various induction methods. Neuro-
surgical induction approaches are discussed by Kling (1968).

The most prevalent animal model for depression prior to the
advent of the social induction methods was that produced by reserpine in the rat. Reserpine was tested in a more complex social
system in rhesus monkeys and the effects included decreased activity
and locomotion as well as increased social withdrawal and huddling
as long as the drug was being administered. No cumulative effect or
tolerance was noted (McKinney et al., 1971).

The role of dopamine, norepinephrine, and serotonin in the regulation of primate social behaviors is being explored through the
utilization of agents which block the synthesis of these compounds.
Parachlorophenylalanine, an inhibitor of serotonin synthesis (Koe
and Weissman, 1966), produces no major behavioral changes when given
to stumptail or rhesus monkeys (Redmond et al., 1971; McKinney et
al., in preparation). Alpha-methyl-para-tyrosine, a blocker of norepinephrine synthesis through inhibition of tyrosine hydroxylase
(Spector et al., 1965), produces a syndrome similar to that of the
reserpinized animal in the rhesus monkey, again dependent on time
and dose (Redmond et al., 1971; McKinney et al., in preparation).

In 1970, 6-hydroxydopamine, when given centrally, was reported
to destroy the central noradrenergic neurons without affecting either

the peripheral noradrenergic system or the serotonergic system (Breese and Taylor, 1970; Breese et al., 1972). The ability to selectively deplete the brain noradrenergic system (Schildkraut, 1970), has permitted the beginning study of the effects of this depletion on both social behaviors and urinary metabolites after intraventricular 6-hydroxydopamine (Kraemer et al., 1975). This study revealed 50-60% depletions of norepinephrine with normal levels of urinary metabolites, including 3-methoxy-4-hydroxy-phenylglycol which has been postulated to be a peripheral indicator of brain norepinephrine metabolism (Schanberg et al., 1968). These relationships are being studied and will be reported in future publications.

IV. THE ENVIRONMENT OF REHABILITATION

These studies fulfill McKinney and Bunney's criteria that a treatment modality effective in the reversal of human psychopathology should also be effective in reversal of the behavioral changes seen in animals. Social rehabilitative methods can be clearly applied to socially-induced behavioral states and potentially to biologically-induced states of altered behavior. Biological rehabilitation may, of course, also be used with either induction technique.

Throughout much of this volume, "therapeutic environment" is considered equivalent to enrichment. This is postulated throughout the literature, both popular and professional, as an almost magical cure-all. However, a less connotative word, or an awareness that enrichment is not always therapeutic, must be kept in mind. The hyperactive child or the person suffering an acute manic episode is not aided by additional sensory or social input (see also Greenough, this volume). With regard to learning, isolate monkeys differ from those monkeys raised in enriched environments only in ability on the oddity learning set (Gluck et al., 1973). The only noted comparison was that isolates required a more prolonged period of adaptation to the learning set procedure (Harlow et al., 1969). Responses to social versus nonsocial stimuli were described by Baldwin and Suomi (1974). Isolate monkeys respond less to social stimuli; this is thought to be due to a learning deficit from a lack of interaction with social stimuli (Sackett, 1966; Sackett et al., 1965).

Emergence from an enclosed isolation chamber is associated with various phenomena. Fuller (1967) felt that abnormalities in dogs were related more to stress in the complex new environment rather than the stress of isolation. However, nonsocial adaptation of subjects during the isolation period to test situations which would be used following removal from isolation had little effect (Mitchell and Clark, 1968). Some authors have reported decreased post-isolation disturbance and depression following pre-exposure to the new environ-

ment (Fuller and Clark, 1966) but this has not prevented the appearance of aberrant post-isolation social behaviors (Mitchell, 1970).

A. Rehabilitation: The Social Environment

   Until recently, reversal of the isolation syndromes had met with
little success whether the attempt involved aversive conditioning
(Sackett, 1968a) or adaptation through pairing isolates (Suomi,
1973a). The feasibility of rehabilitating isolates through social
means became apparent following observation of changing maternal behavior of "motherless mother" monkeys. These are animals who have
been raised in social isolation, exhibit inappropriate and infrequent
adult sexual behavior, and require unusual methods for impregnation
(Allen et al., 1967). Maternal behavior with the first infant was
characterized by physical brutality or indifference with the infants
exhibiting greater frequencies of self-mouthing and cooing vocalizations than infants of normal mothers (Seay et al., 1964). The
motherless mothers were subsequently reported to treat their second
infant with less brutality and with greater adequacy than their first
(Harlow et al., 1966). This improvement had been postulated to be
related to the greater social responsiveness of isolate-reared mothers
to immature strangers (Mitchell and Clark, 1968) and to the observation that infants who survived the behavior of their mothers had made
efforts to maintain maternal body contact (Harlow et al., 1966).

   The first successful social rehabilitations of six-month isolation-reared animals were reported by Harlow and Suomi (1971; Suomi
and Harlow, 1972; Suomi et al., 1972). "Monkey psychiatrists,"
three-month-old surrogate and peer-reared females, all exhibiting
age-appropriate social development, were the "therapists." They were
three months younger than the isolate subjects, and, at age three
months, exhibited no aggressive responses. Their social interactions
were characterized by clinging behaviors and the initial manifestations of simple play without any abnormal behaviors. The process of
therapy, as shown in Figure 11, involved the isolates responding initially by huddling in a corner and the therapists first responding
by approaching and clinging to the isolate. After three weeks, the
isolates reciprocated the clinging and the therapists were attempting
to initiate play with the isolates. By nine weeks of therapy the
isolates began to initiate play activity with corresponding decreases
in self-disturbance data. By one year of age the isolates and therapists were virtually indistinguishable from one another. Twelve
month isolates treated in this manner also showed similar results
(Novak and Harlow, 1975). The results of these studies and the
generalization of behavior to other social situations were consistent with the position that the isolation syndrome involved deficits
in learning and inconsistent with critical period or emergence trauma
explanations of isolation effects.

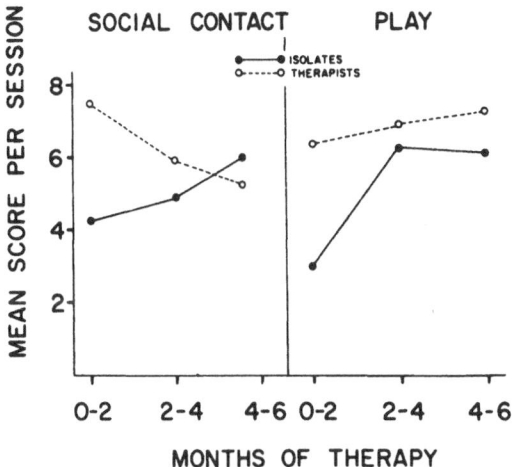

Fig. 11. Reflection of the therapeutic process in regard to social contact and play behaviors between the monkey "therapists" and isolate "patients."

In further work on social rehabilitation it has been reported that in monkeys who have had the opportunity to develop social affection prior to separation or isolation, later isolation produces less severe deficits (Harlow and Novak, 1973). Continuing work in this area is providing information as to the stability of the social rehabilitation procedures (Cummins, 1973).

B. Rehabilitation: The Biological Environment

The social therapies, as one method of rehabilitation, proved successful but also again proved that rehabilitation is not a simple task. Human therapists, in their attempts to correct aberrant early development, are familiar with the inherent difficulties of this task. The use of social therapies in humans also often requires the adjunctive use of biologic methods and, in some cases, these are of primary importance.

The first successful pharmacological treatment of social isolated rhesus monkeys was reported by McKinney et al. (1973c). Self-disturbance behaviors which had been predominant in the subjects for at least a half year were improved dramatically by the administration of chlorpromazine. Sociability scores were not significantly increased and this was probably a reflection of the less complex and less advanced patterns of interaction characteristic of isolates lacking experience with normal monkeys. Baysinger (1975) noted that

chlorpromazine decreased disturbance behavior of total isolate subjects. This was not due to suppression of motor activity and it was
noted that no facilitory effect on pituitary-adrenal function was
caused by the drug, a finding at variance with reports in the rat
(DeWeid, 1967; Maickel et al., 1974).

Diazepam, an antianxiety agent, was used following the premise
that a decrease in anxiety would effect rehabilitative changes
(Noble et al., 1975). In comparison to chlorpromazine, diazepam
more consistently led to increases in social and aggressive behaviors
and increases in environmental exploration. The effectiveness of
this drug in therapeutic change, and the fact that chlorpromazine
is not the only agent for rehabilitation of isolates, argues against
a premature acceptance of the social isolation syndrome as a model
for human psychosis. Again we caution against the premature attachment of clinical labels to abnormal behaviors in animals, before clear
and comprehensive mechanism and rehabilitation studies are completed.

Electrically-induced convulsions (EIC) remain a valuable therapeutic tool in the treatment of serious depression. Convulsive
treatment of rhesus isolates caused a general activation effect in
isolate monkeys together with decreased self-disturbance behaviors.
A control group, who received sham convulsive treatment (administration of neuromuscular blocking agents and anesthetic without the
actual convulsion) had a general lessening of activity (Lewis and
McKinney, 1975).

In a series of experiments, the effects of the antidepressant
imipramine were studied on the peer separation syndrome. Imipramine
alleviated the symptoms of the separation syndrome, thus again supporting the possibility that a usable model of depression can be
created.

V. DYSFUNCTIONAL ENVIRONMENT: A SUMMARY STATEMENT

The use of primate animal models, as seen from this chapter, has
contributed to the understanding of the production and maintenance
abnormal behavior. Emphasis on the interaction of biologic and behavioral environments in both the induction and rehabilitation of
abnormal behaviors in primates completed this chapter. These are
summarized in Figures 12 and 13. It is important to remember that
the interactions in both induction and rehabilitation involve all
aspects of the environment.

The biologic induction methods focus primarily on observation
of behavior in the animal following experimental alterations of peripheral and/or brain amine levels. Alpha-methyl-para-tyrosine, a
blocker of norepinephrine synthesis, has produced in the rhesus
monkey behaviors such as decreased locomotion, decreased active

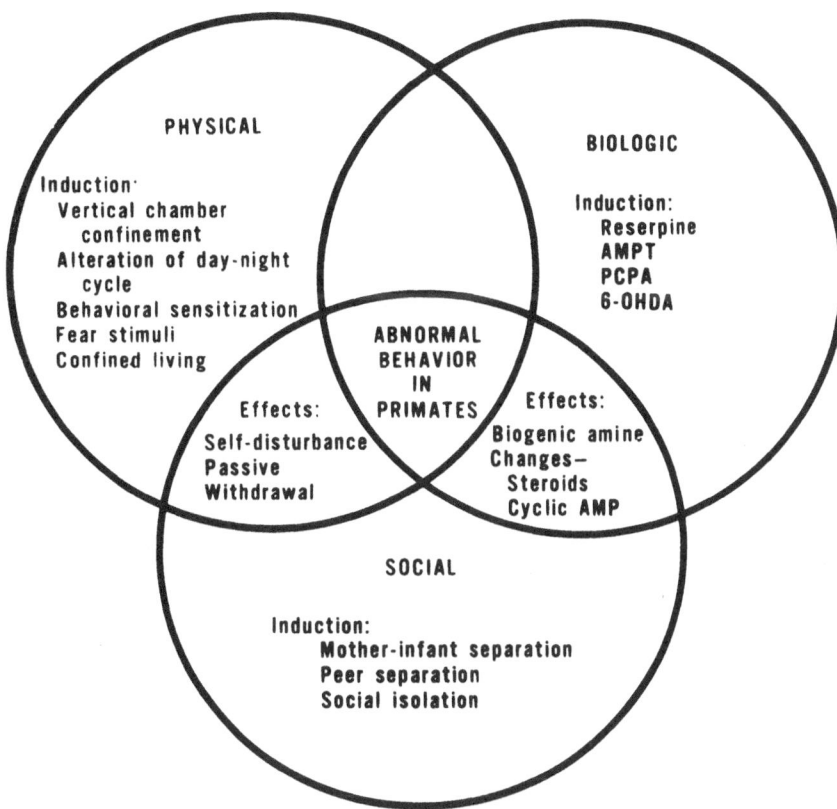

Fig. 12.   Interactive environments in the induction of psychopathology in primates and their major effects on behaviors.

social behaviors, increased passive behaviors and huddling. A serotonin synthesis inhibitor, parachlorophenylalanine, has not been
found to produce major behavioral changes. Reserpine, a depletor of
both catecholamines and indoleamines in the periphery and brain, also
produces behaviors similar to those exhibited by separated animals
in the despair stage of separation. Specific techniques designed
to effect changes in the brain but not in the periphery include the
use of intraventricular application of drugs. 6-Hydroxydopamine,
thought to specifically destroy noradrenergic nerve terminals in the
brain, is currently being studied to assist in clarifying the role
of central and peripheral amines in the regulation of urinary metabolite excretion and social behavior.

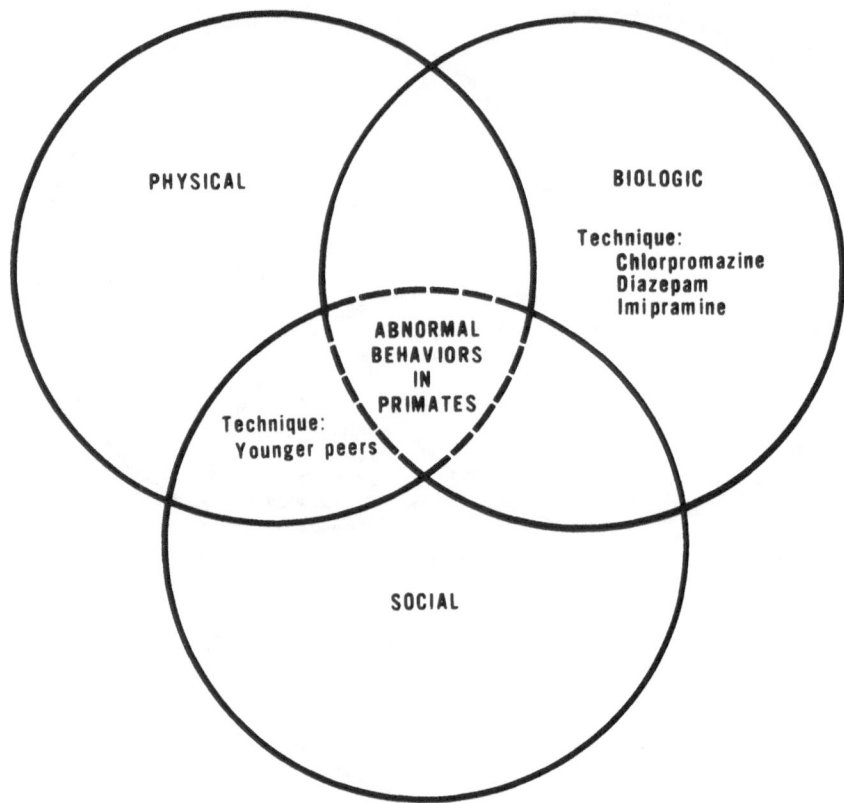

Fig. 13.   Interactive environments in rehabilitation of psychopathology in primates and the primary techniques of inducing change.

       Social techniques of induction involve alterations in the early
social environment and its subsequent effect on the development of
social competency. The various rearing conditions in use in the
Wisconsin Primate Laboratory involve surrogates only, peers only,
mother-peer, mother only and nuclear family. Generally, the more
complex the social rearing environment, the more complex the social
behaviors exhibited by the animals. Disruption of affectional bonds,
or separation, has been studied in primates. Separation from peers
is a possible animal model for depression. Repetitive separation of
peers provides potential for crossover designs, repeated treatments
and the evaluation of antidepressant and antianxiety medications.
Partial social isolation, preventing the monkey from physical contact
with others but allowing visual and auditory contact, produces a

syndrome of stereotyped behavior, excessive self-orality and self-clasping behaviors and decreased social initiations. Total social isolation, denying the infant visual or tactual contact with others but providing adequate nutrients, results in severe behavioral abnormalities. These differ not only in degree from the partial social isolates but also in the persistence of deficits. Varying periods of total isolation for up to six months increases the duration and degree of abnormality. Developmental stages, age, sex, and early experience with prior separations are important variables to be considered in the production of psychopathology. Infants show both protest and despair responses while adolescent age monkeys show no despair stage. Separations of adults from the nuclear family with subsequent individual housing lead to reactions similar to those of infants raised in isolation. Male subjects show greater personal behavior disturbances than females and are less responsive to the post-isolation environment, either inanimate or social. Previous separations seem to predispose the subject to a more severe depressive reaction.

Biologic alterations accompanying separation are being studied. Turnover rates of biogenic amines and concentration of amines in various brain regions are a focal point of these investigations.

Following induction of a syndrome and fulfilling the criteria of McKinney and Bunney relevant to animal models and the syndrome produced, the task turns to reversal of these behavioral changes. The techniques used in rehabilitation of the abnormal behavior of animals are similar to those used in reversal of depressive symptomatology in humans. Social or biological rehabilitative methods are paired with either biological or social induction techniques. "Monkey psychiatrists," three months of age, are paired with six month social isolate animals. At one year of age the isolates are virtually indistinguishable from their "therapists." Chlorpromazine, diazepam and electrically-induced convulsions are at least partially successful biologic reversal techniques, while imipramine has been of value in alleviation of the symptoms of peer separation.

The value of animal models to clarify the interactions between biologic and social systems should not be underestimated. Most frequently, this has occurred when writers discard the basic premise that commonality of observable behavior does not imply commonality of mechanisms or meanings of those behaviors. The equation of primate and man, albeit tempting, is a fallacy not representative of the scientific work in progress in the field of animal models of human psychopathology. Of equal import is the zeal with which other authors deny any relevance of animal models to the conditions in humans. It is obvious that neither of these positions permit the incorporation of these theories into an improved understanding of human behavior and its development. The acceptance of these phenomena as basic to the understanding of behavior can only be done with careful and qualified discussion. Ultimately, the concern of all scientists is their subjects' behavior, with all its physical, social and biologic concomitants. The interactional model posed throughout this chapter facilitates our understanding of behavioral events without imposing a simplistic solution or explanation for its concepts. The relevance of animal models is best summed up in its readily apparent contribution to the study of interactions and to its future importance in delineation of the processes of adaptation and maladaptation seen in man.

REFERENCES

Akiskal, H. S., and McKinney, W. T. 1973. Depressive Disorders: Toward A Unified Hypothesis. Science 182:20-29.

Akiskal, H. S., and McKinney, W. T. 1975. Overview of Recent Research in Depression. Arch. Gen. Psychiat. 32:285-305.

Alexander, B. K. 1966. The Effects of Early Peer-Deprivation on Juvenile Behavior of Rhesus Monkeys. Unpublished doctoral dissertation, University of Wisconsin.

Allen, J. R., Schiltz, K. A., Ripp, C., Eisele, S. C., and Johnson, L. C. 1967. Laboratory Procedures. Regional Primate Research Center and Laboratory, Madison: University of Wisconsin.

Arling, G. L., Ruppenthal, G. C., and Mitchell, G. D. 1969. Aggressive Behavior of the Eight Year Old Nulliparous Isolate Female Monkey. Anim. Behav. 17:109-113.

Baldwin, D. V., and Suomi, S. J. 1974. Reactions of Infant Monkeys to Social and Non-Social Stimuli. Folia Primatol. 22:307-314.

Baysinger, C. M. 1975. Effects of Chlorpromazine on Rhesus Monkeys Reared in Social Isolation. Unpublished master's thesis. University of Wisconsin, Madison, Wisconsin.

Berkson, G., Mason, W. A., and Saxon, S. V. 1963. Situation and Stimulus Effects on Stereotyped Behaviors of Chimpanzees. J. Comp. Physiol. Psychol. 56:786-792.

Birch, J. 1961. The Pertinence of Animal Investigations for Science of Human Behavior. Amer. J. Orthopsychiat. 31:267.

Blomquist, A. J., and Harlow, H. F. 1961. The Infant Rhesus Monkey Program at the University of Wisconsin Regional Primate Research Center and Laboratory. (Association for Laboratory Animal

Science.) Proc. Anim. Care Panel II, No. 2, 57-64.

Boelkins, R. C. 1963. The Development of Social Behavior in the
    Infant Rhesus Monkey Following a Period of Social Isolation.
    Unpublished master's thesis, University of Wisconsin.

Boelkins, R. C., and Heiser, J. F. 1970. Biological Bases of Ag-
    gression, pp. 15-52. In D. N. Daniels, M. F. Gilula, and
    F. M. Ochberg (eds.). Violence and the Struggle for Existence.
    Little Brown, New York.

Bowden, D. M., and McKinney, W. T. 1972. Behavioral Effects of
    Peer Separation, Isolation and Reunion on Adolescent Male
    Rhesus Monkeys. Develop. Psychobiol. 5:353-362.

Bowlby, J. 1958. The Nature of the Child's Tie to His Mother.
    Intern. J. Psychoanal. 39:350-373.

Bowlby, J. 1973. Attachment and Loss, Vol. 2. Separation: Anxiety
    and Anger, p. 85. Basic Books, New York.

Breese, G., and Taylor, T. D. 1970. Effect of 6-Hydroxydopamine on
    Brain Norepinephrine and Dopamine: Evidence for Selective De-
    generation of Catecholamine Neurons. J. Pharm. Exp. Ther. 174:
    413-420.

Breese, G. A., Smith, R. D., Meuller, R. A., Howard, J. L., Prange,
    A. J., Lipton, M. A., Young, L. D., McKinney, W. T., and Lewis,
    J. L. 1973. Induction of Adrenal Catecholamine Synthesizing
    Enzymes Following Mother-Infant Separation. Nature New Biol.
    246:94-96.

Breese, G., Prange, A., McKinney, W., Lipton, M., Bowman, R., Howard,
    J., and Bushnel, P. 1972. Behavioral and Biochemical Effects
    of 6-Hydroxydopamine in Rhesus Monkeys. Symposium on Catechol-
    amine Metabolism and Affective Disorders. American Psychiatric
    Association, Dallas, Texas.

Broadhurst, P. L. 1953. Abnormal Animal Behavior, pp. 153-222.
    In J. Wortis (ed.). Basic Problems in Psychiatry. Grune and
    Stratton, Inc., New York.

Carpenter, C. A. 1942. Societies of Monkeys and Apes. Biol.
    Sympos. 8:177-204.

Clark, D. L. 1968. Immediate and Delayed Effects of Early, Inter-
    mediate, and Late Social Isolation in the Rhesus Monkey.
    Doctoral dissertation, University of Wisconsin.

Cross, H. A., and Harlow, H. F. 1965. Prolonged and Progressive Effects of Partial Isolation on the Behavior of Macaque Monkeys. J. Exp. Res. Per. 1:39-49.

Cummins, M. S. 1973. Behavioral Stability of Rhesus Monkeys Following Differential Rearing. Unpublished master's thesis. University of Wisconsin, Madison, Wisconsin.

DeWeid, D. 1967. Chlorpromazine and Endocrine Function. Pharm. Rev. 19:2.

Dilger, W. C. 1960. The Comparative Ethology of the African Parrot Genus Agapornis. Z. Tierpsychol. 17:649-685.

Dollard, J., and Miller, N. E. 1950. Personality and Psychotherapy, p. 133. McGraw-Hill, New York.

Fabricius, E. 1962. Some Aspects of Imprinting in Birds. Sym. Zool. Soc. Lond. 8:139-148.

Foley, J. P., Jr. 1934. First Year Development of a Rhesus Monkey (M. mulatta) Reared in Isolation. J. Genet. Psychol. 45:39-105.

Foley, J. P., Jr. 1935. Second Year Development of a Rhesus Monkey Reared in Isolation. J. Genet. Psychol. 47:39-105.

Forgays, D. G., and Forgays, J. W. 1952. The Nature of the Effect of Free-Environmental Experience on the Rat. J. Comp. Physiol. Psychol. 45:322-328.

Fuller, J. L. 1967. Experimental Deprivation and Later Behavior. Science 158:1645-1652.

Fuller, J. L., and Clark, L. D. 1966. Genetic and Treatment Factors Modifying the Postisolation Syndrome in Dogs. J. Comp. Physiol. Psychol. 61:251-257.

Goldfarb, W. 1955. Emotional and Intellectual Consequences of Deprivation in Infancy: A Re-evaluation, pp. 105. In P. H. Hoch and J. Zubin (eds.). Psychopathology of Childhood. Grune and Stratton, Inc., New York.

Gluck, J. P., Harlow, H. F., and Schiltz, K. A. 1973. Differential Effects of Early Enrichment and Deprivation on Learning in the Rhesus Monkey (Macaca mulatta). J. Comp. Physiol. Psychol. 84: 598-604.

Harlow, H. F. 1958. The Nature of Love. Amer. Psychologist 13: 673-685.

Harlow, H. F., and Harlow, M. K. 1971. Psychopathology in Monkeys, pp. 203-229. In H. D. Kimmel (ed.). Experimental Psychopathology: Recent Research and Theory. Academic Press, Inc., New York.

Harlow, H. F., and Novak, M. A. 1973. Psychopathological Perspectives. Perspect. Biol. Med. 16:461-478.

Harlow, H. F., and Suomi, S. J. 1970a. Nature of Love - Simplified. Amer. Psychologist 25:161-168.

Harlow, H. F., and Suomi, S. J. 1970b. Induced Psychopathology in Monkeys. Engineer Sci. 33:8-14.

Harlow, H. F., and Suomi, S. J. 1971. Social Recovery by Isolation Reared Monkeys. Proc. Nat. Acad. Sci. 68:1534-1538.

Harlow, H. F., and Zimmerman, R. R. 1959. Affectional Responses in the Infant Monkey. Science 130:421-432.

Harlow, H. F., Rowland, G. L., and Griffin, G. A. 1964. The Effect of Total Social Deprivation on the Development of Monkey Behavior. Psy. Res. Rep. 19:116-135.

Harlow, H. F., Harlow, M. K., Dodsworth, R. O., and Arling, G. I. 1966. Maternal Behavior of Rhesus Monkeys Deprived of Mothering and Peer Associations in Infancy. Proc. Amer. Phil. Soc. 110:58-66.

Harlow, H. F., Schiltz, K. A., and Harlow, M. K. 1969. Effects of Social Isolation on the Learning Performance of Rhesus Monkeys, p. 25. In C. R. Carpenter (ed.). Proc. 2nd Int. Con. Primat., Vol. 1. Karger, New York.

Harlow, H. F., Suomi, S. J., and McKinney, W. T. 1970. Experimental Depression in Monkeys. Mainly Monkeys 1:6-12.

Harlow, M. K. 1971. Nuclear Family Apparatus. Behav. Res. Meth. Instru. 3:301-304.

Heath, R. G. 1972. Electroencephalographic Studies in Isolation-Reared Monkeys With Behavioral Impairment. Dis. Nerv. Syst. 33:157-163.

Hebb, D. O. 1947. Spontaneous Neurosis in Chimpanzees. Psychosom. Med. 9:3-16.

Hebb, D. O. 1949. Organization of Behavior. Wiley, New York.

Hebb, D. O., and Thompson, W. R.   1954.   The Social Significance of
    Animal Studies, pp. 532–561.   In G. Lindzey (ed.).   Handbook
    of Social Psychology, Vol. 1, Theory and Method.   Addison-
    Wesley, Cambridge.

Hess, E. H.   1959.   Imprinting.   Science 130:133–141.

Hinde, R. A.   1974.   Biological Basis of Human Social Behavior.
    McGraw-Hill, New York.

Hinde, R. A., and Spencer-Booth, Y.   1971.   Effects of Brief Sepa-
    ration From Mother on Rhesus Monkeys.   Science 173:111–118.

Hinde, R. A., Thorpe, W. H., and Vince, M. A.   1956.   The Following
    Response of Young Coots and Moorhens.   Behavior 9:214–242.

Hofer, M. A.   1972.   Physiological and Behavioral Processes in Early
    Maternal Separation.   In CIBA Symposium, No. 8, Physiology,
    Emotion and Psychosomatic Illness.   Elsevier, Amsterdam.

Hofer, M. A.   1975.   Studies on How Early Maternal Separation Pro-
    duces Behavioral Changes in Young Rats.   Psychosom. Med. 3:
    245–264.

Hollos, M., and Cowan, P. A.   1973.   Social Isolation and Cognitive
    Development: Logical Operations and Role-Taking Abilities in
    Three Norwegian Social Settings.   Child Dev. 44:630–641.

Jaynes, J.   1958.   Imprinting: The Interaction of Learned and Innate
    Behavior: IV. Generalization and Emergent Discrimination.
    J. Comp. Physiol. Psychol. 51:238–242.

Jennings, K.   1975.   People Versus Object Orientation, Social Be-
    havior and Intellectual Abilities in Preschool Children.   Dev.
    Psychol. 11:511–519.

Kaufman, I. C., and Rosenblum, L. A.   1967.   The Reaction to Sepa-
    ration in Infant Monkeys: Anaclitic Depression and Conserva-
    tion-Withdrawal.   Psychosom. Med. 29:648–675.

Kling, A.   1968.   Amygdalectomy in Free Ranging Vervet.   Read be-
    fore the Psychiatric Research Society, New Haven, Connecticut.

Koe, B. K., and Weissman, A.   p-Chlorophenylalanine: A Specific
    Depleter of Brain Serotonin.   J. Pharm. Exp. Ther. 154:499–516.

Konrad, K. W., and Bagshaw, M.   1970.   Effect of Novel Stimuli on
    Cats Reared in a Restricted Environment.   J. Comp. Physiol.
    Psychol. 70:157–164.

Kraemer, G., McKinney, W. T., Breese, G., and Howard, J. 1975. Effects of 6-Hydroxydopamine in the Rhesus Monkey. Paper presented at American Psychiatric Association Annual Meeting, Anaheim, California.

Kubie, L. A. 1939. The Experimental Induction of Neurotic Reactions in Man. Yale J. Biol. Med. 11:541-545.

Levy, D. M. 1952. Animal Psychology in Its Relation to Psychiatry. In F. Alexander (ed.). Dynamic Psychiatry. University of Chicago Press, Chicago.

Lewis, J. L., and McKinney, W. T. 1975. Mother-Infant Separation in Rhesus Monkeys: A Reconsideration. Arch. Gen. Psychiat. In press.

Lewis, J. L., and McKinney, W. T. 1975. The Effect of Electrically Induced Convulsions on the Behavior of Normal and Abnormal Rhesus Monkeys. In preparation.

Lewis, M., and Rosenblum, L. A. 1974. The Effect of the Infant on Its Caregiver. The Origins of Behavior, Vol. 1. John Wiley and Sons, New York.

Lorenz, K. 1935. Der Kumpan in der Umwelt des Vogels. J. f. Ornith. 83:137-213.

Lorenz, K. 1971. Studies in Animal and Human Behavior, Vol. 2. Harvard University Press, Cambridge, Massachusetts.

McCulloch, T. L., and Haslerud, G. M. 1939. Affective Responses of an Infant Chimpanzee Reared in Isolation from Its Kind. J. Comp. Psychol. 28:437-445.

McKinney, W. T. 1974a. Animal Model of Depression: Current Status of the Field. In J. Westermeyer (ed.). Anthropology and Mental Health. Mouton Publishers, The Hague.

McKinney, W. T. 1974b. Animal Models in Psychiatry. Perspec. Biol. Med. 17:529-541.

McKinney, W. T. 1974c. Primate Social Isolation. Psychiatric Implications. Arch. Gen. Psychiat. 31:422-426.

McKinney, W. T. 1975. Psychoanalysis Revisited in Terms of Experimental Primatology. In E. T. Adelson (ed.). Sexuality and Psychoanalysis. Brunner Mazel, New York.

McKinney, W. T., and Bunney, W. E. 1969. Animal Model of Depres-

sion: Review of Evidence Implications for Research. Arch.
Gen. Psychiat. 21:240-248.

McKinney, W. T., Eising, R. G., Moran, E. C., Suomi, S. J., and
Harlow, H. F. 1971. Effects of Reserpine on the Social Behavior of Rhesus Monkeys. Dis. Nerv. Syst. 32:735-741.

McKinney, W. T., Suomi, S. J., and Harlow, H. F. 1971. Depression
in Primates. Am. J. Psychiat. 127:1313-1320.

McKinney, W. T., Suomi, S. J., and Harlow, H. F. 1972a. Vertical
Chamber Confinement of Juvenile Age Rhesus Monkeys. Arch.
Gen. Psychiat. 26:223-228.

McKinney, W. T., Suomi, S. J., and Harlow, H. F. 1972b. Repetitive
Peer Separations of Juvenile Age Rhesus Monkeys. Arch. Gen.
Psychiat. 27:200-202.

McKinney, W. T., Kliese, K. A., Suomi, S. J., and Moran, E. C. 1973a.
Can Psychopathology Be Reinduced in Rhesus Monkeys? An Experi-
mental Investigation of Behavioral Sensitization. Arch. Gen.
Psychiat. 29:630-634.

McKinney, W. T., Suomi, S. J., and Harlow, H. F. 1973b. New Models
of Separation and Depression in Rhesus Monkeys, pp. 53-66. In
J. P. Scott and E. C. Senay (eds.). Separation and Depression.
Washington, AAAS Publication Number 94.

McKinney, W. T., Young, L. D., Suomi, S. J., and Davis, J. M. 1973c.
Chlorpromazine Treatment of Disturbed Monkeys. Arch. Gen.
Psychiat. 29:490-494.

McKinney, W. T., Suomi, S. J., Mersky, I. A., and Miller, R. Parachlorophenylalanine and Rhesus Monkeys. In preparation.

Maickel, R., Braumstein, M. C., McGlynn, M., Snodgrass, W. R., and
Webb, R. W. 1974. Behavioral, Biochemical and Pharmacological
Effects of Chronic Dosage of Phenothiazine Tranquilizers in
Rats. Adv. Biochem. Psychopharm. 9:593-602.

Mason, J. W., and Brady, J. V. 1965. The Sensitivity of Psychoendo-
crine Systems to Social and Physical Environment, pp. 4-23.
In P. H. Liederman and D. Schapiro (eds.). Psychobiological
Approaches to Social Behavior. Tavistock, London.

Mason, W. A. 1963. The effects of Environmental Restriction on the
Social Development of Rhesus Monkeys, pp. 161-173. In C. H.
Southwick (ed.). Primate Social Behavior. Van Nostrand, New
Jersey.

Mason, W. A. 1965. The Social Behavior of Monkeys and Apes, pp. 514-543. In I. Devore (ed.). Primate Behavior. Holt, New York.

Mason, W. A. 1968a. Early Social Deprivation in the Nonhuman Primates. Implications for Human Behavior, pp. 70-100. In D. C. Glass (ed.). Environmental Influences. Rockefeller University and Russell Sage Foundation, New York.

Mason, W. A. 1968b. Scope and Potential of Primate Research, pp. 198-213. In J. H. Masserman (ed.). Science and Psychoanalysis, Vol. XII, Animal and Human. Grune and Stratton, New York.

Meldrum, B. S., Chir, B., Horton, R. W., and Toseland, P. A. 1975. A Primate Model for Testing Anticonvulsant Drugs. Arch. Neurol. 32:289-294.

Miller, R. E., Caul, W. F., and Mersky, I. A. 1967. Communication of Affect Between Feral and Socially Isolated Monkeys. J. Pers. Soc. Psychol. 7:231-239.

Miller, R. E., Caul, W. F., and Mersky, I. A. 1971. Patterns of Eating and Drinking in Socially Isolated Rhesus Monkeys. Physiol. Behav. 7:127-134.

Mirsky, I. A. 1968. Communication of Affects in Monkeys, pp. 129-137. In D. C. Glass (ed.). Environmental Influences. Rockefeller University Press and Russell Sage Foundation, New York.

Mitchell, G. D. 1970. Abnormal Behavior in Primates, pp. 196-249. In L. Rosenblum (ed.). Primate Behavior. Academic Press, New York.

Mitchell, G. D., and Clark, D. L. 1968. Long-Term Effects of Social Isolation in Nonsocially Adapted Rhesus Monkeys. J. Genet. Psychol. 113:117-128.

Mitchell, G. D., Raymond, E. J., Ruppenthal, G. C., and Harlow, H. F. 1966. Long-Term Effects of Total Social Isolation Upon Behavior of Rhesus Monkeys. Psychol. Rep. 18:567-580.

Morrison, H. L., and McKinney, W. T. 1976. Models of Human Psychopathology: Experimental Approaches in Primates. In A. Frazer and A. Winokur (eds.). Clinical Neuropsychopharmacology. Spectrum, New York. In press.

Mussen, P. H., and Conger, J. J. 1956. Child Development and Personality, pp. 137-138. Harper, New York.

Newberne, P. M. 1975. Animal Models for Investigation of Latent Effects of Malnutrition. Am. J. Dis. Child. 129:574-577.

Nissen, H. W., Chow, K. L., and Semmes, J. 1951. Effects of Restricted Opportunity for Tactual, Kinesthetic and Manipulative Experience on the Behavior of Chimpanzees. Amer. J. Psychol. 64:485-507.

Noble, A. B., McKinney, W. T., and Mohr, C. 1975. Diazepam Treatment of Socially Isolated Monkeys. Paper presented at American Psychiatric Association Annual Meeting, Anaheim, California.

Novak, M. A. 1975. Social Recovery of Monkeys Isolated for the First Year of Life. II. Test of Therapy. In Preparation.

Novak, M. A., and Harlow, H. F. 1975. Social Recovery of Monkeys Isolated for the First Year of Life. I. Rehabilitation and Therapy. Dev. Psychol. 11:453-564.

O'Connor, N. 1968. Children in Restricted Environments, p. 530. In G. Newton and S. Levine (eds.). Early Experience and Behavior. Charles C. Thomas, Springfield, Illinois.

Prince, J. 1967. The Dominance Hierarchy and the Evolution of Mental Illness. Lancet 2:243-246.

Rall, D. P. 1969. Animal Models for Pharmacotherapeutic Studies. In Animal Models for Biomedical Research. Fed. Proc. 32: 125-132.

Redmond, D. E., Maas, J. W., Kling, A., Graham, C. W., and Dekirmenjian, H. 1971. Social Behavior of Monkeys Selectively Depleted of Monoamines. Science 174:428-431.

Riesen, A. H. 1950. Arrested Vision. Sci. Amer. 183:16-19.

Riesen, A. H. 1965. Effects of Early Deprivation of Photic Stimulation, pp. 61-85. In S. F. Osler and R. E. Cooke (eds.). The Biosocial Basis of Mental Retardation. Johns Hopkins Press, Baltimore.

Riesen, A. H. 1975. The Sensory Environment in Growth and Development, pp. 1-6. In A. H. Riesen (ed.). The Developmental Neuropsychology of Sensory Deprivation. Academic Press, New York.

Reiss, B. F. 1954. The Effect of Altered Environment and of Age on Mother-Young Relationships Among Animals. Ann. N. Y. Acad. Sci. 57:606-610.

Ribble, M. A. 1943. The Rights of Infants. Columbia University Press, New York.

Robertson, T., and Bowlby, J. 1952. Responses of Young Children to Separation From Their Mothers. Cours du Centre International de l'Enfance 2:131-142.

Rosenblum, L. A., and Kaufman, I. C. 1968. Variation in Infant Development and Response to Maternal Loss in Monkeys. Am. J. Ortho. psychiat. 38:418-426.

Rowland, G. L. 1964. The Effects of Total Social Isolation Upon Learning and Social Behavior in Rhesus Monkeys. Unpublished doctoral dissertation. University of Wisconsin.

Ruppenthal, G. C., Harlow, M. K., Eisele, C. D., Harlow, H. F., and Suomi, S. J. 1974. Development of Peer Interactions of Monkeys Reared in a Nuclear Family Environment. Child Dev. 45: 670-682.

Sackett, G. P. 1966. Development of Preference for Differentially Complex Patterns by Infant Monkeys. Psychonon. Sci. 6:441-442.

Sackett, G. P. 1968a. Abnormal Behavior in Laboratory Reared Rhesus Monkeys, pp. 293-331. In M. W. Fox (ed.). Abnormal Behavior in Animals. Saunders, Philadelphia.

Sackett, G. P. 1968b. The Persistence of Abnormal Behavior in Monkeys Following Isolation Rearing. Int. Psychiat. Clin. 6: 3-37.

Sackett, G. P. 1972. Prospects for Research on Schizophrenia. 3. Neurophysiology of Isolation Rearing in Primates. Neurosci. Res. Prog. Bull. 10:388-392.

Sackett, G. P., Porter, M., and Holmes, H. 1965. Choice Behavior in Rhesus Monkeys. Effect of Stimulation During the First Month of Life. Science 147:304-306.

Sackett, G. P., Holm, R. A., and Landesman-Dwyer, S. 1975. Vulnerability for Abnormal Development: Pregnancy Outcomes and Sex Differences in Macaque Monkeys, pp. 59-76. In N. R. Ellis (ed.). Aberrant Development in Infancy. Erlbaum Associates, New Jersey.

Schanberg, S., Schildkraut, J., and Breese, G. 1968. Metabolism of Normetanephrine in Rat Brain: Identification of Conjugated 3-Methoxy-4-hydroxy-phenylglycol as Major Metabolite. Biochem. Pharm. 17:247-254.

Schildkraut, J. 1970. Neuropsychopharmacology and the Affective
    Disorders. Little Brown, Boston.

Seaman, S. F. 1975. Unpublished manuscript.

Seay, B., and Harlow, H. F. 1965. Maternal Separation in the Rhesus
    Monkey. J. Nerv. Ment. Dis. 140:434–441.

Seay, B. M., Alexander, B. K., and Harlow, H. F. 1964. Maternal
    Behavior of Socially Deprived Rhesus Monkeys. J. Abnorm. Soc.
    Psychol. 69:345–354.

Seitz, P. D. 1959. Infantile Experience and Adult Behavior in
    Animal Subjects. II. Age of Separation From the Mother and
    Adult Behavior in the Cat. Psychosom. Med. 21:353–378.

Seligman, M. E. P., Maier, S. F., and Geer, J. 1968. The Allevia-
    tion of Learned Helplessness in the Dog. J. Abnorm. Soc.
    Psychol. 73:256–262.

Senay, E. C. 1966. Toward an Animal Model of Depression: A Study
    of Separation Behavior in Dogs. J. Psychiat. Res. 4:65–71.

Spector, S., Sjoerdsma, A., and Udenfriend, S. 1965. Blockage of
    Endogenous Norepinephrine Synthesis by Alpha-Methyl-Para-
    Tyrosine, An Inhibitor of Tyrosine Hydroxylase. J. Pharm. Exp.
    Ther. 147:86–95.

Spencer-Booth, Y., and Hinde, R. A. 1967. The Effects of Separating
    Rhesus Monkey Infants. J. Child Psychol. Psychiat. Allied Dis.
    7:179–197.

Spitz, R. A. 1946. Anaclitic Depression: An Inquiry Into the
    Genesis of Psychiatric Conditions in Early Childhood. II. Psy.
    Study of Child. 2:313–342.

Suomi, S. J. 1973a. Surrogate Rehabilitation of Monkeys Reared in
    Total Social Isolation. J. Child Psychol. Psychiat. 14:71–77.

Suomi, S. J. 1973b. Repetitive Peer Separation of Young Monkeys.
    Effects of Vertical Chamber Confinement During Separations.
    J. Abnorm. Psychol. 81:1–10.

Suomi, S. J. 1974. Social Interactions of Monkeys Reared in a
    Nuclear Family Environment Versus Monkeys Reared With Mothers
    and Peers. Primates 15:311–320.

Suomi, S. J., and Harlow, H. F. 1969. Apparatus Conceptualization
    for Psychopathological Research in Monkeys. Behav. Res. Meth.
    Instr. 1:1–12.

Suomi, S. J., and Harlow, H. F. 1972. Social Rehabilitation of
    Isolate-Reared Monkeys. Dev. Psychol. 6:487-496.

Suomi, S. J., Harlow, H. F., and Domeck, C. J. 1970. Effect of
    Repetitive Infant-Infant Separation of Young Monkeys. J.
    Abnorm. Psychol. 76:161-172.

Suomi, S. J., Harlow, H. F., and McKinney, W. T. 1972. Monkey
    Psychiatrists. Amer. J. Psychiat. 128:927-932.

Suomi, S. J., Eisele, C. D., Grady, S. F., and Harlow, H. F. 1975.
    Depressive Behavior in Adult Monkeys Following Separation from
    Family Environment. Abnorm. Psy. In press.

Thompson, W. R., and Melzack, R. 1956. Early Environment. Sci.
    Amer. 194:38-42.

Thompson, W. R., and Solomon, L. M. 1954. Spontaneous Pattern Dis-
    crimination in the Rat. J. Comp. Physiol. Psychol. 47:104-107.

Tinkelpaugh, O. L. 1928. The Self-Mutilation of a Male Macacus
    Rhesus Monkey. J. Mammal. 9:293-300.

Waters, R. H., Rethlingshafer, D. A., and Caldwell, W. E. (eds.).
    1960. Principles of Comparative Psychology, p. 437. McGraw-
    Hill, New York.

White, N. F. (ed.). 1974. Ethology and Psychiatry, p. 257. Uni-
    versity of Toronto Press, Toronto, Canada.

Wildt, D. E., and Dukelow, W. R. 1974. The Nonhuman Primate as a
    Model for Human Twinning. Lab. Primate News 13:15-18.

Winnicott, D. W. 1948. Pediatrics and Psychiatry. Brit. J. Med.
    Psychol. 21:229-240.

Yarrow, L. J., Rubenstein, J. L., Pedersen, F. A., and Jankowski,
    J. J. 1972. Dimensions of Early Stimulation and Their Dif-
    ferential Effects on Infant Development. Merr. Palm. Quart.
    18:205.

Yerkes, R. M. 1913. Comparative Psychology: A Question of Defini-
    tions. J. Phil. 10:580-582.

Young, L. D., Suomi, S. J., Harlow, H. F., and McKinney, W. T. 1973.
    Early Stress and Later Response to Separation in Rhesus Monkeys.
    Am. J. Psychiat. 130:400-405.

Zubeck, J. P., Bayer, L., and Shepard, J. M. 1969. Relative Effects
    of Prolonged Social Isolation and Confinement: Behavioral and

EEG Changes. J. Abnorm. Psychol. 74:625-631.

Zubeck, J. P., Hughes, G. R., and Shepard, J. M. 1971. A Comparison of the Effects of Prolonged Sensory Deprivation and Perceptual Deprivation. Can. J. Behav. Sci. 3:282-290.

Zuckerman, S. 1932. The Social Life of Monkeys and Apes. Routlege, London.

NEURAL RESPONSES TO THERAPEUTIC

SENSORY ENVIRONMENTS

Roger N. Walsh
Department of Psychiatry and Behavioral Sciences
Stanford University School of Medicine
Stanford, California 94305
            and
Robert A. Cummins
Department of Physiology
University of Queensland
St. Lucia, Queensland 4067
Australia

INTRODUCTION

While it is widely accepted that the sensory environment can modify behavior, the underlying neural changes are not well understood. However, during the last two decades many studies have demonstrated that brain structure can be modified by sensory stimulation. This suggests that the sensory environment may be used to ameliorate the neurological effects of brain damage. The evidence for this suggestion will be presented under the following headings: experimental variables, the state of the art, physiological mechanisms, and outstanding questions. We will also use the available research data to speculate upon the etiology of both damaging and repair processes.

EXPERIMENTAL VARIABLES

Sensory Environments

Of the many possible types of sensory stimulation, only five appear to have been employed in studies of neural rehabilitation. These five are light versus dark rearing, social rearing versus isolation, complexity (social plus "toys") versus isolation, behavioral training versus no training and active versus passive exploration. Other types of stimulation such as handling and vestibular stimulation do not appear to have been used for neural studies of rehabilitation even though they have proved useful for behavioral studies.

Brain Damaging Agents

A major limitation of the field to date is that with few exceptions, the brain damaging agents employed prior to studies of neural
rehabilitation have been limited to varieties of sensory deprivation
(isolation, dark rearing, etc.). Thus as yet we have little direct
evidence of environmental influences on neural recovery from physical,
nutritional, pharmacological, hormonal or metabolic agents; although considerable behavioral recovery may be evident (see other
chapters in this volume).

THE STATE OF THE ART

Effects of Sensory Stimulation on Normal Subjects

In general, environmental stimulation leads to an increase in
brain weight and size with this increase being most marked in the
cerebrum (Rosenweig et al. 1972; Walsh et al. 1971a). Even
within the cerebrum itself, a degree of regional specificity exists
and in the rat the occipital cortex is most susceptible (Rosenzweig
et al. 1972; Walsh et al. 1969; Walsh et al. 1972). Within the
cortex, the histological components contributing to this increase
include cell bodies and an increased arborization of the dendritic
tree (Diamond et al. 1966; Greenough and Volkmar 1973; Walsh
and Cummins 1975; Walsh et al. 1971b). The number of dendritic
spines is also increased with the magnitude of the increase depending on the type and locality of the dendrite in question (Globus
et al. 1973). Synapses show alterations in size and numbers according to the locality and type of stimulation and there is possibly
an alteration in the numbers of synaptic vesicles (Cragg, 1974). Bio-
chemically, the amounts of both protein and RNA are increased as are
the enzymes associated with the acetylcholine system, namely cholinesterase, acetylcholinesterase and choline acetyl transferase (Rosenzweig et al. 1972). The biogenic amines are also altered but the
effects are less well established (Geller et al. 1965; Riege and
Morimoto 1970). For complexity, social, and isolation reared animals, correlations between the biological parameters of brain weight
and acetylcholinesterase concentrations and problem   solving parameters have been reported but little else in the way of neurobehavioral correlation has been achieved (Rosenweig et al. 1972). For reviews see Rosenzweig et al.(1972), Globus (1975), Greenough (1975)
and Walsh and Cummins (1975). As will be seen, a number of these
changes are opposite to those produced by several brain damaging
processes, and so it is that the heightened stimulation has been
the sensory modification most frequently assayed as a therapeutic
agent. The emphasis on heightened stimulation in this chapter is
not meant to imply that it is always beneficial.

Anatomical Recovery

For the majority of anatomical parameters it would seem that
the effects of prior deprivation can be at least partially revers-

ed by subsequent exposure to heightened stimulation. This has been
well demonstrated for cerebral weight, for not only may stimulation
enhance recovery but it may also afford protection against subsequent deprivation. This was shown in a series of switchover experiments in which rats were reared from weaning in either isolation or
environmental compexity. After various times of exposure, half of
the subjects of each group were switched to the opposite environment for an equal period of time while the remainder continued in
the original environment. This procedure resulted in four groups,
two of which had continuous exposure to either complexity or isolation and two of which were exposed first to one and then the other
(Cummins and Walsh 1975). The results from such a 30 day + 30
day design showed that the exposure to complexity was effective in
increasing final cerebral weight whether this exposure was in the
first or the second 30 days. Animals which experienced both complexity and isolation (switchover groups) in either order, showed
cerebral weights as large as those of animals which remained in
complexity for the full 60 days, and all three of these groups had
significantly greater cerebral weights than those of the animals
which remained in isolation throughout. Interestingly, this experiment
shows not only that complexity was sufficient to overcome the effects
of prior deprivation, but also that earlier exposure to complexity
afforded protection against subsequent isolation.

While in the above study, both primary and secondary environments exerted a significant effect Figure 1 shows that in another
switchover study where the animals were reared for prolonged periods
(60 days in both primary and secondary environments) the effects
of the primary exposure were largely dissipated and the terminal
brain weights were determined only by the secondary environment.
These studies support some findings of Rosenweig et al. (1962)
that 33 days of isolation followed by 48 of enrichment produced
brain weight, and cholinesterase and acetylcholinesterase, concentrations, intermediate between those of the litter-mates who
were maintained for the full 81 days in either complexity or isolation. A later study (Rosenweig et al. 1967) suggested that the
effects of 80 days of complexity or isolation were largely removed
by a subsequent 50-day period in the opposite environment, so that
the terminal values appeared to be largely determined by the secondary environment.

Twenty-one days of Hebb-Williams maze testing was also found to
be effective in overcoming isolation induced cerebral weight and
size reduction (Figure 2: Cummins et al. 1973). In this study
rats were reared under either complexity or isolation for 535 days
and then half of each group was maze tested. For isolates the
testing raised the cerebral values almost to the level of the complexity animals whereas the complexity reared subjects showed no
significant effects of testing. This study suggests that at least
some of the neural effects of deprivation may be maintaimed for con-

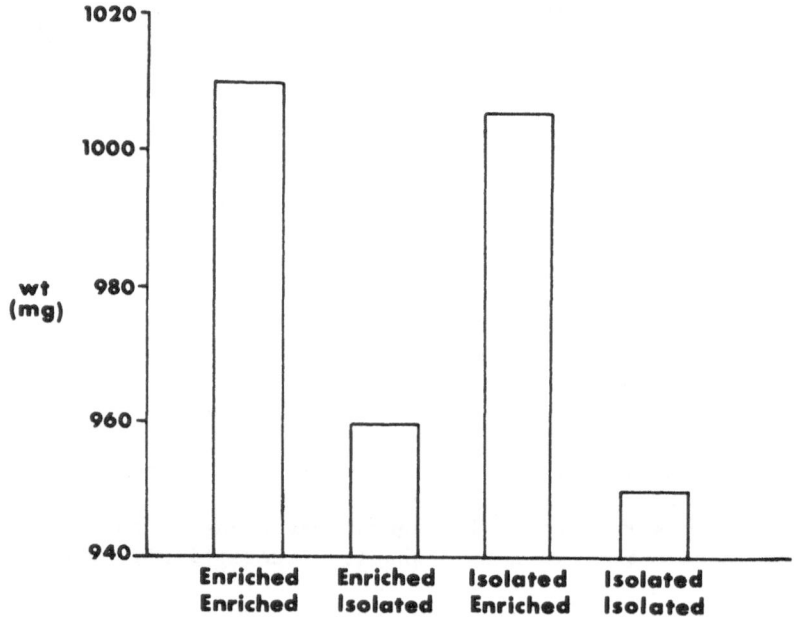

Fig. 1. Effects of 60 days exposure to both primary and secondary environments on cerebral weight. The effect of the secondary environment was significant at the 0.01 level while the primary environment no longer exerted a significant effect, either direct or interactional.

siderable periods, yet may still be reversed with relatively short periods of augmented sensory input; a finding with obvious therapeutic implications.

    In line with the above studies showing a significant but partially transient protection against isolation effects by prior exposure to complexity are some studies by Bennett et al (1974). They initially placed weanling rats in either complexity or isolation after either 30 or 80 days of differential rearing. They transferred some animals from complexity to isolation and kept them there for periods ranging from 7 to 47 days in order to measure the persistence of the complexity effects. The effects of 30 days of differential experience appeared to be less persistent than those of 80 days although it must be noted that the experiments confound the duration of initial rearing and the age at which subjects were placed in the second environment. After an initial 30 days differential rearing period, cortical weight showed a reduction to about 60% of the original complexity value within 7 days and to about 30% within 14 days, while acetylcholinesterase activity showed a somewhat greater persistence. After an initial 80 day differential

rearing period both anatomical and chemical measures once again
exhibited asymptotically declining values but the persistence was greater and remained detectable in the occipital cortex
after 47 days.

Cortical weight persistence = 25%, NS, acetylcholinesterase
activity persistence (65%, $p< 0.05$). In contradistinction to
these trends, cholinesterase activity, which is usually, though
variably reduced by isolation, actually showed an increase after
transfer from complexity to isolation. Thus, with the exception
of cholinesterase, the anatomical and chemical effects of complexity
tend to dissipate when subjects are transferred to isolation but
the degree of dissipation depends on the parameter and brain region
under investigation as well as the duration of prior treatment and
possibly also the age of the subject.

Taken together, these studies suggest that when an animal is
removed from one sensory environment and placed in another, the
cerebral response to the secondary environment is dependent upon
the residual response to the first. Where the period of secondary
exposure is short (30 days or less) the subjects coming from the
condition of stimulus deprivation attain cerebral weight values
close to those of subjects exposed to continuous stimulation.
Subjects removed from complexity, on the other hand, show comparatively little loss during the subsequent deprivation. The basis
for this differential responsivity has not been established but
one possible explanation is provided by the differential arousa-
bility of these subjects. Isolates have been behaviorally observed

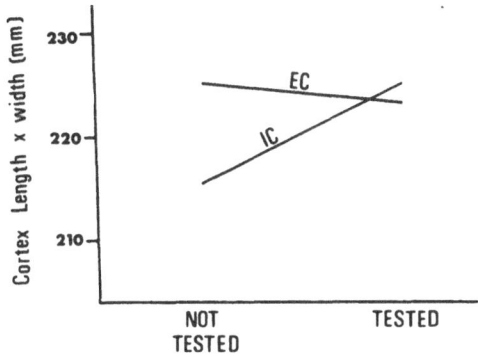

Fig. 2. Testing x environment interaction on the derived parameter
of cerebral length x cerebral width. The environment main effect
was significant ($p<0.02$) while the testing main effect was not.
The interaction effect was significant ($p<0.05$) due to the fact
that testing exerted an effect on the isolated (4.7%, $p <0.5$) but
not on complexity exposed subjects. Reprinted by permission from
Nature (Lond.), 243: 517, (1973).

to be more easily aroused than complexity reared subjects (Konrad
and Melzack 1975; Cummins et al.   1974 ; Walsh and Cummins
1975 ;1976) and the physiological arousal response has been hypothesized as one possible mechanism by which sensory stimulation
elicits brain changes (see the subsequent section on mechanisms).

Further evidence for the therapeutic potential of environmental
complexity has come from the study of neurological recovery after
experimental brain damage. Will et al. (1975 a; b) performed bilateral occipital cortex lesions in rats either at birth or later
in life at 30 days of age. These animals were then reared for
various times in either isolation or environmental complexity. This
differential rearing was followed by a period of maze testing, after
which the rats were killed and their brains examined for evidence
of neurological recovery. The behavioral results reported by these
studies are discussed in the chapter by Greenough et al. in this
volume.

The rats lesioned at birth were differentially reared either
from day 5 for 60 days or from day 25 for 40 days, and after approximately 30 days of behavioral testing, the cerebral length and
width were measured. It was found that while lesioning reduced
both cortical length and width, environmental complexity tended to
increase these cerebral dimensions. As with previous reports
(Walsh et al. 1971a; 1973), the increase attributable to environmental complexity was greater for length than for width. Especially
interesting from a therapeutic standpoint was that the environmental
effect was significantly stronger in the lesioned than in the nonlesioned subjects.

When the animals were lesioned at 30 days of age, the effect
of environmental complexity was not necessarily greatest in the
lesioned subjects. Thus, while environmental complexity tended to
increase both the weight and the RNA/DNA ratio of the cortex, the
weight increase was greatest in the sham-operated controls whilst
the increased RNA/DNA ratio was greatest in the previously lesioned
animals. This indicates a degree of variability in the interaction
between environmental therapy and brain recovery. Thus, while the
overall evidence clearly indicates that environmental stimulation
can aid neurological recovery from non-environmentally induced
deficits, it remains unclear whether this occurs by a direct effect
on the recovery process itself.

Dark rearing evokes a number of anatomical responses analogous
to those induced by isolation but as yet there are few studies of
recovery. Reduced cell size in the lateral geniculate and occipital cortex has often been reported (e.g.Gyllensten et al. 1966;
Guillery, 1972;).Kalil (1975) examined cats which had been dark
reared from birth for 4 and 8 weeks and then light exposed for at
least 3 months. Depth perception, visual avoidance, following

and placing behaviors appeared with only one week of normal vision
and by the end of three months geniculate cell area had normalized.
A decrease in the number of pyramidal cell dendritic spines has been
found after dark rearing although this effect was partially transitory. Thus in animals dark reared from birth there was a tendency
to normalization such that by 50 days only a small, though significant, difference was observed and this normalization was hastened
by exposure to light (Valverde 1967; 1971; Ruiz-Marcos and Valverde 1970).

A number of studies have demonstrated synaptic alterations following dark rearing (Cragg 1967; 1974; Fifkova 1970a;b) but the
extent of possible recovery is less clear. Vrensen and DeGroot
(1974) reared three groups of rabbits: a control group raised under
normal lighting, a deprived group raised in darkness for 7 months
from birth, and a darkness-light group also reared in complete darkness for 7 months but thereafter in normal lighting conditions for
12 months. They measured synaptic length, surface area, number of
synaptic contact zones and the number of synaptic vesicles per terminal. Only the latter showed effects of deprivation, in that dark
reared animals had fewer synaptic vesicles per terminal than normally reared subjects and this deficit persisted in spite of 12 months subsequent light rearing. This contrasts markedly with certain
findings of Cragg (1967; 1974). He reared rats in darkness until
weaning when half were placed under diurnal lighting conditions for
periods varying from 3 hours to 10 weeks. Light exposure resulted
in increased synaptic dimensions in the superficial half of the
cortex with a reversed effect on the lower half. Synaptic numbers
per unit area were increased in the lower cortex but not significantly affected superficially. This was interpreted as due to light
induced synaptogenesis in the deeper layers and synaptic enlarge-
ment superficially in response to light stimulation. Periods of
light exposure as short as 3 hours were sufficient to elicit detectable effects after a further 48 hours of subsequent darkness.
By subjective examination, Cragg could not identify any qualitative
effects on synaptic profiles, vesicles, or regions of apposition.
However, in view of the smallness of the anticipated effects, it
is not surprising that non-quantitative methods were inadequate to
detect them, if indeed they exist. Cragg's findings suggest a considerably greater synaptic response to light after dark rearing than
do the findings of Vrensen and DeGroot. This could reflect a number of factors, especially species differences, differences in duration of exposure and subject age. Unfortunately, Cragg's studies
do not include a group reared continuously in normal diurnal lighting so that it is impossible to know to what extent the changes
he reports represent recovery towards the norm. In any event, it
is apparent that cerebral dendritic spines and synapses of light deprived subjects are susceptible to subsequent light exposure and
that at least for spines, the changes result in a trend towards
normalization.

Chemical Recovery

Chemical studies are few but tend to support the concept of the reversibility of prior experimental deprivation. The effects of environmental complexity on RNA/DNA ratios in lesioned rat brains (Will et al. 1975a; b) have already been discussed. Diaz et al. (1975) claim preliminary results indicating differential effects of complexity and isolation on norepinephrine uptake recovery following lesioning by 6-hydroxydopamine, but full details are not yet available. Investigations of protein percursor uptake have been carried out in rats reared from birth to 50 days of age in darkness and then exposed to light for varying periods (Rose 1967; Rose and Sinha 1974). The incorporation of 3-H-lysine into occipital cortex tissue was initially abnormally great but this persisted for less than 99 hours. Cholinesterase and acetyl cholinesterase activities in rats reared under complexity or isolation showed partial or complete dissipation of effects due to the primary environment when the animals were switched to the opposite rearing conditions (Rosenzweig et al. 1967). Similarly, the effects of isolation on these enzymes are partially dissipated by subsequent problem solving tasks (Rosenzweig et al. 1972), a finding reminiscent of that for cerebral weight in the previously mentioned study by Cummins et al. (1973). Geller (1971) reared rats in either complexity or isolation for 30 days and then re-housed them in pairs for a further 30. Although significant differences in dopamine and norepinephrine concentrations remained, they were smaller than the differences after the original 30 day exposure to differential environments, suggesting that these substances also show at least partial reversibility.

Electrophysiological Recovery

The electrophysiology of recovery from sensory deprivation is better known than either the anatomy or chemistry. Unilateral and bilateral visual deprivation produce very different effects and so will be considered separately.

Dark rearing, a form of bilateral visual deprivation, tends to retard maturation of visual evoked potentials. Evoked potentials in rabbits dark reared from birth exhibited a simple form like those of neonatal animals, were rapidly fatiguable (Fourment & Scherrer 1961: Scherrer and Fourment 1964) and were superimposed on a low level of background electrical activity (Shilyagina 1973). Return to normal lighting resulted in a gradual recovery of both the background activity and evoked potentials towards patterns more characteristic of normal adults (Shilyagina 1973). Meisami and Timiras (1971) have used the electroshock seizure threshold (the minimum current capable of eliciting evidence of clonic convulsion) as a measure of the development of excitatory-inhibitory balance under differential light exposure. Both continuous lighting and darkness delayed development in the young rat and both ultimately resulted in a lowered threshold. However, dark but not light reared subjects showed a tendency to normalization beginning about day 34 and this was hastened by exposure to normal diurnal lighting.

The interneuronal connections of the visual system are directed by innate mechanisms. However, these connections are highly vulnerable to stimulus deprivation in early postnatal life especially since retinofugal fibers compete with their homologous contralateral counterparts for innervation of higher order neurons within the lateral geniculate and the occipital cortex. The magnitude of the competition varies across species but in the cat, in which it is most evident, early unilateral deprivation upsets it so that the deprived pathways not only suffer from a form of disuse atrophy, but appear to be suppressed by the non-deprived competing pathways such that recovery is minimal (Guillery 1972; Sherman and Sanderson 1972).

The electrophysiological effects of monocular deprivation are detectable at several levels of the visual system. They are less marked in the lateral geniculate than in the occipital cortex in spite of the fact that the geniculate exhibits greater histological evidence of atrophy. Thus, three months of unilateral deprivation from birth in the kitten did not preclude normal concentric receptive field organization in affected geniculate layers even though the deprived neurons were significantly smaller. However, some fields had abnormally large centers and contained a reduced number of active cells as well as some cells which reacted sluggishly (Wiesel and Hubel 1963a).

In the occipital cortex the changes in unit activity were dramatic (Wiesel and Hubel 1963b; Ganz et al. 1968; Hubel and Wiesel 1970; Wilson and Sherman 1975). Some neurons ceased to respond altogether. In the normal cat, about 80% of the striate cells can be driven by both eyes (Hubel and Wiesel 1962) but this percentage is greatly reduced by unilateral deprivation and those few cells which remain binocularly driven are dominated by the non-deprived eye. Neurons dominated by the same eye tend to be arranged in columns, ocular dominance columns, and following unilateral deprivation the columns of the deprived eye shrank in size, while those of the non-deprived eye expanded to fill a larger proportion of the cortex. In cells which the deprived eye could still trigger, the response tended to be more sluggish and to fatigue more rapidly. These cells also failed to display the normal

response selectivity to oriented lines stimuli, i.e., they were
circular in receptive field and unselective to form or motion.
The fact that these effects were less marked with bilateral eye
closure (Wiesel and Hubel 1965a) was one of the first suggestions
of the possibility of competition between axon terminals from the
two sides for control of the postsynaptic cell.

The degree of physiological and behavioral recovery which is
possible after such insults depends on the animals' age, duration
of deprivation, and the method of treatment. If deprivation is
maintained throughout the entire sensitive period, which lasts from
birth to about three months in the cat, then simply opening the
deprived eye has little effect. However, with shorter periods of
deprivation, varying degrees of recovery are possible. This recovery is enhanced by closure of the control eye at the same time
as the occluded one is opened.

Within the cat lateral geniculate, almost no electrophysiological recovery occurs although eye closure reversal elicits a degree
of histological rehabilitation. Within the occipital cortex, reversal of electrophysiological deficits is more marked provided,
of course, that the initial period of deprivation is considerably
less than the sensitive period. This recovery is most evident as
a decrease in the number of unresponsive cells although the number
of binocularly driven cells shows only a minimum change. The number
of monocular cells driven by the formerly deprived eye increases
and as it does so, there are concomitant changes in the size of the
corresponding ocular dominance columns (Movshon and Blakemore
1975). Whether this recovery represents simply the activation of
formerly ineffective synapses, as has been noted in other regions
of the CNS (e.g., Wall and Egger 1971; Merril and Wall 1972), or
an actual formation of new connections is unknown, but there seems
no reason to presume that both do not occur.

Periods of deprivation extending throughout the total duration
of the sensitive period almost preclude any significant degree of
physiological recovery. This suggests that once unilateral innervation of the visual cortex neurons is effected then competition for
the postsynaptic cells greatly reduce the chance of functional recovery of the deprived pathways. However, while there was little
or no physiological recovery of animals deprived throughout the
sensitive period, reversal of eye closure was found to aid behavioral rehabilitation (Dews and Wiesel, 1970; Chow and Stewart, 1972).
This behavioral recovery in the absence of neurophysiological correlates may seem surprising but appears to be based on the learning
of alternative cues for the solving of perceptual problems, an
example of behavioral substitution. For example, visually deprived cats have been found to move their heads along the contours
of stimuli thus translating the configurational cues of a discrim-

ination task into a combination of visual flux, visual reaffer-ence, and proprioception (Rizzolatti and Tradari 1971; Ganz and Haffner 1974). However, discriminations such as these are more precarious and easily disrupted by any change in the sensory en-vironment, thus considerably reducing the generality, transfer-ability and behavioral reserve of the animal.

Auditory evoked potentials have been used to investigate the effects of deprivation and subsequent recovery within the auditory system. Rats reared for the first eight weeks of life in a sound attentuated environment exhibited raised auditory thresholds. How-ever, exposure to normal ambient sound resulted in partial recovery within 48 hours and complete recovery within three weeks. (Batkin et al. 1970). The extent of electophysiological recovery from long term sensory deprivation in humans is unknown, but it is of more than academic interest that prisoners, especially those sub-jected to solitary confinement, exhibit slowing of the EEG (Gend-reau et al. 1972).

SUMMARY

In general, the effects of bilateral sensory deprivation can be at least partially reversed by provision of the missing stimuli. At least for gross anatomical parameters in rodents, these does not seem to be much in the way of a critical period limiting the reversibility of environmentally induced brain changes. However, as yet there has been little investigation of more discrete vari-ables, and it remains possible that recovery of size of preexisting structures such as increased nuclear and cell body dimensions, may occur more readily than the formation of new cell constitutents, e.g., new dendritic branches and synapses. The brains of deprived animals show a more rapid response to stimulation than do non-deprived subjects, but this effect is transient. As yet there has been almost no success in finding neurobehavioral correlations in these types of recovery studies and some researchers have called the worth of neural studies into question because of this. This seems premature since the complexity of the brain is such that one can rarely expect recovery of even a relatively simple behavior to correlate with any one brain parameter.

These comments have referred to recovery from bilateral depriv-ation. Recovery from the effects of unilateral deprivation seems more difficult largely because of competitive functional suppression. Cells within the retino-cortical system compete with their contra-lateral homologues for post-synaptic cells and once the competitive balance has been upset, it is extremely difficult to reverse. Phy-siological recovery of the deprived eye and its projections is therefore extremely limited even though there may be considerable apparent behavioral recovery. This physiological-behavioral dis-

sociation is due to the ability to compensate for lost function
by using alternative cues.

Future research efforts will doubtless aim at enhancing recovery and several lines of attack seem possible. Closure of the
control eye aids recovery and it may be that this effect can be
potentiated. Long acting local anesthetics applied to the dominant visual pathways might reduce competitive inhibition while
application to corticofugal systems, which are partially inhibitory (Sherman, 1974) perhaps at the level of the visual cortex,
might be helpful. Antich olinesterase agents and anti-inhibitors
such as strychnine (see the subsequent section on mechanisms and the
chapter by Greenough et al.) could also prove useful. Active
exploration and visual reafference have proved helpful in retention of pattern discrimination in rats subjected to two stage
lesions of the visual cortex (Dru et al. 1975). and might
prove helpful in visually deprived animals (see the chapter by
Greenough et al.).

The monocular deprivation paradigm may prove to be a useful
experimental model for a number of significant clinical problems.
It has been suggested that humans develop the capacity for speech
in both cerebral hemispheres, but that one is subsequently suppressed (Milner 1973; Geschwind 1974). The variable degree of
recovery from aphasia which follows damage to the domiment hemisphere would thus reflect the varying degrees of contralateral
depression. Similarly, while the limbs are normally activated
by ipsilateral corticospinal pathways they can sometimes be usefully innervated by contralateral tracts when the ipsilateral
ones are damaged (Nathan and Smith 1973) due once again, perhaps, to the release of competitive inhibition. If this is so,
then the therapeutic task in these cases becomes one of maximizing the recovery from competitive inhibition, a task for which
the monocular deprivation paradigm may prove an excellent model.
In any event, because its anatomy and physiology are so well known
and because the behavioral effects of pathology can be detected with
precise perceptual parameters, the visual system will doubtless continue to be an excellent model for the study of environmentally induced damage and recovery. Finally, the studies by Will et al.
demonstrating environment - lesion interactions present an excellent
model for studies of rehabilitation following nonsensorilly induced
brain damage.

MECHANISMS MEDIATING RECOVERY

To date, there has been little empirical evidence and even less
speculation on the mechanisms which mediate environmentally induced recovery. This should come as little surprise since the mechanisms involved in the induction of environmental effects on normal brains are very much in question. This section examines the

mechanisms thought to mediate both environmentally induced brain changes and recovery after damage. It will also introduce the concept of a function limiting factor, consider interactions between sensory and nonsensory deficiencies and examine environmentally induced recovery from a reinforcement perspective.

Conceptualization of the mechanisms mediating recovery has traditionally emphasized the physiological approach, although in fact the transduction of sensory stimulation into neural changes probably involves many mechanisms operating at a variety of levels in a complex interdependent manner. The physiological mechanisms classically thought to underlie recovery are four in number (Luria et al. 1969; see the Greenough et al. chapter for a more detailed discussion including behavioral mechanisms).

1. Functional recovery of damaged neurons
2. Functional takeover by adjacent or contralateral analogous structures.
3. Reorganization of neural functional systems
4. Disinhibition of adjacent functionally inactivated neurons.

Functional takeover by undamaged tissue is a much debated mechanism which assumes the possibility of latent vicarious function. This concept is closely related to that of redundancy which assumes that some systems so overlap in their properties that they are partially interchangeable. However, it is apparent that systems vary widely in their recovery potential and this potential appears to be closely related to the diffuseness and overlap of the system's afferent and efferent anatomical projections (Goldberger 1974). A host of other factors are doubtless also involved but remain to be identified. Functional takeover has long been thought to occur more readily in younger subjects (Geschwind 1974) though this is debated by some (e.g. Isaacson 1974), and the extent of this takeover and the role of sensory input are still uncertain.

The concept of the functional reorganization of neural tissue is by no means universally accepted and some workers such as Le Vere (1975), maintain that recovery is the result of the continued normal operation of spared neural mechanisms. However, among those who accept it, the concept appears to have been used in slightly different ways by Western and Russian workers. Both imply a permanent change in function of the undamaged responsible parts of the nervous system rather than the expression of latent function. However, recent Western thinking has emphasized factors such as collateral sprouting and denervation supersensitivity (Goldberger, 1974) whereas the Russians have continued to emphasize variations in the nature and sequencing of functional components in the restoration of complex functions (Luria et al. 1969). The latter has been much used therapeutically and here sensory input of a particular kind is

essential; namely, instructional and feedback information from a
therapist.

Russian physiologists have made much of the concept of disinhibition in recovery. Following damage, adjacent and contralateral
tissue is often found to be functionally depressed due to so called
protective inhibition, and a decreased ratio of acetycholine to
acetycholinesterase in these areas has been postulated (Gazzaniga
1974). In accordance with this suggestion, is the finding that
anticholinesterase agents are sometimes therapeutically useful.
Functional restoration, for example, of motor activity or speech,
may occur following anticholinesterase administration even in cases
where the duration of the disorder is measured in years (Luria et
al., 1969). This therapeutic effect develops rapidly, is often
detected immediately after the first administration and may even
be permanent after a single injection. Sensory stimulation increases the enzymes of the acetylcholine system and may also increase the acetylcholine to acetycholinesterase ratio (e,g,
Rosenzweig et al., 1962). It might therefore, be expected that
appropriate sensory input would also be effective in causing disinhibition and that sensory input and exercise would therefore,
produce additive or synergistic effects when combined with anticholinesterases. This has, in fact, been observed (Luria et al.
1969); for example, in a case where initial exercise therapy was
ineffective in motor recovery from brain damage, a single injection of anticholinesterase elicited partial recovery which thereafter, increased with exercise.

The fact that drug-exercise combinations may elicit recovery
where either component alone proves ineffective suggests the possibility of some kind of therapeutic threshold in which initial
disinhibition may require massive stimulation after which maintenance is relatively easily obtained. Such a possibility suggests
that some types of brain damage may benefit from an initial vig-
orous multimodality therapeutic assault rather than the graduated
rehabilitation which is the norm. It also calls into question
the therapeutic nihilism which holds that rehabilitation programs
have little effect on speech or motor recovery following a stroke
(Sarno 1970; Stern et al. 1971) and which has inclined Western
neurologists not to attempt therapeutic trials using anticholinesterases.

The arousal response has been advanced as a physiological
mechanism mediating both environmentally induced changes and
brain damage recovery (Walsh and Cummins 1975). Reafferent stimuli and stimulus novelty may be particularly important in inducing
effects by virtue of their arousal eliciting nature. There are
a number of tantalizing reports of amphetamines facilitating recovery of discriminative behavior in rats (Braun et al. 1966)

as well as both accelerating and making more complete, the recovery of motor function in monkeys while in other monkeys, sedatives such as barbiturates had the opposite effect (Watson and Kennard 1945).

If the arousal mechanism does represent a common link between environmentally induced changes and recovery from brain damage, or if arousal mediates the production of environmentally induced changes which compensate for brain damage, then the study of arousal induced changes in normal brains should be relevant to the therapeutic situation. For example, it is known that the effects of environmental complexity on brain weight and enzymes of the cholinesterase system are enhanced by stimulant drugs; simultaneous presentation of social and nonsocial stimuli, stimulation during the most behaviorally aroused part of the diurnal rhythm (Rosenweig et al. 1972) and stimulus novelty (Brown and King 1971). Effects are dependent on direct contact with stimulus objects (Ferchmin et al. 1975) and reafferent stimulation may be particularly important (Walsh and Cummins 1975). Indeed, active, as opposed to passive exploration has been found to be important for recovery from occipital cortex lesions in rats (Hein 1970; Dru et al., 1975). The combination of stimulants or social grouping together with nonsocial stimulation has been found to prolong behavioral activity and exploration in rodents (Rosenzweig and Bennett 1972). Similarly, the variety and kind of objects available to the normal human infant may enhance arousal and cognitive development (Yarrow et al. 1972; Korner and Thoman 1972; Ainsworth 1973; see also Hunt this volume) though there is evidence to suggest that it is only when they become incorporated into a social interaction that they exert significant effects (Williams and Scarr 1971; Clark-Stewart 1974). These findings suggest a number of principles which might be used to guide research and clinical practice in the therapy of brain damage. Perhaps, therefore, in optimal therapeutic regime might include direct and reafferent stimulation of a novel or changing nature, given in a social context which gave feedback and rewarded high stimulation levels at times of the day at which arousal was maximal, perhaps aided by stimulant drugs.

A large number of anatomical changes occur within the brain both during recovery from damage and following sensory stimulation and it is possible to conceptualize these as mediating mechanisms for environmentally facilitated recovery, although at the present time this is almost purely speculative. For example, aberrant major fiber tracts may develop following certain types of brain damage in young subjects. In the newborn kitten, monocular enucleation results in the axons from the remaining eye spreading to layers of the lateral geniculate from which they are normally excluded (Kalil 1973). In the newborn rat, unilateral damage to the cortico-spinal tract results in the hyperthrophy of an uncrossed corticospinal

pathway (Hicks and D'Amato 1970; Castro 1975) and it is possible
that this might be the neural basis for the finding that animals so
damaged at birth are sometimes capable of greater recovery than ones
damaged later in life.   The functional significance of these aberrant fiber tracts is unknown (Dejerine (1914) reported a similar
phenomenon in humans with infantile hemiplegia, but it seems quite
feasible to expect that sensory stimulation might be capable of
modifying the extent of their functional development.

A second possible anatomical mechanism is that of axonal sprouting. Typically, this has been considered a regenerative response
of proliferation and migration of axon collaterals into areas deprived of their normal input, although it is possible that the
brain undergoes ultrastructural remodelling throughout life (Sotelo and Palay 1971). The axonal sprouting may occur from trans-
sected neurons or as collateral sprouting from intact cells,
although only the former has been examined in detail in the CNS
(for reviews see Guth 1974; Moore 1974). The implicit assumption has often been that such sprouting aids recovery by replac-
ing lost input. However, the value of this replacement, which
may even be from another system entirely, is uncertain. Indeed,
preliminary studies by Isaacson (1974) suggested that chemical
inhibition of sprouting actually ameliorated some of the usual
consequences of brain damage.

The possibility of future pharmacological interventions to
therapeutically modify this sprouting seems a very real possibility. However, in view of Isaacson's findings, it is uncertain
whether the optimal modification will entail increasing or de-
creasing sprouting or possibly both. Conceivably, stereotactic
injection might allow a highly selective regionally specific
modification of the sprouting process so as to ensure regenerative input from one particular system in those areas where regeneration from inappropriate systems is likely to occur, e.g.
the hippocampus (Lynch et al. 1974; 1975). Agents that have been
found to enhance axonal regeneration include triiodothyronine and
nerve growth factor, while concanavlin A (a lectin that binds to
glycoproteins) appeared to reduce adjacent microcavitation (Bjork-
lund and Stenevi 1972; Fertig et al., 1971). The dynamic nature
of the remodelling of the damaged nervous system is suggested by a
study of Bernstein et al. 1975) who found that the number of bou-
tons terminaux on spinal cord neurons below the level of a lesion,
declined for the first 20 postoperative days, recovered for the
next 10 and then exhibited a secondary decline for a further 30
days. This suggests the possibility of a critical, or at best, sensitive, period for optimal therapeutic intervention.

Although sprouting has typically been considered a regeneta-
tive phenomenon, it seems possible that it may occur continuously

throughout life as a consequence of an ultrastructural dynamic
equilibrium with which the brain responds to functional demands.
Consequently, it may also possibly occur following sensory stimulation alone since the latter may certainly increase dendritic and
synaptic numbers. It seems, therefore, reasonable to suggest that
sensory environments may modify axonal sprouting in both damaged and
undamaged neurons and that this may be one of the mechanisms mediating environmentally facilitated recovery.

A number of authors have reported modification of dendritic
length, arborization, spatial orientation, and dendritic spines
following sensory stimulation and deprivation (Globus _et al_. 1973;
Greenough et al. 1973).   Valverde (1967) found that the spatial
orientation of visual cortex dendrites following enucleation of the
eye was altered in such a way as to reduce the number of dendrites
in the functionally deprived layers and increase them in others. It
seems possible that the mechanisms of dendritic and axonal reorganization might form a basis for functional takeover by perifocal tissue.
Whether the effectiveness of this takeover might be enhanced by sensory stimulation remains to be determined.

One further possible anatomical mechanism remains but must be
regarded as highly speculative at the present time. This is the
postnatal formation of new neurons. Altman et al. (1968) have
demonstrated that at least in the rodent, neuron formation continues
after birth in the anterior cerebrum and the dentate gyrus. Both
these areas have proved morphologically sensitive to environmental
complexity (Walsh et al. 1973; 1974) and it seems possible that this
may reflect an environmental modification of the neurogenesis. If
so, then modification of this process might also occur in environmentally facilitated rehabilitation at least in younger subjects.

The Function Limiting Factor

The basic tenet of this discussion has been that the nature and
amount of sensory stimulation may set a limit to the function and
development of the brain. Obviously this is only one example of
a large range of other factors (genetic, nutritional, hormonal,
etc.) any one of which may determine the limits of functioning in
the normal brain or may limit recovery after brain damage. In other
words, the functional ceiling will be determined by the most deficient factor; what we might call "The Function Limiting Factor".
Orthomolecular psychiatry with its emphasis on providing supplements
of assumed function limiting molecules may be seen as one derivative
of a function limiting factor concept, though the latter includes
the nonmolecular factors of sensory stimuli. Since diminished neuronal metabolic activity would be a common end point for several
types of deficiencies, this function-limiting factor hypothesis
helps to explain certain similarities in the brains of animals

suffering from diverse types of deficiencies. For example, the
reduced neuronal size, RNA to DNA ratio, amounts of protein and
less extensive dendritic arborization can be seen as the resultants
of a final common pathway metabolic slow-down produced by any one
of a number of limiting factors, both sensory and nonsensory.

The concept of a function-limiting factor raises several important therapeutic questions. The first of these concerns the
nature of the interaction between two or more limiting factors. Presumably the interaction can be additive or interactive so that the
effects of one factor exacerbate or protect against the effects of
another. Where neural insults follow one another sequentially, it
is important to know the nature of this interaction for the preventive purposes of identifying subjects at particular risk following
exposure to the first trauma. For example, if infants with a history of perinatal trauma or malnutrition subsequently exhibit reduced tolerance to variations in sensory input, then obviously
their environments and upbringing will require specific precautions
(see the chapters by both Richardson and Beckwith in this volume).

The nature of this interaction may be even more important when
we come to individuals subject to simultaneous risk factors. If
the nature of the interaction is additive, that at times of risk,
we must be particularly aware of subjects exposed to two or more
risk factors. However, if the nature of the interaction is protective, i.e. if the presence of deficiency A protects against the
effects of deficiency B, then intervention with Factor A prior to
remedying deficiency of factor B may be disastrous. Such situations
are not uncommon in medicine as for example, in the alcoholic undergoing withdrawal who is susceptible to both glucose and thiamine
deficiencies. If glucose is administered without thiamine, then the
increase in metabolic demands may precipitate life-threatening
central nervous system manifestations of thiamine deficiency. It
seems quite possible that a similar situation could occur where one
of the deficient factors is sensory stimulation. Perhaps stimulation should be kept to a minimum during the acute phases of malnutrition, hypothyroidism, trauma etc., in order to minimize metabolic
demands on marginally functioning neurons even though stimulation
in the post-acute rehabilitative phase might be extremely helpful.
There is some indirect evidence to support this concept. Following
brain damage, the disordered system may fail to respond at all to
stimulation, but during recovery, may evince a paradoxical response
known as supramarginal inhibition (Luria et al. 1969). During this
phase, weak stimuli elicit adequate responses whereas normal and
strong stimuli evoke no reaction, presumably due to functional overload of the neurons' reduced metabolic capacity.

Another question concerns the nature of the function limiting
factor in an apparently normal or recuperating brain without evidence

of nutritional, hormonal or sensory deficiencies. Presumably if
the nature of this factor could be determined, then its addition
would both hasten and increase the ceiling of development. Mathies
et al. (1973) have suggested that the rate limiting factor for RNA
synthesis, which is one of the initial stages in the proposed chemical mechanisms (Walsh and Cummins 1975) mediating the transduction of sensory stimulation into altered brain structure, is
pyrimidine precusor availability. A worthwhile experiment would
be to determine the effects of precursor administration on recovery
from brain damage. It may also be possible to extend the concept of
limiting factor interaction to the therapeutic use of anesthetic
agents and other brain activity inhibitors during acute brain damage
situations. For example, perhaps brief anesthesia during the acute
phase of thromboembolic stroke or perinatal anoxia would reduce the
metabolic demands of the oxygen deprived tissue to a level where
some additional neurons would survive until the insulting agent could
be removed. This is not to be confused with the approach of Ivanow-
Smolenski (1954), who anesthetized war trauma victims after the brain
injury in an effort to reduce Pavlovian inhibition which he felt to
be responsible for many behavioral deficits.

Effective Stimuli and a Reinforcment Perspective

A major question for studies of environmentally facilitated
recovery concerns the precise nature of the facilitating stimuli.
If this is known, then an orthosensory environment or therapeutic
regime can be designed. However, as yet all we have is some preliminary data concerning the stimuli which are most potent in
eliciting environmental complexity effects in normal brains. It
is apparent that subjects must interact physically with the stimuli
and it seems that reafferent stimulation may be particularly important (Ganz 1975; Walsh and Cummins 1975; Ferchmin et al. 1975;
Dru et al. 1975). The power of reafferent stimulation raises two
important points. Firstly, that the individual serves largely as
his own stimulus source, and secondly, that feedback information
may be especially valuable.

Feedback may be even more important in therapeutic situations.
Certainly it is one of the major functions of a therapist during
clinical rehabilitation (Luria et al. 1969). A possible important
future source of a special type of reafference may be biofeedback
which, in preliminary studies has proved promising for a variety
of brain dysfunctions ranging from the motor to the electroeceph-
alographic. In the presence of a therapist or biofeedback each
performance becomes a source of further corrective information and
reinforcement aimed specifically at the function under consideration. Ultimately performance and perceptual sensitivity may be
increased to a level at which feedback augmentation by therapist,
or instrumentation, are no longer necessary.

If reafferant input is important, and the individual serves largely as his own stimulus source, then the effects of environmental stimulation may be mediated by stimulation from the behavioral changes with which the individual responds to the environment. Thus, in addition to exerting a direct physiological effect on the nervous system, the sensory environment may also elicit recovery via its potential for eliciting therapeutic behavior. This raises the possibility of a whole new conceptual framework within which to view the effects of environmental stimulation on recovery; namely a reinforcement framework. Within such a framework, the therapeutic task becomes one of identifying the nature and magnitude of the behaviors associated with recovery and designing environments which are optimally reinforcing to them, that is, which tend to sustain or increase the frequency of appropriate behaviors.

The reinforcement framework allows a new perspective on one of the major, and most neglected, therapeutic problems, that of maintenance of therapeutic gains (Thoresen & Mahoney, 1974; Walsh et al., 1976. Intervention programs to date have emphasized the provision of short term stimulation to the subject. Where this leads to behavior which is intrinsically reinforcing (e.g. walking) then it is likely that these behaviors will generalize to other environments. However, as Hunt notes in this volume, other behaviors such as intellectual stimulus seeking may not be reinforced in home environments, a fact which may account for the transient nature of the intellectual gains found in programs such as Head Start. Once again, therefore, the therapeutic task becomes one of identifying therapeutic and therapy sustaining behavior and designing optimally reinforcing environments.

IMPLICATIONS, QUESTIONS AND FUTURE RESEARCH

The study of neural responses to therapeutic environments is obviously at an early stage. Relatively few factors have been investigated as yet and one of the immediate priorities must be to extend studies across a wider range of variables. The first of these variables is the nature of the lesion. Its pathophysiological form (trauma, endocrine, etc.) and acuity of onset are both important and there is already evidence to suggest that the sensory environment is important in determining the extent of the behavioral deficit which follows staged lesions (Isaac 1964; Worthington and Isaac 1967; see Greenough et al. this volume). The site of the lesion will obviously determine the nature and extent of the behavioral deficit and presumably the optimal variety of sensory input. In fact, future clinical studies will doubtless move in the direction of the more precise neuropsychological assessment of deficits in order to determine the precise nature of the optimal rehabilitative input.

The genetic, developmental and experiental history of the

individual must also be investigated since it is already apparent that there are wide individual differences in the behavioral sequelae of brain damage and sensory stimulation (Walsh and Cummins 1976). Presumably, similar differences in therapeutic reponsiveness will also be identified and comparison of responders and non-responders may provide some insight into the therapeutic process. Differential responsiveness according to age remains an unresolved question but studies, such as those of Cummins et al. (1973) indicate a far greater degree of cerebral plasticity in geriatric animals than previously thought possible and argue against the therapeutic nihilism which has so often permeated thinking about geriatric rehabilitation.

The brain regions and parameters under investigation also need extension. While changes within the focal area of damage are important, the Russian emphasis on perifocal protective inhibition and therapeutic disinhibition suggests that investigation of perifocal areas could be fruitful. The effects of rehabilitation on non-related neural areas have been accorded little importance. However, recent studies have revealed the gradual development of widespread ipsilateral brain atrophy following localized cerebral damage (Isaacson 1974; Will et al. 1975a;b) or lobotomy (Geschwind 1974). In the case of lobotomized patients, this atrophy parallels a slow decline in intellectual function (Hamlin 1970) and it may be that some behavioral sequalae of brain damage thought to be due to changes in the primary focus may actually reflect this type of secondary atrophy. On the other hand, compensatory hypertrophy is a possibility. It has been suggested as a basis for the hypertrophy of the auditory cortex in mice (Gyllensten et al. 1966; Ryugo et al. 1975) and somesthetic cortex in rats reared from birth in the dark to compensate for the reduced occipital cortex (Bennett, Rosenzweig and Krech 1964). Finally, of course, it is obvious that we need information on a wider range of anatomical, physiological and chemical parameters, preferably obtained from the same subjects and in conjunction with behavioral studies. As always, it is easier to suggest than to do such studies but it is hoped that the huge amount of information and the greater significance for meaningful interpretation which such studies afford, plus their potential for clinical application, may prove sufficiently rewarding to seduce some experimenters.

It is important to learn to what extent the findings derived from studies of environmental stimulation on normal brains are applicable to the brain damaged. For example, if the effects and mechanisms are similar then optimal treatment programs can be rationally planned on the basis of what is already known concerning normal brains. It also seems possible that some of the deprivation recovery studies already performed on the visual system may serve as useful clinical models. For example, monocular deprivation may serve as a model for aphasia rehabilitation following damage to the dominant speech center.

Another line of questioning concerns the temporal characteristics of recovery. The question of when to intervene may be very important in view of the preceding discussion on possible interactions between function limiting factors. Similarly, if we accept the hypothesis that initial therapeutic stimulation must exceed a certain threshold level to be effective, then in some situations it might be appropriate to apply simultaneous, multimodality stimulation rather than a graduated sequential program. Since certain cerebral effects of stimulation are partially transient, the question of maintaining gains arises. Presumably this could involve a number of "booster" sessions (reinstatement) or more effectively by reinforcement of those behaviors such as stimulus seeking, which are themselves effective in assisting recovery.

Assuming that environmental recovery programs continue to prove effective then one of the future research foci will doubtless be how to augment such recovery. One of the possibilities relates to the nature of the stimuli employed? To date a small range of therapeutic environments have been employed and a number of other sensory modalities such as vestibular stimulation (Korner 1973; Korner and Thoman 1972) may prove effective in some dysfunctions. Another approach may be to more precisely match the type of stimulus to the neuropsychological deficit. Other approaches will doubtless try to determine and treat the function limiting agent for each individual case, while combinations of sensory and pharmacological interventions may also prove useful.

Finally, an effort must be made to educate researchers and clinicians alike of the sensitivity of the nervous system both normal and damaged to its sensory environment. It took decades for reseachers to begin to appreciate the extent and sublety of environmental influences on behavior and one wonders how many of the now classic psychobiological controversies and multiple irreproducable results can be attributed to the fact that a wide range of rearing and experimental procedures have formerly been relegated to the role of maintenance routines. It has taken us even longer to appreciate the plasticity of brain anatomy and chemistry. Similarly, environmental sensory influences on the damaged brain have been almost completely ignored in the past, but we continue to do so at our own risk.

ACKNOWLEDGMENTS

Experimental work contributed by the authors and preparation of this manuscript was assisted by the Foundation Fund for Psychiatric Research and the Australian Research Grants Committee. We are grateful for the helpful comments of Dr. William Greenough, Dr. Tom Horvath and Professor Otto Budtz-Olsen.

REFERENCES

Ainsworth, M.D.S. 1973. The development of infant-mother attach-
    ment. In B.M. Caldwell and H.N. Riccuiti (Eds.). Review of
    Child Development Research, Vol. 3. University of Chicago
    Press, Chicago.

Altman, J., Wallace, R.B., Anderson, W.J., and Das, G.D. 1968.
    Behaviorally induced changes in length of cerebrum in rats.
    Develop. Psychobiol., 1:112-117.

Batkin, S., Groth, H., Watson, J., and Ansberry, M. 1970. Effects
    of auditory deprivation on the development of auditory sensit-
    ivity in albino rats. Electroenceph. Clin. Neurophysiol. 28:
    351-359.

Bennett, E.L., Rosenzweig, M.R. and Krech, D. 1964. Effects of
    postweaning blinding and light deprivation on retinas and
    brains of rats. Fed. Proc., 23:384.

Bennett, E.L., Rosenzweig, M.R., Diamond, M.C., Morimoto, H., and
    Herbert, M. 1974. Effects of successive environments on brain
    measures. Physiol. Behav., 12:621-631.

Bernstein, J.J., Gelderd, J., and Bernstein, M.F. 1975. Alteration
    of neuronal synaptic complement during regeneration and axonal
    sprouting of rat spinal cord. Exp. Neurol. (In Press).

Bkordlund, A. and Stenevi, V. 1972. Nerve growth factor: Stimu-
    lation of regenerative growth of central noradrenergic neurons.
    Science, 175: 1251-1253.

Braun, J.J., Meyer, P.M., and Meyer, D.R. 1966. Sparing of a bright-
    ness habit in rats following visual deterioration. J. Comp.
    Physiol. Psych. 61: 79-82.

Brown, C.P. and King, M.G. 1971. Developmental environment: Vari-
    ables important for later learning and changes in cholinergic
    activity. Develop. Psychobiol. 4: 275-286.

Castro, R.J. 1975. Ipsilateral corticospinal projections after
    large lesions of the cerebral hemisphere in neonatal rats.
    Exp. Neurol., 46: 1-8.

Chow, K.L. and Stewart, D.L. 1972. Reversal of structural and
    functional effects of long-term visual deprivation. Exp.
    Neurol., 34: 409-433.

Clarke-Stewart, K.A. 1974 . Interactions between mothers and their
    young children. Characteristics and consequences. Monographs
    Soc. Res. Child Develp. 38: (6-7, Serial No. 153).

Cragg, B.G. 1967. Changes in visual cortex on first exposure of
    rats to light: Effect on synaptic dimensions. Nature 215:
    251-253.

Cragg, B.G. 1974. Plasticity of synapses. Brit. Med. Bull.,
    30: 141-145.

Cummins, R.A. and Walsh, R.N. 1976. In preparation.

Cummins, R.A., Walsh, R.N., Budtz-Olsen, O.E., Kostantinos, T.,
    and Horsfall, C.R. 1973. Environmentally induced changes
    in the brains of old rats. Nature, 243:516-517.

Cummins, R.A., Budtz-Olsen, O.E., Walsh, R.N., and Worsley, A.
    1974. Testosterone, early experience and behavioral arousal
    in a novel environment. Horm. Behav., 5: 283-288.

Déjérine, J. 1914. Sémiologie des Affections de Systeme Nerveaux.
    Victor Masson et fils, Paris.

Dews, P.B. and Wiesel, T.N. 1970. Consequences of monocular de-
    privation on visual behavior in kittens. J. Physiol. 206:
    437-455.

Diamond, M.C., Law, F., Rhodes, H., Lindner, B., Rosenzweig, M.R.,
    Krech, D. and Bennett, E.L. 1966. Increases in cortical depth
    and glial numbers in rats subjected to enriched environments.
    J. Comp. Neurol. 128: 117-126.

Diaz, J., Ellison, G. and Masuoka, D. 1975. CNS response to injury
    in enriched and impoverished environments: A behavioral and
    neurochemical study in plasticity. Soc. Neurosci. Abst. 1:511.

Dru, D., Walker, J.P. and Walker, J.B. 1975. Self produced loco-
    motion restores visual capacity after striate lesions. Science.
    187: 265-266.

Fertig, A., Kierman, J.A. and Seyan, S. 1971. Enhancement of axonal
    regeneration in the brain of the rat by corticotrophin. Exp.
    Neurol. 33: 372-385.

Ferchmin, P.A., Bennett, E.L. and Rosenzweig, M.R. 1975. Direct
    contact with enriched environment is required to alter cere-
    bral weights in rats. J. Comp. Physiol. Psych. 88: 360-367.

Fifková, E. 1970a. The effect of monocular deprivation on the
    synaptic contacts of the visual cortex. J. Neurobiol., 1,
    285-294.

Fifková, E. 1970b. Changes of axosomatic synapses in the visual
    cortex of monocularly deprived rats. J. Neurobiol., 2, 61-
    71.

Fourment, A. and Scherrer, J. 1961. Responses electrocorticales
    du lapin élévé dans l'obscurité. J. Physiol. (Paris), 53:
    340-341.

Ganz, L. 1975. Orientation in visual space by neonates and its
    modification by visual deprivation, pp. 171-210.   In
    A.H. Riesen (Ed.). The Developmental Neuropsychology of
    Sensory Deprivation. Academic Press, New York.

Ganz, L. and Haffner, M.E. 1974. Permanent perceptual and neuro-
    physiological effects of visual deprivation in the cat. Exp.
    Brain Res., 20: 67-87.

Ganz, L., Fitch, M. and Satterberg, J.A. 1968. The selective
    effect of visual deprivation on receptive field shape deter-
    mined neurophysiologically. Exp. Neurol. 22:614-637.

Gazzaniga, M.S. 1974. Determinants of cerebral recovery. In
    D.G. Stein, J.J. Rosen and N. Butters (Eds.). Plasticity
    and Recovery of Function in the Central Nervous System.
    Academic Press, New York.

Geller, E., Yuwiler, A. and Zolman, J.F. 1965. Effects of environ-
    mental complexity on constituents of brain and liver. J.
    Neurochem. 12: 949-955.

Geller, E. 1971. Some observations on the effects of environmental
    complexity and isolation on biochemical ontogeny. pp. 277-
    296. In M.B. Sterman, D.J. McGinty and A.M. Adinolfi (Eds.).
    Brain Development and Behavior. Academic Press, New York.

Gendreau, P., Freedman, N.L., Wilde, G.J.S. and Scott, G.D. 1972.
    Changes in EEG alpha frequency and evoked response latency
    during solitary confinement. J. Abnorm. Psych. 79: 54-59.

Geschwind, N. 1974. Late changes in the nervous system: An over-
    view, pp. 467-508. In D.G. Stein, J.J. Rosen and N. Butters
    (Eds.). Plasticity and Recovery of Function in the Central
    Nervous System. Academic Press, New York.

Globus, A. 1975. Brain morphology as a function of presynaptic
    morphology and activity. In A.H. Riesen (Ed.). The Devel-
    opmental Neuropsychology of Sensory Deprivation. Academic
    Press, pp 9-92.

Globus, D., Rosenzweig, M.R., Bennett, E.L. and Diamond, M.C.
    1973. Effects of differential experience on dendritic
    spine counts in rat cerebral cortex. J. Comp. Physiol.82:
    175-181.

Goldberger, M.E. 1974. Recovery of movement after CNS lesions in
    monkeys. pp 265-338. In D.G. Stein, J.J., Rosen and N.
    Butters (Eds.). Plasticity and Recovery of Function in the
    Central Nervous System. Academic Press, New York.

Greenough, W.T. 1975. Experimental modification of the developing
    brain. Amer. Scientist, 63: 37-46.

Greenough, W.T. and Volkmar, F.R. 1973. Pattern of dendritic branch-
    ing in rat occipital cortex after rearing in complex environ-
    ments. Exp. Neurol. 40: 491-504.

Greenough, W.T., Volkmar, F. and Juraska, J.M. 1973. Effect of rear-
    ing complexity on dendritic branching in frontolateral and
    temporal cortex of the rat. Exp. Neurol. 41: 371-378.

Guillery, R.W. 1972. Binocular competition in the control of gen-
    iculate cell growth. J. Comp. Neurol. 144: 117-130.

Guth, L. 1974. Axonal regeneration and functional plasticity in
    the central nervous system. Exp. Neurol. 45: 606-654.

Gyllensten, L., Malmfors, T. and Norrlin, M. 1966. Growth altera-
    tion in the auditory cortex of visually deprived mice. J.
    Comp. Neurol. 126: 463-470.

Hamlin, R.M. 1970. Intellectual functions 14 years after frontal
    lobe surgery. Cortex, 6: 299-307.

Hein, A. 1970. Recovering spatial motor coordination after visual
    cortex lesion. pp. 163-175. In D.A. Hamburg, K.H. Pribram,
    and A.J. Stunkard (Eds.). Perception and Its Disorders.
    Williams and Wilkins, Baltimore.

Hicks, S.P. and D'Amato, C.J. 1970. Motor-sensory behavior after
    hemispherectomy in newborn and mature rats. Exper. Neurol.
    29: 416-438.

Hubel, D. and Wiesel, T.N. 1962. Receptive fields, binocular
    interaction and functional architecture in the cat's
    visual cortex. J. Physiol. 160: 106-154.

Hubel, D. and Wiesel, T.N. 1970. The period of susceptibility
    to the physiological effects of unilateral eye closure in
    kittens. J. Physiol. 206: 419-436.

Isaac, W. 1964. Role of stimulation and time in the effects of
    spaced occipital abalations. Psychol. Rep. 14: 151-154.

Isaacson, R.L. 1974. Recovery "?" from early brain damage. Paper
    presented at the National Conference on Early Intervention
    with High Risk Infants and Young Children. Chapel Hill.

Ivanow-Smolenski, A.G. 1954. Srundzuge der pathophysiologie der
    holeren Nerventatigkeit. Akademic Verlag. Berlin.

Kalil, R.E. 1973. Formation of new retino-geniculate connections
    in kittens: Effects of age and visual experience. Anat. Rec.
    175: 353.

Kalil, R.E. 1975. Recovery from dark rearing: Behavioral and ana-
    tomical observations. Soc. Neurosci. Abstr. 1: 85.

Konrad, K. and Melzack, R. 1975. Novelty enhancement effects
    associated with early sensory-social isolation. In A.H.
    Riesen (Ed.). The Developmental Neuropsychology of Sensory
    Deprivation. Academic Press, New York, pp 253-276.

Korner, A. 1973. Early stimulation and maternal care as related
    to infant capabilities and individual differences. Early
    Child Development and Care 2: 307-327.

Korner, A.and Thoman, E.B. 1972. The relative efficacy of con-
    tact and vestibular proprioceptive stimulation in soothing

neonates. Child Development. 43: 443-453.

LeVere, T.T. 1975. Neural stability, sparing and behavioral recovery following brain damage. Psych. Bull. 82: 344-358.

Luria, A.R., Naydin, V.L., Tsvetkova, L.S. and Vinarskaya, E.N.
  1969. Restoration of higher cortical function following
  local brain damage. pp. 368-433. In P.J. Vinken and G.W.
  Bruyer (Eds.). Handbook of Clinical Neurology, Vol. 3.
  North-Holland Publishing Co. Amsterdam.

Lynch, G., Stanfield, B., Parks, T. and Gotman, C.W. 1974.
  Evidence for selective postlesion growth in the dentate
  gyrus of the rat. Brain Res. 69: 1-11.

Lynch, G., Smith, R. and Cotman, C.W. 1975. Recovery of function
  following brain damage: A consideration of some neural
  mechanisms. In A. Tobias and A. Buerger (Eds.). The Neurophysiological Basis of Rehabilitative Medicine. Thomas
  Springfield, Ill.

Marcos, A.R. and Valverde, F. 1970. Dynamic architecture of the
  visual cortex. Brain Res. 19: 25-39.

Mathies, H., Lossner, B., Ott, T., Pohle, W. and Rauca, C. 1973.
  The intraneuronal regulation of neuronal connectivity.
  Proc. 5th Internat. Cong. Pharmacol. 4: 29-38.

Meisami, E. and Timiras, P.S. 1971. Influence of early visual
  input on development of brain excitability in the rat.
  Amer. J. Physiol. 220: 233-238.

Merrill, E.G. and Wall, P.D. 1972. Factors forming the edge of a
  receptive field: The presence of relatively ineffective
  afferent terminals. J. Physiol. 226: 825-846.

Milner, B. 1973. Hemispheric specialization: Scope and limits,
  pp 75-89. In F.O. Schmitt and F.G. Worden (Eds.). The
  Neurosciences: Third Study Program. M.I.T. Press, Cambridge, Mass.

Moore, R.Y. 1974. Central regeneration and the recovery of function: The problem of collateral reinnervation. In D.C.
  Stein, J.J. Rosen and N. Butters, (Eds.). Plasticity and
  the Recovery of Function in the Central Nervous System.
  Academic Press, New York. pp 111-128.

Movshon, J.A. and Blakemore, C. 1975. Functional reinnervation in
  kitten visual cortex. Nature, 251: 504-505.

Nathan P. and Smith, M. 1973. Effects of two unilateral cordotomies
  on the motilities of the lower limbs. Brain 96: 471-494.

Reige, W.H. and Morimoto, H. 1970. Effects of chronic stress and
  differential environments upon btain weight and biogenic
  amine levels in rats. J. Comp. Physiol. Psych. 71: 396-404.

Rizzolatti, F. and Tradari, V. 1971. Pattern discrimination in monocularly reared cats. Exp. Neurol. 33: 181-194.

Rose, S.P.R. 1967. Changes in visual cortex on first exposure to light: Effect on incorporation of tritiated lysine into protein. Nature 215: 233-235.

Rose, S.P.R. and Sinha, A.K. 1974. Incorporation of 3H-Lysine into a rapidly labelling neuronal protein fraction in visual cortices is suppressed in dark reared rats. Life Sci., 15: 223-230.

Rosenzweig, M.R. and Bennett, E.L. 1972. Cerebral changes in rats exposed individually to an enriched environment. J. Comp. Physiol. Psych. 80: 304-313.

Rosenzweig, M.R., Krech, D., Bennett, E.L. and Zolman, J.F. 1962. Variation in environmental complexity and brain measures. J. Comp. Physiol. Psych. 55: 1092-1095.

Rosenzweig, M.R., Bennett, E.L. and Diamond, M.C. 1967. Effects of differential environments on brain anatomy and brain chemistry. Proc. Amer. Psychopath. Assn. 56: 45-56.

Rosenzweig, M.R., Bennett, E.L., Diamond, M.C. 1972. Chemical and anatomical plasticity of brain: Replications and extensions. In J. Gaito (Ed.). Macromolecules and Behavior. 2nd edition. Appleton-Century-Crofts, New York, pp 205-278.

Ruiz-Marcos, A. and Valverde, F. 1970. Dynamic architecture of the visual cortex. Brain Res. 19: 25-39.

Ryugo, D.K., Ryugo, R., Globus, A. and Killachey, H.P. 1975. Increased spine density in auditory cortex following visual or somatic deafferentation. Brain Res. 90: 143-146.

Sarno, M.T. 1970. Speech therapy and language recovery in severe aphasia. J.S.H.R. 13: 607-625.

Scherrer, J. and Fourment, A. 1964. Electrocortical effects of sensory deprivation during development. In W. Himwich and H. Himwich (Eds.). Progress in Brain Research, Vol. 9, Elselvier Amsterdam, pp 103-112.

Sherman, S.M. 1974. Monocularly deprived cats: Improvement of the deprived eye's vision by visual decortication. Science, 186: 267-269.

Sherman, S.M. and Sanderson, K.J. 1972. Binocular interaction on cells of the dorsal lateral geniculate nucleus of visually deprived cats. Brain Res. 37: 126-131.

Shilyagina, N.N. 1973. Electrical activity of the cortical and subcortical parts of the rabbit brain following early visual deprivation. J. Higher Nerv. Act. I. Pavlov, 5: 1066-1073.

Sotelo, C. and Palay, S.L. 1971. Altered axons and axon terminals in the lateral vestibular nucleus of the rat. Lab. Invest. 25: 653-671.

Stern, P., McDowell, F., Miller, J.M. and Robinson, M. 1971. Factors influencing stroke rehabilitation. Stroke, 2:213-218.

Thoreson, C.E. and Mahoney, M.J. 1974. Behavioral Self-Control Holt, Rinehart and Winston, New York.

Valverde, F. 1967. Apical dendritic spines of the visual cortex and light deprivation in the mouse. Exp. Brain Res. 3: 337-352.

Valverde, F. 1971. Rate and extent of recovery from dark rearing in the visual cortex of the mouse. Exp. Brain Res. 33:1-12.

Vrensen, G. and deGroot, D. 1974. The effect of dark rearing and its recovery on synaptic terminals in the visual cortex of rabbits. A quantitative electron microscopic study. Brain Res. 78: 263-278.

Wall, P.D. and Egger, M.D. 1971. Formation of new connections in adult rat brain after partial deafferentation. Nature 232: 542-545.

Walsh, R.N. and Cummins, R.A. 1975. Mechanisms mediating the production of environmentally induced brain changes. Psych. Bull. 82: 986-1000.

Walsh, R.N. and Cummins, R.A. 1976. The Open Field Test: A critical review, Psych. Bull. (In Press).

Walsh, R.N., Budtz-Olsen, O.E. Penny., J.E. and Cummins, R.A. 1969. The effects of environmental complexity on the histology of the rat hippocampus. J. Comp. Neurol. 131: 361-365.

Walsh, R.N., Budtz-Olsen, O.E., Torok, A. and Cummins, R.A. 1971a. Environmentally induced changes in the dimensions of the rat cerebrum. Develop. Psychobiol. 4: 115-122.

Walsh, R.N., Cummins, R.A., Budtz-Olsen, O.E., O'Rourke, G., Brown, H. and Cameron, J. 1971b. Effects of environmental enrichment and deprivation on cerebral histology and composition. Proc. Austral. Soc. Med. Res. 2: 478.

Walsh, R.N., Cummins, R.A., Budtz-Olsen, O.E. and Torok, A. 1972. Effects of environmental enrichment and deprivation on rat frontal cortex. Internat. J. Neurosci. 4: 239-242.

Walsh, R.N., Cummins, R.A. and Budtz-Olsen, O.E. 1973. Environmentally induced changes in the dimensions of the rat cerebrum: A replication and extension. Develop. Psychobiol. 6:3-8.

Walsh, R.N., Cummins, R.A., Budtz-Olsen, O.E., Lee, A.S., Davidson, P.G. and Davidson, B.J. 1974. Alterations in neuronal pleomorphism within the dentate gyrus following environmental sensory stimulation: An indication of increased postnatal neuron formation? Paper presented at the Internat. Soc. Develop. Psychobiol. Ann. Meet. St. Louis, October.

Walsh, R.N., McAllister, A., Taylor, B. and Ferguson, J. 1976. The Smoking Therapies. Plenum, New York (In Press).

Wiesel, T.N. and Hubel, D. 1963a. Effects of visual deprivation on morphology and physiology of cells in the cats lateral geniculate body. J. Neurophysiol. 26: 978-993.

Wiesel, T.N. and Hubel, D. 1963b. Single cell response in striate cortex of kittens deprived of vision in one eye. J. Neurophysiol. 26: 1003-1017.

Wiesel, T.N. and Hubel, D. 1965a. Comparison of the effects of unilateral and bilateral eye closure on cortical unit reponses in kittens. J. Neurophysiol. 28: 1029-1040.

Will, B.E., Rosenzweig, M.R.,and Bennett, E.L. 1975a. Effects of differential environments on recovery from neonatal brain lesions, measured by problem solving scores and brain dimensions. (In preparation).

Will, B.E., Rozenzweig, M.R., Bennett, E.L., Herbert, M. and Morimoto, H. 1975b. Relatively brief environmental enrichment aids recovery of learning capacity and alters brain measures after postweaning brain lesions in rats. (In preparation).

Williams, M. and Scarr, S. 1971. Effects of short term intervention on performance in low birth weight disadvantaged children. Paediatrics. 47: 289.

Wilson, J.R. and Sherman, S.M. 1975. Effects of monocular deprivation on cat striate cortex. Soc. Neurosci. Abstr. 1:86.

Worthington, C.S. and Isaac, W. 1967. Occipital ablation and retention of a visual conditioned avoidance response in the rat. Psychol. Sci. 8: 289-290.

Yarrow, L.S., Rubenstein, F.J., Pederson, F.A. and Jankowski, J.J. 1972. Dimensions of early stimulation and their differential effects on infant development. Merrill-Palmer Quarterly, 18: 205-218.

ENVIRONMENTAL PROGRAMMING TO FOSTER COMPETENCE AND PREVENT MENTAL

RETARDATION IN INFANCY[1]

J. McVicker Hunt

Department of Psychology
University of Illinois
Champaign, Illinois 61820

The idea of arranging environmental encounters in the care of infants to promote competence and good character is as old as the classical thought of the Greeks. In the Laws (Book VII, 788ff), Plato has his Athenian stranger contend that lawgivers should stress the importance of nurture and education in achieving citizens with characters appropriate for the good of the state. On the other hand, this idea is also new. From the time of Plato until the beginning of the twentieth century, exceedingly few of the philosophers who concerned themselves with education and the development of moral character considered nurture and experience during infancy and early childhood to be of significance in the adult outcome of human development. Aries (1960) has described the gradual discovery through the centuries of childhood in the institutional practices of the family and the school. This evolving discovery has continued into the twentieth century, as the age when causal significance attributed to the environments encountered has been extended downward to birth and even to the emotional and nutritional state of the maternal host at conception and during gestation (see Hunt, 1969, Chap. 7).

Programming the environment in child care has been conducted under such rubrics as nurture, child-rearing practices, and early

1 The work underlying what is summarized here has been supported by grants from the Russell Sage Foundation, the Carnegie Corporation, the Commonwealth Fund, the United States Public Health Service (MH-18567, MH-08468, MH-10226, and MH-16074) and the Office of Child Development (SRS-OCD-CB-03) and the writing of this paper by USPH MH-11321.

education. This chapter will focus on such programming to foster
competence and to prevent mental retardation. Here mental retardation should not be confused with hereditary mental deficiency which
does exist in a small portion of the population. In this paper, I
shall first identify the conceptual fictions[2] that have guided early
educational practice and provided the historical roots for the
several traditions in the investigation of early development.
Second, I shall indicate the nature of the various lines of evidence
that weakened the faith in predeterminism and built sufficient faith
in environmental influence to permit the launching of Project Head
Start. Third, I shall describe why Project Head Start failed to
fulfill the unrealistic hopes for it. Fourth, I shall summarize the
research on how to foster psychological development and the attempts
to uncover relationships of specific competencies to antecedent
experiences. Finally, I shall indicate the possibilities of early
education with illustrations of the range of reaction in certain
phenotypic measures.

I. CONCEPTUAL FICTIONS

The conceptual fictions concerning the nature of early development, and the role of experience (or encounters with environmental
circumstances) in development can be grouped under four main headings: (1) preformationism, (2) predeterminism, (3) environmentalism,
and (4) interactionism.

A. Preformationism

Development has always been puzzling. Especially puzzling has
been that occurring between the conception and the birth of an
infant mammal or that metamorphosis occurring between the egg and
the adult forms of an insect. Once men began to distinguish reality
from the appearance of things, they found it hard to believe what
they seemed to observe in embryological development. Thus,
Anaxagoras asserted that "hair could not come from not-hair nor
flesh out of not-flesh" (Cornford, 1930). Later, Hippocrates
claimed that, "Everything in the embryo is formed simultaneously.
All the limbs separate themselves at the same time and so grow, none
comes before or after other, but those which are naturally bigger
appear before the smaller, without being formed earlier" (Needham,
1959, p. 34). When Van Leeuwenhoek, the inventor of the compound
microscope, and others, began using it to examine the ova and semen
of various species, they first reported seeing animalcules resembling
the species concerned. It was not until after the middle of the
eighteenth century that the Russian investigator, C. F. Wolff,
finally disposed of the fiction of preformationism in embryology
with his classic demonstrations of an epigenesis in the development
of the circulatory system and the intestines in chick embryos (see
Needham, 1959).

Despite the demise of this fiction of preformationism in embryology, its corollaries in epistemology, probably originating with Plato, and theology continued in various versions of nativism to be of influence. One version was the doctrine of innate ideas held by such philosophers as Descartes, Spinoza, and Leibnitz. It was against this doctrine that John Locke (1690) took his stand in his famous Essay Concerning Human Understanding. Another version from Immanuel Kant's Critique of Pure Reason contended that the central factor in knowing is the synthetic power of the mind achieved through such inherent organizing categories as object, causality, space, and time, for sense perception and as quantity, quality, and relation, for judgment. It is for such categories that Piaget (see e.g., 1937 and Inhelder and Piaget, 1955) has been at pains to show a developmental epigenesis growing out of a child's informational interaction with his physical and social environment. Yet another version has persisted in the Gestalt view of perception (Koehler, 1929), and other nativistic views of perception persist (Pastore, 1960).

Theological nativism in the doctrine of original sin has helped to justify through history the practice of punishing children for misbehavior. After Martin Luther's reformation made learning to read important not only as a source of knowledge but as an avenue to salvation, universal education was a consequence. Calvin later blamed the inattentiveness of young children to the Biblical text that served as a primer, on their inherent depravity. Schools were therefore typically rough places through the seventeenth, eighteenth, and much of the nineteenth centuries (see Aries, 1960).

A major transition began with Rousseau. In opposition to this idea of original sin and to the corollary notion that the arts and sciences improve man, Rousseau proclaimed his doctrine of the innate goodness of man or the superiority of the noble savage over civilized man, and the damaging effects of social institutions. In his novel, Emile ou l'education, Rousseau (1762) embraced the idea of a developmental epigenesis in the minds of children. His views spread like wildfire. They influenced such educational reformers as Pestalozzi, who was perhaps the first modern educator to give voice to the importance of an individual's own nature and needs in the educational process. Although Pestalozzi was perhaps the first of the educational psychologists, it was Johann Friedrich Herbart (1806) who first attempted to write a science of education. Rousseau's influence extended through Pestalozzi and Herbart to Friedrich Froebel who launched the kindergarten movement. Froebel postulated a divine unity in each child that would unfold as he encountered situations appropriate to his development. Froebel's (1838) Education by Development shows clearly the beginnings of an appreciation of the ongoing organism-environment interaction in development. Thus, Rousseau precipitated a reaction against preformationism that ultimately spawned one of the major institutions

of early education, the kindergarten, with its emphasis on providing educational situations matched to the child's level of
development.

B. Predeterminism

As he disposed of the doctrine of preformationism with his
classic demonstrations of the epigenesis in the circulatory and
intestinal systems of chick embryos, C. F. Wolff attempted to
explain the course of epigenetic changes of structure he had
observed by borrowing Leibnitz's idea of a monad developing into
an organism through its own inherent force and direction. This
set the stage for the fiction of predeterminism. The course of the
epigenesis might be attributed to a Leibnitzian monad, to God, as
it was in Calvinistic theology, or to heredity, as it came to be
by Herbert Spencer, Charles Darwin, and most of the biological
thinkers in the nineteenth century. When Francis Galton (1869)
wrote Hereditary Genius, he embraced the fiction of predeterminism
by attributing class differences and race differences almost
completely to heredity. Assuming that education would be futile
as a means of improving man's lot, moreover, he founded the
eugenics movement. He also invented the coefficient of correlation
and founded an anthropometric laboratory to give tests. When his
test measures of such simple functions as reaction time and the
speed of tapping failed to correlate with indices of eminence,
Galton was disappointed. Nevertheless, he carried on with his
eugenics movement.

It was Alfred Binet who invented the kind of tests that
established the psychometric tradition. Binet had been asked to
seek the basis for the failures of many children in the Paris
schools. With his collaborators, Victor Henri and Theodore Simon,
he began testing more complex functions such as judgment, memory,
and reasoning. The resulting test performances did correlate with
teachers' valuations of the quality of the students' academic performances. When Binet and Simon (1905) hit upon the notion of
mental age, they launched the psychometric tradition. The fact
that success on any item of the test could substitute for that on
any other item rendered mental age also a way to hide the details
of development. It failed to hide them completely as studies of
scatter on the Stanford-Binet scales (see Harris and Shakow, 1938)
and discrepancies between scores on language tests and performance
tests (Babcock, 1930) have shown. Binet's tests of judgment,
memory, and vocabulary, clearly called for information deriving
from experience. Binet saw no harm in this because he contended
that, "the intelligence of children may be increased. One increases
that which constitutes the intelligence in a school child, namely,
the capacity to learn, to improve with instruction" (Binet, 1909,
p. 55). Yet, when Wilhelm Stern (1912) divided each child's mental
age by his chronological age to obtain the IQ, this ratio provided

a number that appeared to assess a fixed measure of a child's
competence, his intelligence. From an operational standpoint,
this ratio represents a kind of average rate of achieving abilities
and information. The fact that the IQs of school age children
exhibited considerable validity in predicting the quality of their
performances in school fit Galton's purposes better than Binet's.
Thus, with the fiction of predeterminism dominating the conceptual
climate of the day, the IQ came to represent not only the achieved
competence of an individual, but a constant, predictive index of
his potential level of competence as well.

Another important adherent of predeterminism who indirectly
influenced both the interpretation of test performances and the
strategy of investigating children's development was G. Stanley
Hall, a self-proclaimed "Darwin of the Mind" (Pruette, 1926).
Because he viewed early behavioral development as preprogrammed
recapitulation of man's evolutionary history, Hall considered that
special efforts at nurture and education, especially in the early
years, could only hamper development. Hall taught by means of
parables. One of his favorites was that of the tadpole's tail.
If one amputates the tail of a frog-tadpole, the hind legs fail to
develop. Hall used this as a metaphor of behavioral development to
imply that disciplinary interference with a child's activity could
only hamper the appearance of the new phase predetermined to emerge
from the punished activity. Hall went on to establish the child-
study movement in America, and his teachings constitute the earliest
basis for what later became laissez-faire child-rearing.

Hall also founded Clark University, modeled on the graduate,
research universities of Germany. Among his early students were
three of the most influential in the establishment of the intelligence testing movement in America, H. H. Goddard, Franz Kühlmann,
and Lewis M. Terman. Another of these early students, Arnold L.
Gesell, exploited the normative approach to child development,
which consists of describing the characteristics of children at
each age, and which was the dominant tradition to at least 1950.
In view of this history, it can be no surprise that the conceptual
fiction of predeterminism has dominated not only the intelligence-
testing movement, but psychometrics in general, and has until
recently, controlled the strategy of investigating psychological
development.

Despite Sigmund Freud's preoccupation with inherited motivational systems, or drives, it is perhaps not unfair to say that he
launched the modern concern with early experience in opposition to
predeterminism. In the second of his Three Contributions to the
Theory of Sex, Freud (1905) wrote, "It is quite remarkable that
those writers who endeavored to explain the qualities and reactions
of the adult have given so much more attention to the ancestral
period than to the period of the individual's own existence --

that is, they have attributed more influence to heredity than to
childhood." Freud then described "infantile sexuality," wherein
he introduced the theory of psychosexual development. This theory
assumed that the sex drive, the libido, was ready-made at birth.
In the course of the first three to five years, this drive was
sequentially localized in the mouth, the anus, and the genitals.
Either too much gratification or too little gratification (frustration) would fixate the infant's development at the stage concerned.
Thus, early in the oral phase, what Erikson (1950) has called an
"incorporative mode" or a passive acceptance of conditions, is
dominant. An infant fixated at this phase adopts not only that form
of obtaining gratification, but the attitude of vapid optimism in
which the world as a whole is seen as analagous to an ever flowing
breast. Each successive zone similarly involved an early and a late
phase, each with its own metaphorical mode of adaptation. Fixation
at any level and mode would lead to later difficulties in adapting
to the real world. Despite the difficulty of assessing the antecedent condition of excessive gratification or excessive frustration,
this theory of psychosexual development served as a conceptual guide
to a majority of the empirical studies of personality development
and socialization until the 1950s, and it continues to provide the
conceptual framework for a good many.

C. Environmentalism

Environmentalism has its historical roots in the empiricism of
John Locke. When Locke (1690) asserted, "There exist no innate
ideas," he was expressing his moral defiance of the medieval fiction
of preformationism. The positive side of this assertion led Locke
(Book II) to postulate, "mind to be, as we say, white paper, void
of all characters, without ideas." Locke then asked how mind comes
to be furnished, and he answered, "From experience." Experience,
for Locke, included the information obtained through the senses and
that deriving from reflection on sensory input.

The modern counterpart of Locke's "white paper" may be seen in
the multiplicity of reflexes implicit in Thorndike's (1898) early
theory of animal intelligence and explicit in Watson's (1926)
Behaviorism: A Psychology Based on Reflexes. Investigators of
infant development took great pains in describing in detail this
reflexive base of original human nature (see Dennis, 1934). Since
each of these reflexes could presumably come to be evoked by a great
variety of receptor inputs through classical conditioning and could
come to be sequentially combined, or changed, in an infinite variety
of ways, the variations of possible outcomes of development in levels
of competence and in personal inclinations would appear to be
essentially unlimited.

This extreme environmentalistic fiction of psychological development did, however, include a place for maturation. The reflexes

which became classically conditioned and sequentially chained were presumed to be unlearned. They emerged automatically with the maturation of somatic and neural anatomy. Learning, at least in the early phase of such theorizing, consisted chiefly in connecting unlearned units with new stimuli and with each other (see Thorndike, 1913a, 1913b; Watson, 1916, 1917).

This connectionist theory was shared in its essentials by Thorndike and Watson but was later modified by Clark Hull. A kind of synthesis between the motivational aspect of Freud's (1915) psychoanalytic drive theory with behaviorism became Hullian learning theory (Hull, 1943; Miller and Dollard, 1941). Another modification came via Skinner (1938) who classified encounters with the environment under two types: Type I, or "operant conditioning," and Type II, the classical conditioning of Pavlov. Operant conditioning involved what Thorndike had included under trial-and-error learning and what Hull (1943) called "instrumental learning." What made any behavioral pattern "operant" was its appearance without specifiable stimulation. The likelihood of any given operant response occurring under given stimulation could be increased through reinforcement. Skinner defined reinforcement in circular fashion as an outcome which increases the frequency with which an operant is emitted. Reinforcement for Hull (1943), on the other hand, required a reduction in the drive. In Skinnerian "shaping," the form of the action, or response, is progressively altered toward a prescribed form by reinforcing each modification that more closely approximates the prescription. In taking such a radical empirical stance, the Skinnerians neglect the origin of the reinforcements they use and thereby relegate their enterprise to the status of a technology, albeit a powerful and sometimes very useful technology.

Throughout this twentieth century, the dominant conceptions of psychological development have been predeterminism and environmentalism. Predeterminism has dominated the psychometric branch of the discipline and environmentalism has dominated the experimental psychology of learning. Predeterminism, as expressed in the normative approach of Arnold Gesell (1954), has also dominated child psychology until the late 1950s when investigators began in force to seek infants and young children as subjects in learning experiments. A major exception to this statement is to be found in those studies of personality development stemming from Freud's (1905) theory of psychosexual development. One consequence of having a science operate with two such antithetical conceptual fictions of development has been a continuing debate over which is the more important. Another consequence has been a relative absence of concern for how hereditary ontology or maturation interacts with the sequence of environmental encounters to produce a variety of phenotypic outcomes even though lip-service was often given to the necessity for both heredity and environment and for their interaction (see e.g., Woodworth's Textbook of Psychology).

D. Interactionism

The concept of interactionism has its historical origin
within this century. The concept was introduced by Wilhelm Ludwig
Johannsen, the Dutch botanist who coined the term gene -- disting-
uished the genotype -- the hereditary constitution of the individual from the phenotype -- the observable and measurable characteristics of the individual. Through his own research he discovered
that the same genotype may give rise to various phenotypic characteristics under differing environmental circumstances and that the same
environment may have differing effects upon different genotypic
strains within a given species (Johannsen, 1909). A major share of
the investigations of interaction have utilized plants and insects
as subjects. Thus, for instance, the relative acidity of the soil
may influence the colors of flowers one observes in sweet peas, and
the effect of a given pH value may vary with the genotype of the
peas. Similarly, in snow-pool mosquitoes common to northern lati-
tudes, raising the temperature to which the eggs and larvae are
exposed during development to $29^{\circ}C$ results in 100 rather than in
50 per cent of adult mosquitoes with phenotypic female anatomy
(Horsfall and Anderson, 1961). A great variety of such genotype-
environmental interactions have been reported (see Dobzhansky,
1951, Ch. 2).

A mere listing of such interactions, however, fails to recognize the full implications of interactionism for anatomical and
behavioral development over an extended period of time and through
an extended series of environmental encounters. From a developmental standpoint, original nature exists only in the zygote.
Certain traits such as the blood groups are irrevocably fixed by
the genotype comprising the zygote, but others, such as emotional
and intellectual development, are susceptible to substantial phenotypic variation through adaptive modifications of ready-made sensorimotor organizations, skills, and conceptions. Development for such
traits is a dynamic process in which the infant or child brings to
each environmental encounter the competencies he has already
achieved. If the environmental circumstances in the encounter call
only for ready-made competencies, the child uses them and no development occurs. Repetitions of such encounters lead to boredom and
ultimately withdrawal or apathy. If the circumstances encountered
call for competencies beyond the child's temporary adaptive capacity,
they evoke frustrative distress, withdrawal, and no development.
If, on the other hand, the circumstances call for modifications in
the child's repertoire of competencies of which he is capable, they
typically evoke both interest and growth (see Hunt, 1965). For an
environmental encounter to produce such growth, it must match the
competencies of the child and his capacity for adaptive modification.
The amount of phenotypic variation that a life's series of such
encounters can produce in a given genotype deserves far more study,
particularly in human beings, than it has heretofore received.

This question of amount of variation, or range of reaction, will
be taken up later in the chapter.

In his presidential address to the American Psychological
Association, Cronbach (1957) described psychometrics and the
psychology of learning as the two disciplines of scientific
psychology, and recommended a synthesis. Ideally, a psychometric
test should provide a prescription of educational treatment. On
the whole, the efforts to bring about such a synthesis have largely
failed. This failure, I believe, results from the norm-referenced
nature of nearly all psychometric tests. Instead of defining the
attainments of an individual along the ordinal hierarchies in the
various branches of development, they serve merely to compare
individuals and to indicate where within a normative sample an
individual falls on the measure of a trait, a skill, or of information. Psychometric scores have little in common either with the
concrete attainments of information and competence or with the
concrete criteria of success in given learning tasks. The typical
psychometric strategy of measuring individual differences is, thus,
poorly adapted to the task Cronbach gave to psychometric tests in
his hoped-for synthesis of the two disciplines of scientific psychology.

The observations and theorizing of Jean Piaget (1936, 1937,
1945) suggest an alternative approach to developmental assessment
that may ultimately be more successful in predicting the outcome
of educational treatments. Thus far, this approach has been
realized only for the sensorimotor phase of development. Uzgiris
and Hunt (1975) have devised a set of scales that identify steps
of developmental achievement along seven branches of sensorimotor
development. These scales are ordinal in character, and evidence
is accumulating that this ordinality represents sequential achievements. The seven branches concern object permanence, methods of
obtaining desired environmental events, gestural imitation, vocal
imitation, operational causality, object relations in space, and
schemes for relating to objects. Rearing conditions interacting
with individual differences affect the rate of achieving the
successive steps on these scales, as discussed later in this
chapter. Thus, performance on these scales can be utilized as
an aid in selecting sequential variations in environmental circumstances to promote the development of the individual child as well
as to assess the effects of various kinds of child-rearing.

II. LINES OF EVIDENCE DISSONANT WITH PREDETERMINISM

The political philosophy expressed in the Declaration of
Independence and the Constitution of the United States has tended
to keep alive in America a faith in environmental influence.
Nevertheless, for the first half of this century, anyone

entertaining the idea of increasing the "natural" competence of
human beings by arranging the environmental circumstances to be
encountered was regarded as an unrealistic do-gooder by authorities
in psychometrics and education. The psychometricians in the
intelligence testing movement considered intelligence to be fixed
in an essentially constant IQ. Moreover, comparisons of the correlations between the IQs from pairs of individuals with differing
proportions of genes in common led to estimates that from 80 to 90
per cent of the variance in the IQ was due to heredity, leaving no
more than 20 per cent attributable to the environment (see revival
of this view by Jensen, 1969). Moreover, the predeterministic
fiction helped justify the prevailing normative approach to the
investigation of development epitomized in the work of Arnold
Gesell. So long as these fictions of fixed intelligence and predetermined development prevailed, the observed characteristics of
races, classes, and individuals were considered to be inevitable.
So long as such fictions ruled the climate of expert scientific
opinion, launching anything like Project Head Start was unthinkable.
The role of education was limited to the inculcation of academic
skills. By the early 1960s, however, several lines of evidence
dissonant with these fictions had combined to make such a project
realistically hopeful.

A.   Institutional Infant-Rearing

Long before the turn of the twentieth century, various physicians and others had noted the poor anatomical development, the
apathy, and the retardation in the behavior of infants and young
children being reared in understaffed orphanages (see Bowlby, 1951).
For the most part, these developmental deficiencies were explained
in terms of defective heredity for the fiction of predetermined
development prevailed. Here and there, however, physicians noted
that the effects could be reversed merely by transferring infants
from orphanages to homes. Even as early as 1908, Chapin, a prominent pediatrician, devised a foster home system to be used in the
place of orphanages and in 1925, Woolley reported an improvement in
tested intelligence in orphanage children from nursery schooling.
A pioneering study of the effects of transferring infants from an
orphanage to a ward for women in an institution for the mentally
deficient by Skeels and Dye (1939) got ridiculed at the time, but
it has since become a classic. This study was prompted by a
"clinical surprise." Two grossly apathetic and retarded infant
residents of a state orphanage were committed to the institution
for the mentally deficient. There they became pets of the moron
women on the ward. Six months later, they had shown remarkable
development. When retested with the Kühlmann scale, the younger
one, transferred at 13 months, showed an improvement in Developmental Quotient of 31 points (from 46 to 77), and the older one,
transferred at age 16 months, showed a change of 52 points (from
35 to 87). In consequence of this surprise, 11 more infants

aged from seven to 30 months, with DQs ranging from 36 to 89 and
a mean of 64.3 were transferred to such wards for women in the
institution for the mentally deficient. For contrast, 12 other
infants aged from 12 to 22 months, with DQs ranging from 50 to 103
and a mean of 87, were kept in the orphanage for observation. When
these 25 infants were retested following periods ranging from six
to 52 months, all those who had been transferred had gained. The
gains ranged from seven to 58 points. On the other hand, all but
two of those remaining in the orphanage showed a substantial
decrease in DQ. The decreases ranged from eight to 45 points with
five of the 12 exceeding 35 points. Although it would seem ridi-
culous to send infants from an orphanage to an institution for the
mentally deficient to improve their intelligence, and a critic can
readily find fault with this study, the findings clearly suggest
that the apathy, retardation, and smallness of stature in orphanage-
reared infants is a matter of experience. Since then other investigations have confirmed this explanatory view (for reviews, see
Ainsworth, 1962; Stone, 1954; Yarrow, 1961). This study did more.
It also suggested the existence of considerable plasticity in the
rate of behavioral development with environmental circumstances
and that this plasticity could show as either a decrease or an
increase in the rate of development depending upon the nature of
the environmental circumstances with which infants interact.
Furthermore, such an empirically-based suggestion would in turn
imply that the basis for the observed constancy in the IQ for a
majority of children may as well reside in consistency of the development-fostering qualities of the environments in which they live
as in their individual genotypes.

     Some 25 years later, Skeels (1966) investigated the adult
status of these children. The increased rate of development in
those transferred to the women's wards of the institution for
mental deficiency made them more attractive and they were adopted.
At the time of the follow-up, all 13 were self-supporting, 11 of
the 13 had married, and nine of these were parents. In this group,
the median educational attainment was high school graduation. Their
occupations ranged from semi-skilled labor to professional. On the
other hand, the progressive retardation associated with those remaining in the orphanage left them unfit for adoption. At the time
of follow-up, one of these had died in adolescence following continued residence in a state institution for the mentally deficient;
five continued to be wards of state institutions. Of the other
six, only two had married, and one of these had been divorced. For
these 12, the median educational attainment fell short of completing
the third grade. Of the six employed, all but one were in completely
unskilled occupations. Thus, increasing the development-fostering
quality of the environment during the early years produced marked
advancements that left those remaining in the orphanage progressively more retarded by comparison. This finding suggested that the
longer an infant remains in circumstances that either foster his

potential or hamper it, the more resistant his phenotypic competence
is thereafter to substantial change.

B. Empirical Instability of the IQ

When Robert L. Thorndike (1933, 1940) reviewed the test-
retest studies concerned with the stability of the IQs of individuals, he found the size of the test-retest coefficients to be a
substantial function of the time between the testings. Moreover,
a given period, say three years, between the testings results in
lower correlations in younger children than for those older (Ebert
and Simmons, 1943). Correlations of IQs at age 18 with IQs from
testings at successively earlier ages has ranged from over .90 for
reliability coefficients to nonsignificant, negative correlations
for DQs obtained during the first six months (see Jones, 1954, p.
639). Although those defending the fiction of "fixed intelligence"
responded by calling the validity of the infant tests into question,
such results, nevertheless, helped to weaken the force of the
fiction (see Hunt, 1961, p. 21-25).

C. The Effects of Nursery Schooling

The use of nursery schooling to foster the development of
toddlers and young children began in orphanages, probably with a
study by Woolley (1925). This was followed by others in which the
effects were measured as increased DQs or IQs. Such leading child
psychologists as Goodenough (1928) and Hildreth (1928) reported
negative findings from such studies and criticized the findings of
the pioneers. In consequence, most investigators withdrew from the
field, but the group at the Iowa Child Welfare Research Station
under the direction of George Stoddard (1939) persisted. They got
highly suggestive results not only in children being reared in an
orphanage, but in those being reared at home (Skeels et al., 1938).
Why other investigators reported negative results was difficult to
determine because neither proponents nor opponents provided clear
operational definitions of what was supposed to be enriching in
their nursery curricula. Even though the countering negative findings and methodological criticisms greatly decreased their impact,
these studies by the Iowa group undoubtedly helped to weaken the
hold of the fiction of "fixed intelligence" on child psychologists
(see Hunt, 1961, pp. 25-31).

D. The Psychoanalytic Movement

During the second, third, and the fourth decades of this
century, the psychoanalytic theory was spreading a competing set
of fictions in America. As already mentioned in his theory of
psychosexual development, Freud (1905) conceived of an etiology for
personality disorders in the fate of the sex drive during infancy
and early childhood (see also Abraham, 1927; Erikson, 1950; Ribble,

1944). The empirical basis for this theory resided in the free associations and dreams of patients suffering from disorders. The free associations led backward in time to the earliest memories of the individuals concerned. They were then built through speculation into a conceptual framework that was called a theory.

From this theory came inferences resulting in advice to parents on the infant disciplines (see Mowrer and Kluckhohn, 1944). This advice favored (1) breast feeding over bottle feeding, (2) feeding on self-demand by the infant rather than on a predetermined schedule, (3) gradual and late weaning rather than abrupt and early weaning, (4) late and lenient bowel and bladder training geared to the infant's development of capacity to control, to locomote, and to communicate rather than early forced training, and (5) lenience in the management of infantile masturbation coupled with training in capacity to name the organs and feelings rather than severity and reticence in communication about such phenomena. Early tests of the validity of these suggestions, typically less well controlled than the later ones, tended to lend them at least an aura of validity (Hunt, 1946), but as such investigation continued, the findings began to look more and more like random variations (Orlansky, 1949; Caldwell, 1964). Sears, Maccoby, and Levin (1957) attempted to specify those practices in mothers' management of the action patterns related to biological drives responsible for such traits as dependency, aggression, and conscience. Both mothers' practices and the outcomes in children's behavior were obtained through interviews with mothers. Most of the specific antecedent-consequent correlations were in the neighborhood of .10 to .20. These were statistically significant for the sample of 379 mothers, but they could account for no more than four per cent of the variance in the reports of consequences. Combining measures of two or more practices sometimes increased the influence; for example, the combination of punishment and permissiveness for aggressive behavior accounted for about 20 per cent of the reported aggressiveness of five-year-olds. Thus, the upshot of such investigation was to demean the importance of the specific advice while leaving important certain aspects of the social relationships encountered during infancy and early childhood.

E. Animal Studies Inspired by Psychosexual Theory

The theory of psychosexual development inspired a number of animal studies of effects from infantile experiences. Assuming an instinctive need for sucking, Levy (1934) put four Scottie puppies of a litter on controlled bottle-feeding. The two that sucked briefly through nipples with large holes were observed to suck all kinds of objects between feedings while the two having to suck longer through nipples with small holes played with the same objects without sucking them. Assuming an instinctive need for pecking, Levy (1938) also reported that chicks reared on wire, which limited

opportunity for pecking, showed more pecking at the wall, at dropp-
ings, and at other chicks than those of the same genetic stock
reared in a pen with an earthen floor.

While Levy limited his concern to consequences observable in
infancy, I introduced experimental control of the life history.
Rats fed irregularly, beginning at 24 days of age, for 15 days,
during which they went without food several times for as much as
36 hours, hoarded as adults, following a period without food, 2.5
times as many food pellets as their littermate controls always on
free feeding until the period without food as adults. The fact
that pups for which the infantile frustration began at age 32 days
failed to hoard more than their littermates suggested that the
feeding schedule that was effective for the younger group may have
been insufficiently severe to condition the hunger drive of those
older. I explained the finding in terms of conditioned drive. The
mild hunger of the adult period without food was supposed to evoke
the intense arousal of the infantile hunger to energize the hoarding
and eating (Hunt, 1941).

World War II halted this program and interfered with reporting
completed studies. Repetitions showed that infant feeding-frustra-
tion increased the rate of eating as well as or in lieu of increasing the amount of hoarding (Hunt et al., 1947). Such other investigators as Marx (1952) failed to confirm the effects of infantile
feeding frustration on hoarding, but did confirm that on the rate
of eating. My conditioned-drive interpretation was apparently
wrong. In unreported studies, the infantile frustrates neither ran
more in activity wheels when hungry nor had shorter starting times
for food in a runway as had been expected from the conditioned
drive interpretation. Instead of energizing adult activities
associated with food, experiences of deprivation of such homeostatic
needs as food or water seem to sensitize animals to cues that lead
them to whatever they were deprived of (Christie, 1952) and/or
increase the reward-value of whatever they were deprived of
(Denenberg and Naylor, 1957; Renner, 1966, 1967). Such interpretations are hardly consonant with Freud's (1915) theory of instinctive drive. While experiences of homeostatic need in infancy appear
to endure to influence adult behavior, the fact that Friedman (1957),
one of my students, found an increased rate of drinking following
repeated experiences without water beginning at ages well beyond 32
days indicates that such experiences probably have the same effect
on later behavior whether they occur in infancy or later.

F.   Evidence Dissonant with the Fiction of Infantile Trauma

Anxiety holds a central position in psychoanalytic theory;
symptoms arise and persist through reducing anxiety. According to
Freud (1926), anxiety originates in the traumata of infancy. These
traumata he believed consist of experiences of either strong

homeostatic need or intense pain, and leave the individual prone to anxiety later in life. Essentially this same notion became central in the behavior theory of acquired drives as applied to social behavior (Miller and Dollard, 1941) and personality development (Dollard and Miller, 1950). According to this theory, later proneness to anxiety comes about because a multiplicity of cues may be present when high levels of arousal are evoked in infancy, and these become the conditional stimuli that evoke anxiety later in life.

Without admitting it in publication, Levine, Chevalier, and Korchin (1956) set out originally to demonstrate the validity of this theory in rats. The pups that they shocked daily during their first 20 days of life turned out as adults, however, to be less emotional in an open field and to be more efficient in avoidance learning than those littermate controls left unmolested in the nest or than those petted during their first 20 days. This unexpected result prompted a substantial series of investigations that confirmed the original finding and extended the significance (see Denenberg, 1962; Levine, 1962). Instead of making animals prone to anxiety, as both psychoanalytic and Hullian behavior theories predict, encountering painful situations, even only briefly during early infancy, appears to desensitize animals to pain and to render them less emotional and less fearful of strange places (Salama and Hunt, 1964). Such findings have paved the way for a broader acceptance of Helson's (1964) theory of the adaptation-level and indicated the nature of a role for it in psychological development. Moreover, where both the psychoanalytic theory and the behavior theory of anxiety considered the effects of experiences of strong homeostatic need and experiences of pain to have equivalent consequences, the studies of feeding and drinking frustration in combination with these studies of early experiences of pain clearly indicate that the consequences are very different. Where early experiences of homeostatic need appear to increase the value of what was needed, those of early trauma appear to decrease sensitivity to pain. Yet other studies appear to show that encounters with natively unpleasant inputs decrease their capacity to evoke withdrawal or to reinforce avoidance behavior (see Hunt and Quay, 1961).

III. CATHEXIS AND THE PSYCHOANALYTIC THEORY OF ATTACHMENT

Emotional attachment to objects, persons, and places was termed cathexis by Freud. Early he expressed the view that "releases of pleasure and pain automatically regulate the course of the cathectic processes" (Freud, 1900, p. 515). The theory of oral primacy, based in part on the obvious strength of the sucking response in newborns, led psychoanalysts to consider maternal attachment to be chiefly a result of the pleasure associated with early sucking behavior (see

Ribble, 1944). Hullian behavior theorists were more likely to
consider maternal attachment a result of hunger gratification.
When Harlow (1958) found infant monkeys seeking solace on their
padded surrogate mothers rather than on the ones where they had
satisfied hunger when he introduced frightening objects into the
cages, he was led to attribute more importance to contact comfort
than to hunger gratification in the formation of such cathexes.

The ethologists introduced the distance receptors into the
formation of such attachments. Since hatchling birds acquire a
relatively permanent attachment to the first object perceived,
normally their mothers, Konrad Lorenz (1937) explained attachment
in terms of what he called "imprinting." Even though Lorenz
emphasized "perceptual releasers" in his theory of instincts, and
even though Ekhard Hess (1959) has emphasized the effort of following the imprinted model in determining the percentages of choices
for that model in his tests, all imprinting procedures appear to
require repeated experiences of seeing and/or hearing the object to
be imprinted before the following response occurs. Thus, it would
appear that recognitive familiarity for the object followed figures
strongly in the motivation of the following behavior (Hunt, 1970).
If this be true, one would infer that human infants will show visual
preference for scenes with which they are becoming recognitively
familiar before they show such preference for those new and novel.
Several investigations have confirmed this inference (Greenberg et
al., 1970; Hunt and Uzgiris, 1964; Weizmann et al., 1971; Wetherford
and Cohen, 1973). Moreover, Friedlander (1968, 1970) has reported
that infants show preference for auditory inputs of high redundancy
before they come to prefer those of low redundancy. Taken together,
such evidence would indicate that maternal attachment is a function
of a variety of experiences that combine and include recognitive
familiarity, the pleasures of sucking and the satisfaction of hunger
(Bowlby, 1958; Ribble, 1944), contact comfort (Bowlby, 1958; Harlow,
1958) and effort (Hess, 1959). This evidence of a role for recognitive familiarity in maternal attachment also suggests that the
cognitive aspect of early experience participates in the motivation
and attachment and probably in other motivation as well. Such consideration calls into question the validity of the traditional
separation of mind into cognition, emotion, and motivation. Moreover, all three sublines of evidence inspired by psychoanalytic
theory have served to reduce the credibility of the fiction of predetermined development.

A. Evidence Stemming from the Theorizing of Hebb and Hydén

A line of evidence indicating that early perceptual and cognitive experience influences adult competence in solving maze problems has stemmed from Hebb's (1949) theoretical solution to the
problem arising from the inability of Gestalt psychology to deal
with learning and the converse inability of behavioristic psychology

to deal with perception. Hebb suggested that both perception and
learning depend upon the gradual formation, through perceptual
encounters during the primary learning of infancy, of complex
neuronal networks that he termed "cell assemblies." He conceived
of primary learning as a slow and prolonged process. Adult learning,
on the other hand, tends to be prompt and to become possible when
sensory inputs set off well-organized "phase sequences" that serve
to recombine familiar perceptions or patterns of movement mediated
by the "cell assemblies" from early experience. Postulating such
neurological entities as cell assemblies led to studies of the
importance of early perceptual experience for adult competence in
solving maze problems (Hebb and Williams, 1946). In the first of
such studies, which involved both perceptual and motor experience,
Hebb had his daughters rear seven rats at home as pets while 25
others of the same colony strain were reared in laboratory cages.
When the pets were tested as adults in the Hebb-Williams maze-test,
"all seven scored in the top third of the total distribution of
cage-reared and pets (Hebb, 1949, p. 298)." Moreover, the pets
progressively improved their relative standing over those cage-
reared animals, thereby demonstrating that their richer early
experience had made them better able to profit by new experiences
at maturity. Later studies by Hymovitch, the Forgays, and Forgus
confirmed these effects of early perceptual experience on later
maze-learning in rats (for references see Hunt, 1961, pp. 99-103).
Other experiments with Scottie dogs as subjects produced even more
pronounced effects of early experience on later maze learning (see
Thompson and Heron, 1954; Thompson and Melzack, 1956).

     This stream of evidence has been enlarged by an extended
program of investigations at the University of California by
Bennett, Diamond, Krech, and Rosenzweig (1964). In these studies,
rats reared in environments containing a variety of objects for the
animals to perceive and manipulate and a variety of spaces to be
explored were not only superior to their cage-reared littermates in
maze-learning, but they had heavier and thicker brain cortices with
higher levels of acetylcholinesterase activity than their cage-
reared littermates.

     The perceptual part of Hebb's (1949) neuropsychological
theorizing prompted Riesen (see 1958) to rear two chimpanzees in
the dark for 16 to 18 months. These animals exhibited not only
such perceptual defects as absence of the blink response, failure
to recognize visually even such highly familiar objects as a nursing
bottle, as was to be expected from Hebb's theorizing, but also
displayed defective neural maturation in their retinae. The perceptual defects proved to be irreversible. When the animals were
sacrificed after some six years in full daylight, histological
examination uncovered a paucity of Mueller fibers in the ganglion-
cell layer of the retinae (Rasch et al., 1961).

Such investigation has another basis in Hydén's (1943) biochemical theory that memory and learning involved the metabolism
of ribonucleic acid (RNA) in the interaction between neural and
glial cells. This theory prompted Brattgård (1952) to rear rabbits
in the dark. Histochemical analysis revealed a lower level of RNA
production in the cells of the retinal ganglion in the dark-reared
rabbits than in their light-reared littermates. Evidence has accumulated that dark-rearing results in neuroanatomical and neurophysiological defects beyond the retinae in the cell areas of the
lateral geniculate bodies of the thalami of kittens (Wiesel and
Hubel, 1963) and even in synaptic spines on the branches of the
dendrites from the pyramidal cells of the occipital cortex in mice
(Valverde and Esteban, 1968). More recent studies by Greenough and
his collaborators have shown that environmental complexity influences
the amount of dendritic branching in the occipital cortex of rats
(Volkmar and Greenough, 1972) and in the temporal cortex as well
(Greenough et al., 1973).

Inasmuch as the evidence in this stream, much of it more
extensively reviewed elsewhere in this book, (see especially the
chapter by Walsh and Cummins) comes from the animal laboratory
where the adequacy of controls is greater than that obtainable with
human subjects, it has carried considerable weight in weakening the
fictions of fixed intelligence and predetermined development. Moreover, it has indicated a role for experience in neuroanatomical
maturation that was, until quite recently, considered to be completely under the control of heredity, and it has indicated that an
infant's informational interaction with the environment through its
eyes and ears and muscular systems is considerably more important
than either the traditional predeterminism or the psychoanalytic
view would hold. Perhaps the most important influence of early
experience is cognitive in character.

B. Motivation in Information Processing and Action

Cognition and motivation are interrelated. Evidence from a
variety of sources indicates that there is a system of motivation
inherent within information processing and action (Hunt, 1963).
Moreover, there appears to be an epigenesis in the development of
such motivation during the first two years of infancy (Hunt, 1965).
In this epigenesis, the orienting response appears to be ready-made
at birth (Sokolov, 1963). As patterns of sight and sound acquire
recognitive familiarity through repeated encounters, they appear to
become for a time, attractive. Then, attraction shifts to what is
new, novel, and challenging. Once interest in novelty and challenge
has developed, interest is evoked by an optimal discrepancy between
what is already recognitively familiar and what is encountered perceptually in the environment, or between what has already been
mastered in adaptive action and what is called for by a model or
situation. If what is seen or heard is already highly familiar, it

becomes as uninteresting as a detective story being read for the
third time. If imitative models and situations call only for
actions and copings already mastered, they are not only boring, but
they lack the challenge that promotes adaptive growth. On the
other hand, scenes too strange become a source of fear (Hebb, 1946a,
1946b), and challenges beyond the coping capacity of a child can
only produce distressful frustration. Such considerations lead to
what this writer likes to call "the problem of the match" (Hunt,
1961, pp. 267-268; 1965). The problem exists for the parent or
teacher who would foster development. When an infant encounters
a situation with which he cannot cope, he withdraws. But when the
love and approbation of parents and teachers are made contingent
upon his coping, such encounters not only destroy self-confidence
and self-esteem and produce distress, they can also become a major
source of psychopathology. Since so little detailed knowledge of
the development of perception and action exists, the most likely
and efficient solution of this problem of the match for those who
would foster the development of competence in the young is to rely
on the behavioral signs of interest in the materials or models the
child encounters. The ordinal scales of Uzgiris and Hunt (1975)
enable caretakers and parents to estimate from the kinds of materials that interest a child at any given time what kinds will shortly
be of interest to him. So long as the child is free to accept or
withdraw from the situations he encounters, little damage can be
done.

C. Learning in Infancy

With the resumption of investigative effort in the behavioral
sciences after World War II, the conviction with which the fictions
of predeterminism and its corollaries were held had so weakened
that two quite novel approaches to the study of psychological
development appeared. In the first of these, investigators under-
took to try out the traditional paradigms of learning with human
infants and young children. Some of these studies aimed at determining the age at which each of the several kinds of learning
(classical aversive conditioning, classical appetitive conditioning,
and operant learning) became possible. Moreover, the adaptation-
habituation phenomenon, in which there is a diminution of response
to repetitive presentations of unconditioned stimuli, that had been
studied in lower animals, was found to be present in newborn infants.
Lipsitt's (1963) first review of such studies noted that even though
they were few, they had demonstrated "that learning occurs within
the first three weeks of human life, probably within the first few
days, but experimental procedures for a stable establishment have
not been explored fully or refined sufficiently." Within a decade
of Lipsitt's first review, an extended body of systematic knowledge
had accumulated to indicate that even newborn infants would modify
their behavior with experience to a wide variety of signals. All
of the various standard forms of conditioning had been demonstrated

in infants of less than a year (Kessen et al., 1970, pp. 339-346).
While these demonstrations illustrated the capacity of infants to
learn, they failed to provide an understanding of how experience
participates in psychological development, of why development is
retarded and abnormal in institutional environments, and of how to
foster development in the young (see also S. White, 1970).

D. Piaget's Interactionism

     The second new approach to the psychological development came
via the rediscovery of the work of Jean Piaget. Piaget's early
works on language and thought, judgment and reasoning, physical
causality, and moral judgment were translated and well disseminated
among American psychologists in the early 1930s. When the elusive-
ness of his evidence, as obtained through the clinical interviews,
resulted in a series of failures to verify the implications of such
notions as "egocentrism," Piaget's work was dropped. Consequently,
his seminal work on the origins of intelligence (Piaget, 1936) and
the construction of reality (Piaget, 1937) failed to get translated
into English until the early 1950s. Shortly thereafter, Berlyne
(1957), Hunt (1961) and Flavell (1963) published synopses of Piaget's
work and theory that helped disseminate them among psychologists of
both Great Britain and the United States. There it has provided a
theoretical orientation which differs substantially from the others
that have been available in developmental psychology. Where Gesell
(1954) and the psychometricians of intelligence (Terman and Merrill,
1960; Wechsler, 1958) had pictured behavioral development as an
unfolding of abilities controlled by hereditary anatomical maturation, Piaget pictured it as a process in which epigenetic changes in
the structure of action and thought come through the infant's adaptive accommodations of existing structures to the demands of the
situations encountered. Whereas S-R behavior theory conceived of
original nature as an abundant repertoire of relatively minute
reflexes, Piaget (1936) found in the human neonate a very limited
number of highly organized sensorimotor systems. These included
sucking, looking, listening, vocalizing, grasping, and various motor
actions of the trunk and limbs. In place of the Freudian and the
S-R behavior view that organisms, including human beings, tend to
be passive and inactive until driven into action by strong stimulation, Piaget (1936, 1937) found his own infants to suck anything
touching the face almost immediately after birth. They were otherwise responsive chiefly to changes in various aspects of the ongoing
environment. Where Skinner (1950) had accepted the existence of
"operants" and "respondents" as given, Piaget's (1936) observations
provided evidence of a rapid epigenetic change in sucking from
"respondent" status to "operant" status. He described interaction-
istic origins of other actions that Skinner would probably call
"operants."

     Reminiscent of the importance of perceptual encounters in the ethologists' imprinting, recognitive familiarity following repeated perceptual exposure appeared to provide motivation for his infants' efforts to retain or to regain perceptual contact with objects, scenes, and actions that were becoming perceptually familiar. Since infants appear to anticipate the outcome of such efforts, their efforts to retain or regain perceptual contact may be regarded, in a sense, as purposive. Skinner's (1938) term, "operant," omits what appears to be the essence of organismic goal striving. When a human infant of only seven or eight weeks looks at a mobile, to which he has already been exposed, newly placed over his crib and begins to shake his body, continuing until the mobile sways and bounces, bringing laughter from the infant, it is difficult to avoid the impression that he anticipates the outcome of his shaking and wants it (Hunt and Uzgiris, 1964; Hunt, 1970).

Piaget's acceptance of purposefulness in action and of a Gestalt "wholeness" of sensorimotor and conceptual structures led him to a view of learning, or change with experience, that differs radically from Thorndike's concept of trial-and-error. When an infant who has achieved purposiveness encounters a new situation, he first applies his existing schemes. When these fail to achieve his ends, he starts a process of accommodative groping. Such groping continues until the infant's goals are achieved or until he gives up in frustration. This groping serves to modify the structure of the sensorimotor organizations that the infant brought to the encounter. In another encounter with the same circumstances under the influence of the same goal, there would be less of the accommodative groping, or, possibly, the infant would bring to the new encounter the scheme as modified in the course of the first successful encounter. Piaget calls this "assimilation" -- an assimilation of the accommodative modification involving the integration of information from the external world into the sensorimotor organization of the infant.

"Accommodation" and "assimilation," then, are two constructs with which Piaget accounts for the effects of encounters with the environment on development. Accommodative failures need not produce frustration, for a child is sensitive to the demands of the situation only when he has already achieved through maturation and the assimilation of past accommodative modifications the sensorimotor or cognitive organizations that enable him to appreciate the situation. "In other words," Piaget (1972) has written, "the sensitivity to the stimulus is the capacity for response, and this capacity for response supposes a scheme of assimilation...The stimulus-response scheme must be understood as reciprocal. The stimulus unleashes the response and the possibility of the response is necessary for the sensitivity to the stimulus. The relationship can also be described as circular which poses the problem of **equilibrium**, an equilibrium between external information serving as a stimulus and the subject's schemes or the internal structures of his activities" (emphasis

added). Thus, Piaget utilizes three constructs in accounting for
the role of environmental encounters in development: (1) accommodation, (2) assimilation, and (3) the equilibrium that exists
between them for the environment encountered to evoke the accommodation. The concept of equilibration resembles what I have called
above "the problem of the match," but where Piaget's concept of
equilibrium is wholly cognitive, mine has emotional and motivational
aspects as well as the cognitive.

The theoretical conceptions and the new evidence stemming from
Piaget's work and theory provide the beginnings of a genuine inter-
actionistic view of development that promises new understandings
which were essentially ruled out by the conceptual fictions of predetermined development and environmentalistic behavior theory.
Piaget has already uncovered a sequential order in development that
he has described under stages. These stages appear to imply a hierarchical structure for intelligence and competence in general. In
this hierarchical structure, abilities and informational structures
would appear to be built one upon another, each with its cognitive
and motivational aspects. Such a conception suggested to me a
radical change in the strategy of assessing development and competence. Where the traditional norm-referenced strategy has sought
the meaning of a child's performances in one index or another of
his rank within the norming population, the new strategy would seek
such meaning in the child's level of achievement within the natural,
ordinal hierarchy of achievements. To date, such scales are available only for the sensorimotor phase of infancy (Uzgiris and Hunt,
1975), but it should be feasible to develop such ordinal scales
through higher levels of development. So far, Piaget's work constitutes but a beginning of what promises to become a genuine inter-
actionistic approach to psychological development. As investigation
continues, both predeterminism and environmentalism should gradually
disappear in the dynamic interplay between them. A dependable educational psychology for infancy and early childhood requires an
accurate and detailed knowledge of this interplay. Piaget's work
appears to be inspiring the wave of the future.

IV.   PROJECT HEAD START

As the seventh decade of this century began, the several lines
of evidence indicated above had severely weakened the fiction of
predeterminism among educators and the students of early development. This released a justified hope that something might be done
about the specter of poverty in the midst of a greater plenty than
had ever been available heretofore. But it is one thing to see that
something can be done and something quite different to know how to
do it. After summarizing the evidence available at that time, I
wrote:

In the light of the evidence now available, it is not
unreasonable to entertain the hypothesis that, with a
sound scientific educational psychology of early experience,
it might become possible to raise the average level of
intelligence as now measured by a substantial degree...
of the order of 30 points of IQ. In a technological
culture...this is an important challenge. At this stage
of knowledge, however, it is still a challenge for
investigation rather than one for application in social
change. (Hunt, 1961, p. 267)

Project Head Start was launched in 1965, however, without the
research and the development of a technology of early education,
and with only the urgency of need and the hope derived from the
evidences of plasticity in development to justify it. The goal was
to enable the children from the poverty sector to catch up with
their middle-class peers before starting school. Many of those
most convinced of plasticity in early psychological development
feared the goal was unrealistic because so little was known about
how to provide compensatory education. Moreover, they were concerned because plasticity cuts both ways. Thus, once the compensatory educational circumstances were withdrawn, the environments
of the public school and the families of poverty would cease to
promote the development of the disadvantaged and those with the
environmental advantages of the middle class would continue to
develop.

For those expecting Head Start to achieve the catch-up for
poor children, Head Start clearly failed. Most of the studies
that compared the gains in achievement scores for participants
with those of nonparticipants from similar backgrounds reported
larger gains for participants than for nonparticipants. But after
a year or two in the public schools, the difference between participating children of poverty and children from the middle class was
as large as ever, or even larger in terms of the IQ ratio. Even
the difference between participants and nonparticipants from similar
backgrounds tended to disappear (see Hunt, 1975).

Those who had never believed the evidence for plasticity in
psychological development quickly revisited predeterminism and the
heritability of intelligence and scholastic achievement to explain
the failure (see Jensen, 1969, 1972). One can readily reject this
explanation and yet find reasons for the limited results of Project
Head Start. For example, the kind of preschool most commonly
deployed in the Project was one with historical roots in the Child
Study Movement of G. Stanley Hall combined with influence of the
psychoanalytic movement. It was developed to release children for
a few hours each day from the over-strict control of their middle
class mothers. The community actions aspect of Head Start programs
often interfered with the planning of even such programs (see Payne

et al., 1973). The educational programs most commonly deployed
were not designed to permit children of poverty to acquire the
knowledge, motivations, and skills missing from their early home
experiences. Also, since plasticity cuts both ways, it was hardly
to be expected that any gains from conditions made especially
favorable for development would persist when those conditions were
removed. Finally, Epstein (1974a, 1974b) has analyzed annual,
biennial, and triennial increments in head circumference, brain
weight, and IQ and found evidence suggesting that there may be
spurts in both the IQ and growth of the brain unassociated with
somatic growth. He claims these spurts come at ages 14-16, 10-12,
6-8, and perhaps at 2-4. If the learning ability of children peaks
during such hypothetical spurts of brain growth, the fact that the
spurts occur before age four and after age six would suggest that
the fifth and sixth years of life would be an especially poor time
to attempt a catch-up.

Project Head Start did have value. Its concern with early
education stimulated reviews of the evidence and new investigations
of class differences in child-rearing, new developments in the
technology of compensatory education, and the exploration of methods
of preventing retardation in children of poverty (see Hunt, 1969,
Chs. 6 and 7). The investigations of class differences revealed
that children of poverty are typically acquainted with a less complex variety of objects, places, and persons, than are children of
the middle class. They also have less opportunity to learn the
spoken symbols for these objects and for such elementary abstractions
as color, position, shape, and number (Hunt and Kirk, 1974) than
their middle-class peers (for omitted sources, see Hunt, 1969, pp.
204-208). Since there is seldom enough of anything to satisfy all
in the households of the poor, it is hardly surprising that children
of poverty prefer immediate reinforcement over delayed reinforcement, and that they have less confidence over the control of their
fate than do children of the middle class (see Hunt, 1969, pp. 208-
214). With both parents all too often absent from home, children
of poverty typically go unsupervised. Thus, the standards of con-
duct that they acquire all too often come down from the adolescents
of the local delinquent gangs (see Hunt, 1969, pp. 214-218). All of
this suggests that compensatory education, to be effective, must
have a therapeutic aspect designed to change attitudes and motivation
as well as to inculcate cognitive and linguistic skills. See also
the discussion of reinforcement and maintenance of therapeutic gains
in the chapter by Walsh and Cummins.

The new developments in compensatory education, pioneered by
Gray and Klaus (1965) have taken several forms. Some, like that of
Bereiter and Engelmann (1966) attempted to teach through supervised
drill the skill shown to be deficient in a test of academic achievement. The effects of such programs have generally been larger than
those of others as measured by those tests of academic achievement.

Other programs, such as that of Weikart (1972, 1975), have been inspired by the work of Piaget and have attempted through manipulations of the environment to inculcate cognitive and linguistic ability in children without formal drill. Several of these compensatory programs have stressed self-directional autonomy and motivation as much as or more than they emphasized the academic skills (Armington, 1968; Hughes et al., 1968; Lavatelli, 1971).

The pioneering efforts of Gray and Klaus (1965) brought the mothers into the classrooms, where they could observe and imitate the teachers and discuss the results. This approach improved test performance not only in the target children who attended the classes, but also in other children of the families concerned (vertical diffusion) and to a lesser degree, in the children of the neighboring families (horizontal diffusion) with face-to-face contact with those in the program (see Miller, 1968). Yet others have shifted the emphasis to the prevention of incompetence and retardation in infants and children under three by attempting to teach the mothers how to foster the psychological development of their infants and toddlers (Karnes et al., 1970; Levenstein, 1970, 1974; Lambie et al., 1974).

Participants four and five years old in programs of compensatory education show gains not found in nonparticipants with the same background, but the gains tend to be substantially smaller than those obtained with three-year-olds or those obtained with children aged six to eight in the various Follow-Through Programs. In the light of Epstein's hypothesis of spurts in brain growth for ages two to four and six to eight, this finding is interesting.

It was early hints of such evidence that suggested extensions of Head Start. In January of 1967, a White House Task Force of which I was chairman, produced a report entitled A Bill of Rights for Children. This report recommended an extension of Head Start up the age scale in the Follow-Through program, and down the age scale in an experimental series of Parent and Child Centers. These recommendations were accepted and implemented. The preliminary summary report by Becker (1974) indicates that those Follow-Through programs most sharply focused on academic skills have shown the largest gains on tests of academic achievement. How permanent these gains are remains to be seen, but the fact that parents are involved in these Follow-Through programs augurs well. In another preliminary report, Milton Goldberg (1974) reported evidence suggesting that Follow-Through in Philadelphia may be influencing more than the scholastic achievement. Participation in the school programs apparently has given parents a feeling of control over their children's education that they value. Whereas approximately 40% of pupils have typically moved each year, this Philadelphia study of Follow-Through shows 72% of the pupils in the Follow-Through classes continuing throughout a four-year period.

No such preliminary evidence of success has eminated from the
Parent and Child Centers. Although the Task Force that recommended
them was concerned chiefly with the fostering of competence in the
children of poor families, it made what now appears to have been a
mistake in emphasizing the involvement of parents in a coordination
of all the services within communities. As a consequence, many
Parent and Child Centers attempted organizational tasks within
communities that were entirely too large. These organizational
tasks interfered with any improvement of child-rearing. Moreover,
these Centers and the whole Head Start Project have suffered from
the lack of dependable knowledge about how to foster the psychological development of infants and very young children. They have
attempted a broad-scale program of early education without the
necessary scientific knowledge of how to foster early psychological
development (for references and more detail, see Hunt, 1975).

A. Investigations of How to Foster Early Psychological Development

Although the literature on infant learning might be expected to
be a major source of information about how to foster early psychological development, such is not the case. The studies of infant
learning so well summarized by Lipsitt (1963, 1967) and by Kessen,
Haith, and Salapatek (1970) have been limited almost entirely to the
immediate effects of conditioning and habituation procedures that
endure but a few minutes. While these have demonstrated the capacity
of even newborn infants for such kinds of learning, they have shown
little about infant-environment interactions that influence the rate
of psychological development and the achievement of various kinds of
competence.

B. Demonstrations in Day-Care

Educational day-care has been one source of evidence. In
America, day care of infants and young children has had an on-off
history. Before and during World War I, day care expanded with
federal assistance especially for the infants of mothers who entered
the labor force, but the influence of psychoanalysis created opposition to such care on the belief that infants and young children
develop best under a consistent relationship with a single mother
figure (Lazar and Rosenberg, 1971). With women increasingly entering the labor force since 1960, the demand for day-care has been
increasing. Moreover, a number of investigators have employed
educational day-care to demonstrate that children of poverty have
more potential for development than they have shown with home rearing.

The recent findings in day-care appear to indicate that the
psychoanalytic claim that multiple mothering is necessarily injurious
is another fiction. What appears to be important is that the infant
have always available adults whom he knows at sight and who, in turn,

know him well enough to recognize the meaning of his attempts to
elicit attention and to indicate his needs. Nearly all those
employing educational day-care to demonstrate the potential of
infants from families of poverty have taken such precautions and
have also attempted to assess any interference of the day-care
experience with maternal attachment (see Caldwell et al., 1970;
Heber et al., 1972; Robinson and Robinson, 1971).

Since the developmental deficits found in children of poverty
have been especially prominent in the domains of cognition and
language, the curricula of educational day-care have emphasized
listening to the sounds from a variety of sources, looking at a
variety of objects, ordering, coordinating, forming concepts, and
solving little problems. Those efforts that have been described
have also been successful at least while children remained in the
programs. Most spectacular, perhaps, is that of Heber and his
collaborators in Milwaukee. In this effort, the mothers of both
the children treated in day-care and those in the contrast group
had IQs of 75 or below. The treatment program continued from the
time the infants were about three months of age until they were
about 66 months of age and ready for school. At that point the
treated group had an average IQ of 125, while those in the contrast
group, who were also examined repeatedly, had an average IQ of about
95. This is an excellent demonstration that even children of mothers
severely retarded (but probably not mentally deficient) have a potential to develop competence well above the average. Yet, even
though Heber et al. (1972) have described their curriculum in considerable detail, their use of the IQ to measure the effects of
their intervention makes it impossible to uncover any relationships
between specific aspects of the intervention and specific achievements. Moreover, how well these children will maintain their
advantaged status once the development-fostering experiences of the
educational day-care are removed remains to be seen. If Jencks'
(1972) evidence that the influence of the family is substantially
greater than that of the school is correct, these children of the
Heber demonstration can be expected to show a gradual but substantial
loss of IQ with time, for those from advantaged families will develop faster than they do. Such a finding will derive from the fact
that the IQ-ratio is a measure of the rate of development. It will
say nothing about the potential of these children, but unfortunately,
it is likely to be misunderstood because many psychometricians still
consider the IQ to be a measure of potential.

C. Efforts to Improve Mothers' Child-Rearing Practices

Efforts to help mothers improve the educational component of
their child-rearing began at about the same time as the launching
of Project Head Start. Gray and Klaus (1965) started by inviting
mothers into the classrooms of compensatory education for their
four- and five-year-olds and then added home visits. Their studies

uncovered the hopeful evidences of vertical and horizontal diffusion of gains. In place of such compensatory efforts, other investigators attempted to help mothers from the poverty sector prevent
the retardation already evident at four.

The most thoroughly tested of these preventive programs is that
of Phyllis Levenstein, based on fostering verbal interaction between
disadvantaged mothers and their toddlers. This program started with
three guiding hypotheses: (1) that language acquisition is funda-
mental for the intellectual development of children from economically
and educationally disadvantaged families, (2) that mothers in such
families can be taught through demonstrations of toys and books,
with mother and child together, to interact verbally with their
children in a fashion that will foster the child's intellectual
and motivational development and also build within the mother a
sense of competence and worth, and (3) that since language development is most prominent during the third and fourth years, such a
program should begin when children are about two years old. The
home visits were made by social workers and paraprofessionals who
had been taught the techniques of verbal intervention which have
been formalized in a Toy Demonstrators' Visit Handbook. The children who start at age two and live through two whole years with
trained mothers have IQs approximating 100 or slightly over by age
four years, averaging between 15 and 20 points above the mean IQ of
children in contrast groups of families of comparable backgrounds
with no mother training. Moreover, apparently because the mothers
have become involved in their children's educational progress, these
gains appear to hold till the children enter school and through the
first grade. I suspect that the mothers would require additional
training to maintain the educational role of their homes in later
grades.

Although all efforts to improve child-rearing have encouraged
mothers to believe that how they interact with their infants makes
a difference in the infant's future, Badger (1971a, 1971b) and
Lambie et al. (1974) have been most explicit about it. Where
Levenstein has focused on language development and started her
intervention at approximately two years of age, Badger, Gordon
(1969) and Lambie have initiated their efforts with mothers while
their infants were in the first year of life. Moreover, Badger
has found it easier to recruit mothers into such a program while
they are still in a lying-in hospital with a new, and particularly
a first, baby. These investigators have typically taught the mothers through "learning games" inspired by Piaget's descriptions of
sensorimotor development or by certain of the infant tests. Badger
and Lambie have been especially explicit about encouraging mothers,
while their infants are very young, to be quickly responsive to
their behavioral indications of distress and of wishes for attention. Badger, moreover, has made an explicit effort to solve the
"problem of the match." She attempts to teach mothers to observe

their infants, in their interaction with play materials or with
models for imitation, for behavioral signs of interest and surprise,
of boredom, and of the distressful frustration that comes in encounters with situations beyond the infant's capacity to cope. Mothers
are then encouraged to provide their infants with materials and
models which bring forth the signs of interest and to leave the
infant free to neglect those that have become boring and to avoid
those that are threatening. Finally, Badger attempts to teach the
mother something about the sequences of developing abilities and
interests to help them choose, on the basis of the materials in
which the infant is already interested, and make available those
materials in which he will shortly become interested.

D. Independence of Development Along Separate Branches

     Gesell's emphasis on the unitary wholeness of development and
Piaget's emphasis on the gestalt-like quality of advances, together
with the long practice of specifying development in terms of mental
ages and IQs combine to foster the view that individual infants and
children develop in toto -- that development of one competence or
along one branch implies corresponding development of other competencies or along other branches. Although I had questioned it, the
evidence that first dissuaded me from acceptance of this fictional
idea came through an accidental observation during a visit to the
laboratory of Burton L. White. White (1967) was investigating the
effects of experience on the development of visually directed reaching. His first, normative study had uncovered a sequence of ten
steps beginning with fisted swiping at a seen object and terminating
with top-level reaching wherein the infant shaped his hand for
grasping as he thrust it toward the object. An enrichment program
that included handling the infants and providing a stabile geared in
complexity to the development of the infants reduced the median age
of achieving top-level reaching from 143 days to 89 days. It was
impressive to find these institution-reared infants attaining this
achievement at an age some six or eight weeks younger than did the
home-reared infants then serving as subjects in the studies that
led to the ordinal scales of Uzgiris and Hunt (1966, 1975). On the
other hand, when I attempted to demonstrate the facial signs of
interest in cooing and babbling sounds and to elicit vocal pseudo-
imitation that I was accustomed to obtaining at between three and
four months in our subjects, I was completely unsuccessful even with
infants of six or more months of age. White had heard infants in
the institution making noise with the saliva in their mouths, and
only when I tried such noises could I get even the facial signs of
interest. Gradually it dawned upon us that we were witnessing
evidence that the rates of progress in eye-hand coordination could
be quite independent of that in vocal imitation and that the rates
of development in the two branches must depend on differing kinds
of infant-environment interactions. The stabiles placed over the
cribs by White elicited both looking and arm-movements and invited

their coordination. Without the vocal play typical of middle-class
mothers, however, White's infants failed to show development along
the branch of vocal imitation. The converse was true of the home-
reared infants in the Uzgiris-Hunt studies. What we were observing
appeared to be a nice illustration of Piaget's aphorism that "use
is the aliment of a scheme" (a scheme is a sensorimotor organization). All this implied that research on psychological development
should consist of a search for relationships between specific kinds
of experiences and specific competencies.

Such experiments as that just synopsized by White (1967) can
be very informative. Unfortunately, they are still scarce. Another example, from my own laboratory, was inspired during the
visit to White's laboratory with the idea that visual accommodation
develops gradually through exercise of looking combined with the
idea that the blink response demands considerable capacity for
visual accommodation. Greenberg arranged to have mobiles placed
over the cribs of ten infants beginning at five weeks of age. He
also got the mothers of ten other infants to agree to postpone
providing mobiles until their infants were at least three months
old. He then measured the blink response in each infant weekly.
Those provided with mobiles blinked to ten of 12 target drops of
11.5 inches at an average of seven weeks, while those with no mobiles failed to achieve this criterion of the blink response until
they were 10.4 weeks of age (Greenberg et al., 1968).

E. Specific Experience-Competence Relationships

Most of the efforts to improve the child-rearing of mothers
have failed to yield evidence of specific experience-competence
relationships because they have used intelligence tests in which
the substitutive averaging to obtain a mental age hides such details. Because the effects of the Badger program have been assessed
with the Uzgiris-Hunt scales, it has begun to yield evidence of
specific relationships.

At the Parent and Child Center of Mt. Carmel, Illinois,
Mrs. Badger taught the mothers in the program who served as caretakers from the program of infant day-care at the Center. In the
first attempt at evaluation, eight consecutive infants born to the
mothers participating in the Center's program entered the day-care
and were examined every other week with four of the seven ordinal
scales. These infants achieved top-level object permanence at a
mean age of 73 weeks. This is nearly half a year younger than the
mean age (98 weeks) at which 12 home-reared infants from predominantly professional families attained this achievement in a study
for other purposes by Uzgiris (Hunt et al., 1975b). It so happened
that the toy that most persistently interested the Mt. Carmel infants was a shape box with five different holes: circular, square,
rectangular, triangular, and irregular, in the top. By using a

ping-pong ball for the round hole, the infants got interested
almost as soon as they could sit up, and with the progressive
complexity provided by the five shapes, they continued to be interested into their second year. It seems likely that this was the
experience so effective in fostering object construction.

This study also brought another bit of evidence of the independence in the rate of development along separate branches. These
eight infants of Mt. Carmel who achieved top-level object permanence
about six months ahead of the 12 Worcester infants from predominantly
professional families were nearly as far behind them in achieving
top-level vocal imitation. This finding illustrates the importance
of assessing separately several branches of psychological development. It also demonstrated for us that the Badger program of
mother training needed to be revised to provide experiences that
would be more effective in fostering vocal imitation.

One of the first attempts to relate specific kinds of experience to specific kinds of development is that of Wachs et al. (1971).
They utilized 72 items from Caldwell's inventory of home stimulation
to assess the environmental circumstances of 102 infants in their
7th, 11th, 15th, 18th, and 22nd months of life and employed six
measures of development from the Uzgiris-Hunt scales. These latter
included (1) object permanence, (2) the development of means of
obtaining desired environmental events, (3) the development of
schemes for relating to objects, (4) vocal imitation, and (5) items
on learning and (6) on foresight. Half of the infants at each age
level came from disadvantaged families of which a majority were
black. The other half came from families of middle class all of
whom were white. The measures of home stimulation were correlated
with the measures of development for each age group.

Two aspects of home environments appear consistently to hamper
development along all branches at all five ages. One of these is
the intensity of auditory noise without signal value to the infant.
It includes such concrete, environmental items as: "noise in the
neighborhood," "high sound level in the home," "inability of the
child to escape noises in the home," and "television on continuously." Since noise is far more characteristic of disadvantaged
homes than homes of middle class, this finding helps to explain the
inattentiveness of children from disadvantaged homes (Deutsch, 1964)
and the fact that such children do a poor job of discriminating
vocal patterns (Clark and Richards, 1966). Repeated encounters with
meaningless sound serve to habituate the attention and arousal of
the orienting response to such sounds. Moreover, as Maltzman and
Raskin (1965) have reported, those kinds of input for which the
orienting response is weak or absent serve poorly as conditional
stimuli or as cues in more complex learning tasks. The second
hampering environmental factor appears to be variety of change in
circumstances. It includes such concrete environmental items as:

"a high level of activity in the home," "mother and child go visiting daily," "neighbors visit the house almost daily." Such findings
are highly dissonant with the view that retardation of development
in children of the poor derives from stimulus deprivation.

Contrariwise, such environmental factors as "an orderly neighborhood," "an orderly decor with a variety of colors," "mother
spontaneously vocalizing to child," "mother naming objects for the
child," and "father playing with the child," are all positively
associated with level of achievement on the ordinal scales. Certain
of these relationships change with the age of the child. Daily
visiting with neighbors shows no correlation with level of achievement at ages either seven or 11 months, but it has a high negative
correlation with competence at 15 and 18 months, when the locomotor
abilities and interests of infants interfere with visiting of the
mothers. The information from this study is highly useful, but its
cross-sectional nature and the way the factors of the home environment are conceptualized does not permit them to be related to the
achievement of specific steps in the scales for object construction,
the development of means, or vocal imitation.

Another investigation deliberately seeking "what kinds of
experience affect which aspects of the developing infant" is that
of Yarrow, Rubenstein, and Pedersen (1974). The strategy again
consists of measuring a variety of antecedent environmental variables
and a variety of consequent behavioral characteristics of the infants, but at only six months of age. The assessments of the specific kinds of experience that constitute the antecedent variables
was based on but two three-hour time-samplings during only two home
visits. The observations of the environments made during these home
visits concerned a large variety of mother-infant interactions and
three aspects (variety, responsiveness, and complexity) of the infants' interaction with the inanimate materials available to them.
The behavioral characteristics of the infant subjects at six months
were assessed with the Bayley Scales of Infant Development. Instead
of utilizing the substitutive averaging to obtain a mental age,
however, they got, in addition to the Mental Development Index and
the Psychomotor Development Index, assessments of eight other aspects that included gross motor development, fine motor development,
social responsiveness, language, goal directedness, secondary circular reactions, reaching and grasping, and object permanence. The
sample consisted of 41 black infants (21 boys and 20 girls) and their
primary caregivers.

Correlating the various kinds of antecedent infant-environment
interactions with these measures of infant development at age six
months reveals a variety of specific relationships too extensive to
report in detail here. Surprising is the fact that both the responsiveness and the variety of the inanimate materials show higher
correlations than do the measures of mother-infant interactions with

such measures of development as the Mental and Psychomotor Development Indices, such cognitive-motivational characteristics as goal-directedness, reaching, secondary circular reactions, and problem-solving. Social responsiveness, on the other hand, is clearly a function of social stimulation and the expressions of positive affect smiling, and play in the mother's interaction with her infant. The amount of vocalization that an infant manifests during exploration is a function of that positive, contingent, maternal response observed to occur with the child's vocalizing. The only antecedent factors among those measured that influence the level of object permanence are the variety of social stimulation and the variety of inanimate materials available. It is also surprising to find measures of antecedent, environmental variables based on only two three-hour home visits showing correlations as high as +.4 and +.5 with measures of infant development at six months. Such high correlations could be obtained only if there is more consistency in the development-fostering quality of home environments than has been suspected. It may well be that a large portion of the empirically-observed constancy in the IQ is a reflection of this consistency in the development-fostering quality of home and neighborhood environments.

Probably the most ambitious and extensive effort "to learn how to structure the experiences of the first six years of life so that a child may be optimally prepared for formal education" is that under the direction of Burton L. White (White and Watts, 1973, p. 4; White, 1974, 1975). The purpose quoted called first for a specification of the nature of human competence at age six. To provide such specification, the first step was to distinguish the 13 most and the 13 least talented children of six years in a sample of 400 from a variety of socioeconomic backgrounds on the basis of some 1,100 protocols of moment-to-moment activities in their homes and institutions. This procedure uncovered a set of eight social abilities that included those to get and hold the attention of adults and to obtain help from them, to express both affection and hostility to adults, and to show pride in accomplishments. It also uncovered four nonsocial abilities that included linguistic and intellectual competencies, executive competence, and capacity for concentration on a task while remaining aware of peripheral happenings. This specification of human competence at age six provided also the basis for an extended list of measures of children's developmental competencies.

As the staff got to know well over 100 young children, they agreed that those well-developed at age three resemble more closely well-developed than poorly developed six-year-olds. This observation, still without quantitative check, served to narrow the focus of the project to the first three years. Moreover, White's group has come to consider most of the first year uncrucial, for "under the variety of early rearing-conditions prevalent in American homes,

divergence with respect to the development of educability and overall competence first becomes manifest during the second year of life"
(White and Watts, 1973, p. 21). As infants aged from eight months
to a year develop locomotion, concern with language, and negativism,
they call upon mothers to give of themselves continuously in active
management. This state of affairs endures until infants are 18 to
20 months old. Thus, White's group considers this period of about
ten to 20 months to be most critical. Moreover, continuous giving
of self is highly stressful. A person depressed, angry with her
fate, or unhappy can hardly take this extra stress. Strong commit-
ments to possessions, meticulous housekeeping, and excessive concern with safety are all likely to damage the development-fostering
quality of maternal care.

A comparison of the infant-environment interactions of the
competent with those of the less competent has shown that as early
as age 12 months, and increasingly thereafter, they differ markedly.
Mothers of competent children interact more with them, engage with
them in more intellectually stimulating activities, encourage them
more, teach them more, initiate activities for them more often, and
are more successful in controlling them than are mothers of less
competent children.

Intellectual competence appears to grow out of unfettered
opportunities to explore and manipulate objects and to ask questions.
Effective mothers fostered development by designing a physical
world full of manipulable and visually-detailed objects, things to
climb and to foster motor interest, and a rich variety of things to
look at. They respond to requests, but spend little time in teaching sessions. Rather, they teach "on the fly" in ten to 30-second
interchanges that are usually initiated by the child. Such responsiveness helps to keep the infant nearby, avoids dangerous use of
locomotor abilities to seek things of greater interest, and helps
to reduce the negativism that is often exaggerated by overt re-
straints and punishments for locomotor explorations. Such responsiveness also helps to foster confidence in getting and holding the
attention of adults and the use of them as resources, and it fosters
pride in their own accomplishments.

Linguistic ability appears to be related to the variety of
objects and situations that the child has encountered and the
frequency with which children's mothers demonstrate and explain
things for them, usually at the infants' instigation rather than
their own. "Mothering," White writes, "is a vastly underrated
occupation."

The Harvard Preschool Project is still in progress. It has
already uncovered a substantial list of hypothetically specific
relationships in a form of value to those who would teach parents
to be better educators of their young. Whether these experience-

competence relationships are specific enough to permit cross-
validation remains to be seen.

F. Evidence From the Orphanage Studies

    Other evidence of specific relationships between antecedent
experiences and consequent achievements of competence are coming
from my orphanage studies. These studies have employed both the
longitudinal strategy, for which only a still unpublished
report exists (Hunt et al., 1975a), and the cross-sectional strategy
(Paraskevopoulos and Hunt, 1971).

    The longitudinal studies have been done in an orphanage of the
Farah Pahlavi Charity Society in Tehran. I was led to this orphanage by Dennis' (1960) report that when he visited it in the middle
1950s, two-thirds of the infants in their second year were still
not sitting up and 85 per cent of those in their fourth year were
not yet walking. Although considerable improvement in caretaking
had been made between the time of the Dennis study and the beginnings of mine in 1968, considerable apathy and retardation were
characteristic of infants reared from birth in them. I am greatly
indebted to the authorities of the Queen Farah Pahlavi Charity
Society for the privilege of conducting my research there.

    The infants who have served as subjects are foundlings. They
were selected before they were a month old from the Municipal
Orphanage of Tehran because they had no parental ties and were
without detectable defects or pathology. For a combination of
ethical and scientific reasons, I avoided the practice of simultaneous treatment and control groups in favor of what one may call
"wave design." In this design, the only intervention for the first,
control wave consisted in examinations with the Uzgiris-Hunt (1975)
scales every other week during their first year and every fourth
week thereafter. Otherwise, the infants were cared for according
to the standard practices of the institution with about ten infants
under each caretaker. The ages at which the infants in this control
wave achieved the successive steps on the seven ordinal scales of
Uzgiris and Hunt served as the baseline against which the effects
of the interventions in the rearing practices for subsequent waves
could be assessed.

    The infants on this first control wave achieved various land-
marks of development on the scales of object permanence and gestural
imitation at ages considerably younger than those examined but once
in the Municipal Orphanage of Athens where the infant-caretaker
ratio was also of the order of 10/1 and where the system of caretaking appeared similar. This finding suggests that these repeated
examinations with the Uzgiris-Hunt scales did not put these children
at risk as certain overly cautious critics have suggested. Rather,
the repeated examinations themselves appear to have had an educa-

tional influence.

The initial experimental intervention for Wave II consisted in a combination of auditory and visual experiences that the infant could control. This intervention was to supplement the customary ministrations of the caretakers who were instructed to give the same care to these infants receiving the extra experience that they gave regularly to others. Unfortunately, this intervention was abortive because the collaborator in charge failed to keep the apparatus working and to change the mother-talk and music available on the tape-recorders. Possibly because the caretakers failed to give the usual care, the infants in this wave actually achieved all but a very few steps on the several scales at ages older on the average than those for the infants in the control wave. An exception to this was the increased proportion of these infants who manifested the facial expressions of interest in the examiner's vocalizations of cooing sounds over the almost complete absence of such interest on the part of the infants in the control wave. Hearing the taped mother talk and music appears to have had some influence on the early phase of development of vocal imitation.

The second experimental intervention for Wave III began about a year after the first. It consisted of human enrichment in which the infant-caretaker ratio was reduced from 10/1 to 3/1, but with no instruction to the caretakers. In addition, student nursery-nurses were invited to play as often as possible with the infants while they were awake. Both caretakers and nursery-nurses did whatever came naturally. The effect of this intervention was limited largely to a very substantial advance in the development of posture and locomotion. Despite the improvements in the care-taking that had been made between the time of Dennis' study and this one of untutored enrichment, the infants in the control wave had seldom begun sitting up before they were nearly a year old, and only one of the 15 managed to pull himself to a standing position in his crib before he was about a year-and-a-half old. These infants with the untutored human enrichment, on the other hand, began sitting alone at between six and eight months of age. Moreover, all but one had pulled themselves up to a standing position and were cruising around their cribs at between 11 and 13 months of age. On the other hand, they were slightly less advanced than those in the control wave in achieving the successive steps of object permanence, of operational causality, and of schemes for relating to objects. They exhibited moderate advances over those in the control wave in achieving the successive steps in the development of means for obtaining desired environmental events and in gestural imitation, but not in vocal imitation. Nevertheless, after the infants were about a year-and-a-half old, a substantially higher proportion of them than of the controls and of Wave II developed some language.

One of the major ways in which the environment can foster development is to provide infants with an opportunity to use their newly ready-made sensorimotor organizations. Although the strategy of this investigation included time-sampling observations to determine what the caretakers and infants actually did, the analyses of these is not yet complete at this writing. What appears from unsystematic observation to have come naturally to the caretakers and nursery-nurses was to carry these infants about and thereby provide them with opportunities to use their balancing mechanisms and to put them in strollers that enabled them to use their legs. The fact that the infant-caretaker ratio was reduced to 3/1 also enabled the caretakers to respond more often and more quickly to the efforts of the infants to elicit attention and interaction. This accounts for the advance in the development of means for obtaining desirable environmental events and perhaps in gestural imitation. Such is the positive side of this first attempt at human enrichment. On the negative side, failure on the part of the caretakers to provide and demonstrate manipulable toys and to encourage vocal imitation appears to account for the retardation in object construction and vocal imitation.

The 20 infants in Wave IV of this program got a combination of audio-visual enrichment that the infants could control and a variety of materials and playthings such as Yarrow et al. (1974) had found to be responsive. Such intervention served gradually to advance later stages of object permanence, to advance markedly the development of means for achieving desired environmental events, to advance somewhat the pseudo-imitation of familiar vocalizations and the later imitation of novel vocal patterns somewhat. It had no effect on the ages of achieving the steps of gestural imitation, of object relations in space, or of schemes for relating to objects. Moreover, postural and locomotor development were nearly as retarded as they had been in the infants of the control wave and of the abortive attempt of audio-visual enrichment.

The 11 infants in Wave V received human enrichment in which the caretakers were tutored in the use of the Badger program for training mothers. Moreover, the Badger program was supplemented with procedures designed to foster vocal imitation. The marvelous development of the infants in this fifth wave has demonstrated that institutional rearing need not be a source of apathy, retardation, or pathology. The 11 foundlings (originally 12) comprising the subjects of this wave, like those in the other waves, were selected by Miss Ghodssi, the Directress of the Orphanage, to be without parental ties and without detectable defects or pathology. For reasons of her own, Directress Ghodssi reduced the infant-caretaker ration to 2/1, instead of 3/1. The nature of the Badger program of mother-training has already been described above. In the supplement designed to foster vocal imitation, the caretakers were shown how to imitate the cooing of their infants and then later, to imitate

the babbling sounds that their infants produced. They were to persist in these imitations until they got vocal games going. Once
these were going, and the caretaker had learned the variety of their
infants' babblings, they were to change the model from one familiar
pattern to another, say, from "ga, ga, ga" to such a one as "boo,
boo, boo." Once their infants got to the level where they would
change their babbling to match that model, the caretakers were encouraged to extend the game to novel vocal patterns. Still later,
they were to introduce the various phonemes of the language. While
this process was under way, the caretakers were to provide experiences designed to foster semantic mastery. For this purpose they
were instructed to accompany their caretaking ministrations with
talk about them. Thus, as a caretaker might be washing an infant's
ear, she was instructed to say the Farsi equivalent of, "Now I'm
going to wash your ear." As she uttered the word ear with vocal
emphasis, she was instructed to touch the ear of the infant with
her washcloth. Such talk was to accompany all kinds of caretaking
activities.

How well these caretakers actually carried out these instruc-
tions will not be known until the observational records have been
analyzed. On the other hand, they must have followed the instruc-
tions quite well for these infants achieved every step on every
scale at a younger average age than did the infants in any of the
other four waves. Moreover, they achieved top-level object construction and vocal imitation at slightly younger mean ages than did
the infants from predominantly professional families of Worcester,
Massachusetts.

These infants reared with tutored human enrichment also acquired
a substantial vocabulary. One could touch the various features of
their face and the various parts of their bodies and the various
pieces of their clothing while asking the Farsi equivalent of, "What
is it?" and get the names for hair, ear, nose, neck, arm, hand, leg,
foot and for the various pieces of clothing. While the examiner was
demonstrating for me that the youngest of the children, 17 months
old, could imitate the names of all of the other children in the
program, she came to Yaz, the name of a child who had already been
adopted and departed. The infant immediately turned her eyes toward
the door, lifted an arm and remarked in Farsi the equivalent of "Yaz
gone." Moreover, at least three of the older infants, aged between
24 and 25 months, knew the names of the four primary colors. They
knew them not only when these colors were asked for in connection
with play with the stacking toy where the children had first learned
them, but also in portions of pictures on the wall. Thus, at least
these three oldest children had achieved semantic mastery for the
elementary abstraction of color. When one considers that about
three-fourths of the four-year-olds in Head Start programs lack such
semantic mastery (Hunt and Kirk, 1974), this must be regarded as no
mean achievement.

Not only were these infants of Wave V competent in terms of their performances on the Uzgiris-Hunt scales, they were lively, socially responsive, and very attractive not only to this investigator, but to people in general. This is attested by the fact that five of the 11 had been adopted by childless couples of upper-middle-class status while the writer was in Tehran during October and November of 1974. In contrast, of the 55 infants in the earlier waves, only two had been adopted, and these were taken before they were six months old because they were attractive looking. If such findings can be repeated with larger infant-caretaker ratios, considerable confidence can be placed in the importance of the combination of vocal imitation and talking about caretaking ministrations for the development of language.

V. THE RANGE OF REACTION

Those revisiting the fictional belief in hereditary predeterminism need reminding that Woltereck identified and named the "norm of reaction" as long ago as 1909 (see Rieger et al., 1968, p. 372). This norm refers to the central tendency of the variations in phenotypic reactions that a genotype can develop in response to life in differing environments. The traditional strategy for estimating the range of reaction for the IQ has been to subtract the percentage of variance attributable to heredity, measured by the heritability index, from 100 on the assumption that sources of variance in the IQ are additive. A strategy for assessing the range of reaction that is much more relevant to educability is to ascertain the difference between the means of phenotypic measures of competence for samples of individuals derived from a given population who have developed under contrasting environmental conditions. Just as the generality of an index of heritability is limited to the population and to the particular set of conditions on which it is based, so is any given measure of the range of reaction. The ultimate range of reaction for measures of competence must, however, be at least as large as the difference obtained between the mean values of measures from samples of individuals, from the same population, who have been reared under a particular pair of differing environments.

Evidence concerning the ranges of reaction for ages of achieving top-level object construction and vocal imitation has come from the cross-sectional studies in my program. The most retarded age of achieving top-level object construction, in which the infant follows a desired object out of sight into a container and then the container through three successive disappearances and retrieves it by going to where the container disappeared last and proceeds in reverse order, came in a cross-sectional study by Paraskevopoulos and Hunt (1971). This sample of infants were those reared in the Municipal Orphanage of Athens where the infant-caretaker ratio approximated 10/1. There were two other samples in this study, one

from Metera Baby Center where the infant-caretaker ratio was of the
order of 3/1 and the other consisted of home-reared infants from
working-class families. The means and standard deviations of the
children at five of the levels on the scale of object construction
appear in the three left-hand bars of each of the five clusters in
Figure 1.

At the Municipal Orphanage, the mean age for the seven infants
at the top-level of object construction was 195 weeks; for those of
Metera Center, the mean was 154 weeks, and for those home-reared,
it was 129 weeks. The difference between the mean age for those
home-reared and the mean age of those of the Municipal Orphanage is
66 weeks for this particular pair of conditions.

The most advanced age of achieving top-level object construction came from a longitudinal study concerned with assessing the
effects of the Badger program for the eight infants in the day-care
program of the Parent and Child Center of Mt. Carmel, Illinois.
These infants achieved top-level object permanence at a mean age of
73 weeks, 25 weeks younger than that (98 weeks) at which the 12
infants from predominantly professional families of Worcester,
Mass., achieved it. (See the two right-hand columns of the right-
most cluster in Figure 1). Since the Athens study employed cross-
sectional strategy, it is necessary to convert the mean age of those
at top-level object-permanence into an estimate of the mean age that
they first achieved it. With the correction, the mean age of achieving this landmark becomes 182 weeks. Thus, subtracting the most
advanced mean age of 73 weeks from the most retarded one of 182
weeks yields an estimate of 109 weeks for the range of reaction in
the age of achieving top-level object permanence. This is five
weeks more than two years.

Since differences between mean ages of achieving developmental
landmarks are unfamiliar, it may be useful for purposes of communi-
cative impact to transform this range of reaction into the terms of
Stern's (1912) IQ ratio for object permanence. When this is done,
the range is of the order of 90 points that extend from a lower
limit of 60 to an upper limit of 150. Strictly speaking, of course,
the children of Mt. Carmel and those of Athens, Greece, do not constitute a population genotype. On the other hand, is there any
reason to believe that the genetic potential of the children largely
from working-class families of Athens is less than that of the children from the parents of greatest poverty in Mt. Carmel, Illinois
(see Hunt et al., 1975b)?

Without giving the data, let me note that the range of reaction
for the age of achieving top-level vocal imitation is every bit as
large as that for object construction. Moreover, as already noted,
the extremes can go in opposite directions for these two branches
of sensorimotor development.

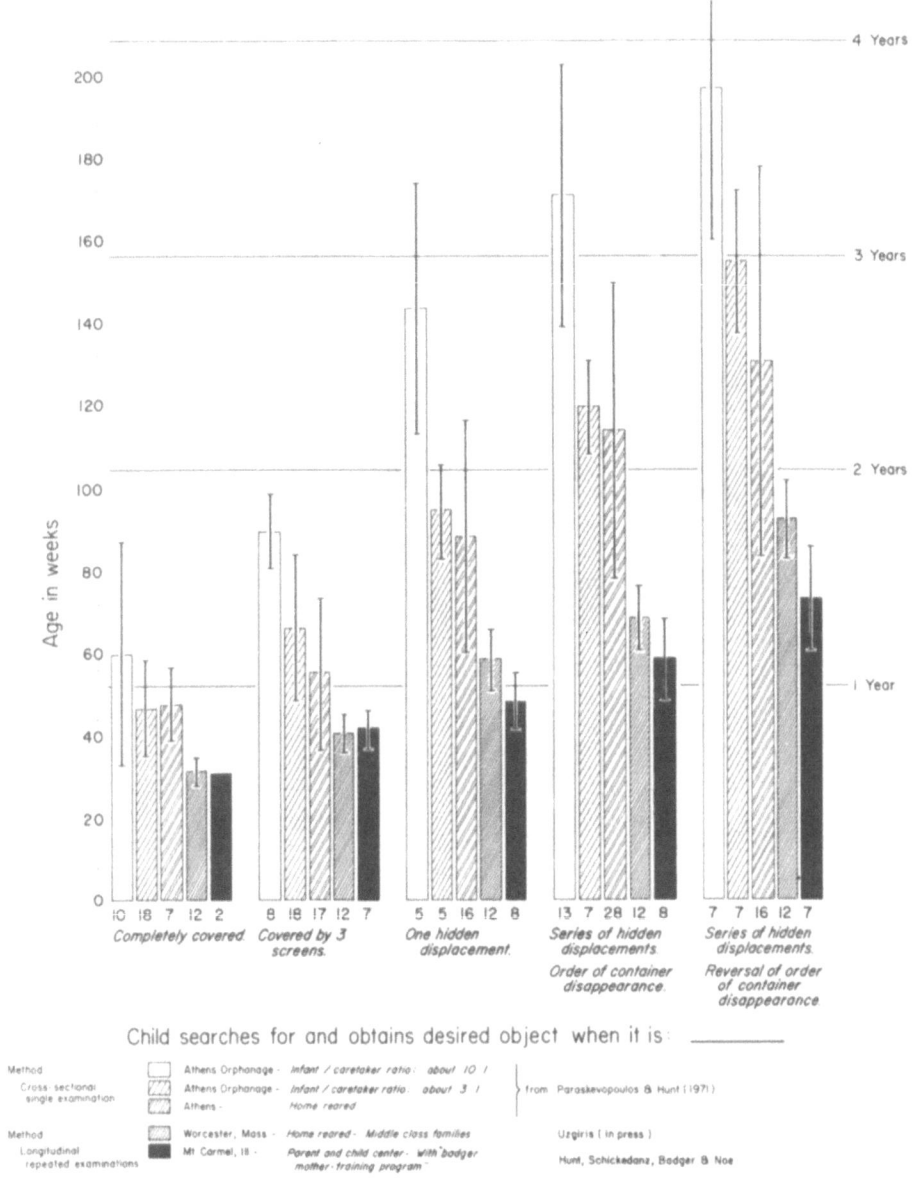

Fig. 1. Object construction under differing conditions of rearing.

Since the data for object construction involve but a single
item, it does violence to the substitutive averaging for the mental
age that serves as the source of an IQ. On the other hand, data
are available in the literature to indicate that this range of
reaction of 90 points may not be abnormally large to any great
degree. Dennis (1966) obtained mean IQs from giving the Goodenough
Draw-A-Man test to samples of typical, healthy children, aged
between six and nine years, who were living in typical family
environments of some 50 cultures over the world. The mean Draw-A-
Man IQs ranged from 124 to 52, giving a range of 72 points, only
18 points short of the 90 for object construction. The high means
came from samples of suburban children in America and England, from
a sample of relatively poor children growing up in a Japanese fish-
ing village, and from a sample of Hopi Indian children who had
almost continuous contact with representative graphic art. The low
means, on the other hand, came from children of nomadic tribes with
almost no contact with graphic art.

While the Draw-A-Man test probably demands a less complex set
of abilities than do the more standard scales, for American children, the IQs from the Draw-A-Man test correspond about as well with
IQs from the Stanford-Binet or the Wechsler Children's Scale as IQs
from these scales correspond with each other.

One can obtain yet another suggestive estimate of the range of
reaction for the IQ at the age of entering school by combining
results from several studies. Two of these, one by Skeels and Dye
(1939) and the other a recent one by Dennis (1973) indicate independently that typical orphanage-rearing results in a retardation
of the order of 50 IQ-points. On the other hand, Garber and Heber
(1973) claim that their educational day-care, described above,
raised the mean Stanford-Binet IQ to 125 for the children at 66
months of age. These results indicate that an intervention has
served to foster, in the offspring of mothers with IQs of 75 or
below, a mean IQ at the age of school entry that is at least 25
points above the norm. Combining the average retardation of 50 IQ-
points with this average advance of 25 IQ-points over the norm
yields an estimate of the range of reaction in standard measures of
the IQ of 75 points.

VI. CONCLUSION

In conclusion, it would appear important that the fiction of
predeterminism should not be allowed to destroy the faith that man
can improve his lot by educational means. The evidence is over-
whelming that there are very substantial effects from the various
kinds of infant-environment interaction on the development of competence and personality. On the other hand, our ignorance of the
details of the relationships between specific forms of antecedent

experiences and later competencies and traits is abysmal. Nevertheless, there are signs of progress, and it should be less than the 2500 years since Plato had his Athenian stranger stress the importance of nature and education before a dependable educational psychology for infancy and early childhood is available.

FOOTNOTES

2. This term _fictions_ is borrowed from Horace Barlow of Cambridge University. In his keynote address at this meeting at the Winter Conference on Brain Research at Steamboat Springs, Colorado, in January of 1975, Dr. Barlow used the term _fictions_ for beliefs that function in the fashion of theory except for their implicit and unanalyzed nature. One message of his address was a plea that fictions should be made explicit for discussion and analysis.

REFERENCES

Abraham, K. 1927. _Selected Papers_. Hogarth, London.

Ainsworth, M.D.S. 1962. The Effects of Maternal Deprivation: A Review of Findings and Controversy in the Context of Research Strategy, pp. 97-165. In _Deprivation of Maternal Care: A Reassessment of its Effects_. World Health Organization, Public Health Paper No. 14, Geneva.

Aries, P. 1960. _Centuries of Childhood: A Social History of Family Life_. (Translation from the French by Robert Burdick). Knopf, New York, 1962.

Armington, D. 1968. _The EDC_ (Educational Development Center) _Head Start Approach_. The Educational Development Center, Newton, Mass.

Babcock, H. 1930. An Experiment in the Measurement of Mental Deterioration. _Arch. Psychol._ 18(117):1-68.

Badger, E. 1971a. _Teaching Guide: Infant Learning Program_. The Instructo Corporation, Paoli, Pa.

Badger, E. 1971b. _Teaching Guide: Toddler Learning Program_. The Instructo Corporation, Paoli, Pa.

Becker, W. 1974. Early Indications of Positive Outcomes. National Follow-Through Sponsor's Presentation, Educational Staff Seminar, February, Washington, D.C.

Bennett, E.L., Diamond, M.C., Krech, D., and Rosenzweig, M.R. 1964. Chemical and Anatomical Plasticity of the Brain. Science 146: 610-619.

Bereiter, C., and Engelmann, S. 1966. Teaching Disadvantaged Children in Preschool. Prentice Hall, Englewood Cliffs, New Jersey.

Berlyne, D.E. 1957. Recent Developments in Piaget's Work. Brit. J. Educ. Psychol. 27:1-12.

Binet, A. 1909. Les Idées Modernes sur les Enfants. Ernest Flamarion, Paris. (Cited from G. D. Stoddard 1939. The IQ: Its Ups and Downs. Educ. Rec. 20:44-57).

Binet, A., and Simon, T. 1905. Méthodes Nouvelles Pour le Diagnostic du Niveau Intellectual des Anormaux. Année Psychol. 11:191-244.

Bowlby, J. 1951. Maternal Care and Mental Health. Monograph Series No. 2. World Health Organization, Geneva.

Bowlby, J. 1958. The Nature of the Child's Tie to his Mother. Internat. J. Psychoanal. 39:1-24.

Brattgård, S.O. 1952. The Importance of Adequate Stimulation for the Chemical Composition of Retinal Ganglion Cells During Early Postnatal Development. Acta Radiologica, Stockholm, Suppl. 96: 1-80.

Caldwell, B.M. 1964. The Effects of Infant Care, pp. 9-87. In M.L. Hoffman and L.W. Hoffman (eds.). Review of Child Development Research, Vol. 1. Russell Sage Foundation, New York.

Caldwell, B.M., Wright, C.M., Honig, A.S., and Tannenbaum, J. 1970. Infant Day-Care and Attachment. Amer. J. Orthopsych. 40: 397-412.

Christie, R. 1962. The Effect of Some Early Experience in the Latent Learning of Adult Rats. J. Exper. Psychol. 43:281-288.

Clark, A.D., and Richards, C.J. 1966. Auditory Discrimination Among Economically Disadvantaged and Nonadvantaged Preschool Children. Exceptional Children 33:259-262.

Cornford, F.M. 1930. Embryology and the Homeomeriety of Anaxagoras. Classical Quart. 24:14-24.

Cronbach, L.J. 1957. The Two Disciplines of Scientific Psychology. Amer. Psychol. 12:671-684.

Denenberg, V.H. 1962. The Effects of Early Experience, pp. 109-138.
    In E.S.E. Hafez (ed.). The Behavior of Domestic Animals.
    Baillière, Tindall, and Cox, London.

Denenberg, V.H., and Naylor, J.C. 1957. The Effects of Early Food
    Deprivation Upon Adult Learning. Psych. Rec. 7:75-77.

Dennis, W. 1934. A Description and Classification of the Responses
    of the Newborn Infant. Psych. Bull. 31:5-22.

Dennis, W. 1960. Causes of Retardation Among Institutional Children:
    Iran. J. Genet. Psychol. 96:47-59.

Dennis, W. 1966. Goodenough Scores, Art Experiences, and Moderniza-
    tion. J. Soc. Psychol. 68:211-228.

Dennis, W. 1973. Children of the Crèche. Appleton-Century-Crofts,
    New York.

Deutsch, C.P. 1964. Auditory Discrimination and Learning Social
    Factors. Merr. Palm. Quart. 10:277-296.

Dobzhansky, T. 1951. Genetics and the Origin of the Species (3rd
    ed.) Columbia University Press, New York.

Dollard, J., and Miller, N.E. 1950. Personality and Psychotherapy:
    An Analysis in Terms of Learning, Thinking, and Culture.
    McGraw-Hill, New York.

Ebert, E., and Simmons, K. 1943. Brush Foundation Study of Child
    Growth and Development: I. Psychometric Tests. Monogr. Soc.
    Res. Child Develop. 8(2), Serial No. 35, 1-113.

Epstein, H.T. 1974a. Phrenoblysis: Special Brain and Mind Growth
    Periods. I. Human Brain and Skull Development. Develop.
    Psychobiol. 7:207-216.

Epstein, H.T. 1974b. Phrenoblysis: Special Brain and Mind Growth
    Periods. II. Human Mental Development. Develop. Psychobiol.
    7:217-224.

Erikson, E.H. 1950. Childhood and Society. Norton, New York.

Flavell, J.H. 1963. The Developmental Psychology of Jean Piaget.
    D. van Nostrand, New York.

Freud, S. 1900. The Interpretation of Dreams. As translated by
    and republished in A.A. Brill 1938. The Basic Writings of
    Sigmund Freud. The Modern Library, New York.

Freud, S. 1905. Three Contributions to the Theory of Sex. In A. A. Brill (Transl. and ed.). 1938. The Basic Writings of Sigmund Freud. Modern Library, New York.

Freud, S. 1915. Instincts and Their Vicissitudes, pp. 60-83. In 1950 Collected Papers, Vol. 4. Hogarth, London.

Freud, S. 1926. Inhibition, Symptom, and Anxiety. H. A. Bunker (Transl.) 1936. The Problems of Anxiety. Norton, New York.

Friedlander, B.Z. 1968. The Effect of Speaker Identity, Voice Inflection, Vocabulary, and Message Redundancy on Infants' Selection of Vocal Reinforcement. J. Exper. Child Psychol. 6:443-459.

Friedlander, B.Z. 1970. Receptive Language Development in Infancy: Issues and Problems. Merr. Palm. Quart. Behav. Develop. 16: 7-51.

Friedman, A. 1957. Drive Conditioning in Water Deprivation. Unpublished doctoral thesis. University of Illinois, Urbana, Illinois.

Froebel, F. 1838. Education by Development. J. Jarvis (Transl.) 1902. Pedagogics of the Kindergarten, Second part. (International Education Series, Vol. 44), Appleton, New York.

Galton, F. 1869. Hereditary Genius: An Inquiry into its Laws and Consequences. MacMillan, London.

Garber, H., and Heber, R.F. 1973. The Milwaukee Project: Early Intervention as a Technique to Prevent Mental Retardation. The University of Conn., National Leadership Institute, Teacher Education/Early Education, Storrs.

Gesell, A. 1954. The Ontogenesis of Infant Behavior. In L. Carmichael (ed.). Manual of Child Psychology. Wiley, New York.

Goldberg, M. 1974. Hopeful Signs for Urban Education. National Follow-Through Sponsor's Presentation to the Education Staff Seminar, February, Washington, D.C.

Goodenough, F.L. 1928. A Preliminary Report on the Effect of Nursery School Training Upon the Intelligence Test Scores of Young Children. Yearbook Nat. Soc. Stud. Educ. 27:361-369.

Gray, S.W., and Klaus, R.A. 1965. An Experimental Preschool Program for Culturally Deprived Children. Child Develop. 36:887-898.

Greenberg, D.J., Uzgiris, I.C., and Hunt, J. McV. 1968. Hastening the Development of the Blink Response with Looking. _J. Genet. Psychol._ 113:167-176.

Greenberg, D.J., Uzgiris, I.C., and Hunt, J. McV. 1970. Attentional Preference and Experience: III. Visual Familiarity and Looking Time. _J. Genet. Psychol._ 117:123-135.

Greenough, W.T., Volkmar, F., and Juraska, J.M. 1973. Effects of Rearing Complexity on Dendritic Branching in Fronto-Lateral and Temporal Cortex of the Rat. _Exper. Neurol._ 41:371-378.

Harlow, H.F. 1958. The Nature of Love. _Amer. Psychol._ 13:673-685.

Harris, A.J., and Shakow, D. 1938. Scatter on the Stanford-Binet in Schizophrenic, Normal, and Delinquent Adults. _J. Abnorm. Soc. Psychol._ 33:100-111.

Hebb, D.O. 1946a. Emotion in Man and Animal: An Analysis of the Intuitive Processes of Recognition. _Psych. Rev._ 53:88-106.

Hebb, D.O. 1946b. On the Nature of Fear. _Psych. Rev._ 53:259-276.

Hebb, D.O. 1949. _The Organization of Behavior._ Wiley, New York.

Hebb, D.O., and Williams, K. 1946. A Method of Rating Animal Intelligence. _J. Genet. Psychol._ 34:59-65.

Heber, R., Garber, H., Harrington, S., Hoffman, C., and Falender, C. 1972. _Rehabilitation of Families at Risk for Mental Retardation._ Rehabilitation Research and Training Center in Mental Retardation, University of Wisconsin, Madison.

Helson, H. 1964. _Adaptation-Level Theory._ Harper and Row, New York.

Herbart, J.F. 1902. _The Science of Education._ H.M. and E. Felkin (Transl.) Heath, Boston.

Hess, E.H. 1959. The Relationship Between Imprinting and Motivation. _Nebraska Symposium on Motivation_ 7:44-77. University of Nebraska Press, Lincoln.

Hildreth, G.H. 1928. The Effect of School Environment upon Stanford-Binet Tests of Young Children. _Yearbook Nat. Soc. Stud. Educ._ 27(1):355-359.

Horsfall, W.R., and Anderson, J.F. 1961. Suppression of Male Characteristics of Mosquitoes by Thermal Means. _Science_ 133:1830.

Hughes, M., Wetzel, R.J., and Henderson, R.W. 1968. The Tucson
    Early Education Model. University of Arizona, College of
    Education, Tucson.

Hull, C.L. 1943. Principles of Behavior. Appleton-Century-Crofts,
    New York.

Hunt, J.McV. 1941. The Effects of Infant Feeding Frustration on
    Adult Hoarding in the Albino Rat. J. Abnorm. Soc. Psychol.
    36:338-360.

Hunt, J.McV. 1946. Experimental Psychoanalysis, pp. 140-156. In
    P. L. Harriman (Ed.). Encyclopedia of Psychology. Philosophi-
    cal Library, New York.

Hunt, J.McV. 1961. Intelligence and Experience. Ronald Press,
    New York.

Hunt, J.McV. 1963. Motivation Inherent in Information Processing
    and Action, pp. 35-94. In O. J. Harvey (ed.). Motivation and
    Social Interaction: The Cognitive Determinants. Ronald Press,
    New York.

Hunt, J.McV. 1965. Intrinsic Motivation and Its Role in Psycholo-
    gical Development. In D. Levine (ed.). Nebraska Symposium on
    Motivation 13:189-282. University of Nebraska Press, Lincoln.

Hunt, J.McV. 1969. The Challenge of Incompetence and Poverty;
    Papers on the Role of Early Education. University of Illinois
    Press, Urbana.

Hunt, J.McV. 1970. Attentional Preference and Experience: I.
    Introduction. J. Genet. Psychol. 117:99-107.

Hunt, J.McV. 1975. Reflections on a Decade of Early Education. In
    D. Wilkerson (ed.). Educating the Children of the Poor: 1975-
    1985. Mediax Associates, Inc., Westport, Conn.

Hunt, J.McV., and Kirk, G.E. 1974. Criterion-Referenced Tests of
    Semantic Mastery in School Readiness: A Paradigm with Illus-
    trations. Genet. Psychol. Monogr. 90:143-182.

Hunt, J.McV., Mohandessi, K., Ghodssi, M., and Akiyama, M. 1975a. The
    Psychological Development of Orphanage Reared Infants: Inter-
    ventions and Outcomes. Department of Psychology, University of
    Illinois (Mimeographed).

Hunt, J.McV., Paraskevopoulos, J., Schickendanz, D., and Uzgiris,
    I.C. 1975b. Variations in the Mean Ages of Achieving
    Object Permanence Under Diverse Conditions of Rearing.
    In B. Z. Friedlander, G. Sterritt, and G. E. Kirk (eds.).
    The Exceptional Infant: Intervention and Assessment, Vol. 3.
    Brunner/Mazel, New York.

Hunt, J.McV., and Quay, H.C. 1961. Early Vibratory Experience and the Question of Innate Reinforcement Value of Vibration and Other Stimuli. Psych. Rev. 68:149-156.

Hunt, J.McV., Schlosberg, H., Solomon, R.L., and Stellar, E. 1947. Studies of the Effects of Infantile Experience on Adult Behavior in Rats: I. Effects of Infantile Feeding Frustration on Adult Hoarding. J. Comp. Physiol. Psych. 40:291-304.

Hunt, J.McV., and Uzgiris, I.C. 1964. Attentional Preference and Cathexis from Recognitive Familiarity: An Exploratory Study. Paper presented at the Symposium to Honor J. P. Guilford, Convention of the American Psychological Association, September. To be published in P.R. Merrifield (ed.). Experimental and Factor-Analytic Measurement of Personality: Contributions by Students of J. P. Guilford. Kent State University Press, Kent, Ohio.

Hydén, H. 1943. Protein Metabolism in the Nerve Cell During Growth and Function. Acta Physiol. Scand. Suppl. 17:1-70.

Inhelder, B., and Piaget, J. 1955. The Growth of Logical Thinking from Childhood to Adolescence: An Essay on the Construction of Formal Operational Structures. Anne Parsons and S. Milgram (Transls.) 1958. Basic Books, New York.

Jencks, C. 1972. Inequality: A Reassessment of the Effect of Family and Schooling in America. Basic Books, New York.

Jensen, A.R. 1969. How Much Can We Boost IQ and Scholastic Achievement? Harv. Educ. Rev. 39:1-123.

Jensen, A.R. 1972. Genetics and Education. Harper and Row, New York.

Johannsen, W. 1909. Elemente der Exakten Erblichkeitslehre. Fischer, Jena.

Jones, H.E. 1954. The Environment and Mental Development. In L. Carmichael (ed.). Handbook of Child Psychology. Wiley, New York.

Karnes, M.B., Teska, J.A., Hodgins, A.A., and Badger, E.D. 1970. Educational Intervention at Home by Mothers of Disadvantaged Infants. Child Develop. 41:925-935.

Kessen, W., Haith, M.M., and Salapatek, P.H. 1970. Infancy, Chap. 5. In P.H. Mussen (ed.). Carmichael's Manual of Child

Psychology, Vol. 1. Wiley, New York.

Koehler, W. 1929. Gestalt Psychology. Liveright, New York.

Lambie, D.S., Bond, J.T., and Weikart, D.P. 1974. Home Teaching
    with Mothers and Infants. High/Scope Educational Research
    Foundation, Ypsilanti, Mich.

Lavatelli, C.S. 1971. A Systematized Approach to the Tucson Method
    of Language Teaching. In C.S. Lavatelli (ed.). Language
    Training in Early Childhood Education. University of Illinois
    Press, Urbana.

Lazar, I., and Rosenberg, M.E. 1971. Day Care in America, Chap. 2.
    In E.H. Grotberg (ed.). Day Care: Resources for Decisions.
    Office of Economic Opportunity, Washington, D.C. Pamphlet
    6106-1.

Levenstein, P. 1970. Cognitive Growth in Preschoolers Through
    Verbal Interaction with Mothers. Amer. J. Orthopsych. 40:
    426-432.

Levenstein, P. 1974. The Mother-Child Home Program. In R.K. Parker
    (ed.). The Preschool in Action (2nd ed.) Allyn and Bacon,
    Boston.

Levine, S. 1962. The Effects of Infantile Experience on Adult
    Behavior, pp. 139-169. In A.J. Bachrach (ed.). Experimental
    Foundations of Clinical Psychology. Basic Books, New York.

Levine, S., Chevalier, H.A., and Korchin, S.J. 1956. The Effects
    of Early Shock and Handling on Later Avoidance Learning.
    J. Person. 24:457-493.

Levy, D.M. 1934. Experiments on the Sucking Reflex and Social
    Behavior in Dogs. Amer. J. Orthopsych. 4:203-224.

Levy, D.M. 1938. On Instinct Satiation: An Experiment on the
    Pecking Behavior of Chickens. J. Genet. Psychol. 18:327-348.

Lipsitt, L.P. 1963. Learning in the First Year, pp. 147-195. In
    L.P. Lipsitt and C.C. Spiker (eds.). Advances in Child Devel-
    opment and Behavior, Vol. 1. Academic Press, New York.

Lipsitt, L.P. 1967. Learning in the Human Infant, pp. 225-247. In
    H.W. Stevenson, R. Hess, and H. Rheingold (eds.). Early
    Behavior: Comparative and Developmental Approaches. Wiley,
    New York.

Locke, J. 1690. An Essay Concerning Human Understanding. Great

Books of the Western World, Vol. 35. Encyclopedia Britannica, Chicago, 1952.

Lorenz, K. 1937. The Companion in the Bird's World. Auk. 54:245-273.

Maltzman, I., and Raskin, D.C. 1965. Effects of Individual Differences in the Orienting Reflex on Conditioning and Complex Processes. J. Exper. Res. Person. 1:1-16.

Marx, M.H. 1952. Infantile Deprivation and Adult Behavior in the Rat: Retention of Increased Rate of Eating. J. Comp. Physiol. Psych. 45:43-49.

Miller, J.O. 1968. Diffusion of Intervention Effects in Disadvantaged Families. Occasional paper. University of Illinois, Coordination Center, National Laboratory on Early Childhood Education, Urbana.

Miller, N.E., and Dollard, J. 1941. Social Learning and Imitation. Yale University Press, New Haven.

Mowrer, O.H., and Kluckhohn, C. 1944. Dynamic Theory of Personality, pp. 69-135. In J.McV. Hunt (ed.). Personality and the Behavior Disorders. Ronald Press, New York.

Needham, J. 1959. A History of Embryology. Abelard-Schuman, New York.

Orlansky, H. 1949. Infant Care and Personality. Psych. Bull. 46:1-48.

Paraskevopoulos, J., and Hunt, J.McV. 1971. Object Construction and Imitation Under Differing Conditions of Rearing. J. Genet. Psychol. 119:301-321.

Pastore, N. 1960. Perceiving as Innately Determined. J. Genet. Psychol. 96:93-99.

Payne, J.S., Mercer, C.D., Payne, R.A., and Davison, R.G. 1973. Head Start: A Tragicomedy with Epilogue. Behavioral Publications, New York.

Piaget, J. 1936. The Origins of Intelligence in Children. Margaret Cook (Transl.) 1952. International Universities Press, New York.

Piaget, J. 1937. The Construction of Reality in the Child. Margaret Cook (Transl.) 1954. Basic Books, New York.

Piaget, J. 1945. <u>Play, Dreams, and Imitation in Childhood</u>.
    C. Gattegno and F.M. Hodgson (Transls.) 1951. Norton, New
    York.

Piaget, J. 1972. Problems of Equilibration, pp. 1-20. In C. F.
    Nodine, J.M. Gallagher, and R.H. Humphreys (eds.). <u>Piaget and
    Inhelder: On Equilibration</u>. Proceedings of the First Annual
    Symposium of the Jean Piaget Society. The Jean Piaget Society,
    Philadelphia, Pa.

Pruette, L. 1926. <u>G. Stanley Hall: A Biography of a Mind</u>. Apple-
    ton-Century-Crofts, New York.

Rasch, E.R., Swift, H., Riesen, A.G., and Chow, K.L. 1961. Altered
    Structure and Composition of Retinal Cells in Dark-Reared
    Mammals. <u>Exp. Cell. Res</u>. 25:348-363.

Renner, K.E. 1966. Temporal Integration: The Effects of Early
    Experience. <u>J. Exper. Res. Person</u>. 1:201-210.

Renner, K.E. 1967. Temporal Integration: Modification of Incent-
    ive Value of a Food Reward by Early Experience with Depriva-
    tion. <u>J. Exper. Psychol</u>. 75:400-407.

Ribble, M.A. 1944. Infantile Experience in Relation to Personality
    Development, Chap. 20. In J.McV. Hunt (ed.). <u>Personality and
    the Behavior Disorders</u>, Vol. 2. Ronald Press, New York.

Rieger, R., Michaelis, A., and Green, M.M. 1968. <u>A Glossary of
    Genetics and Cytogenetics: Classical and Molecular</u> (3rd ed.,
    English). Springer-Verlag, New York.

Riesen, A.H. 1958. Plasticity of Behavior: Psychological Aspects,
    pp. 425-450. In H.F. Harlow and C.N. Woolsey (eds.).
    <u>Biological and Biochemical Bases of Behavior</u>. University of
    Wisconsin Press, Madison.

Robinson, H.B., and Robinson, N.M. 1971. Longitudinal Development
    of Very Young Children in a Comprehensive Day-Care Program:
    The First to Two Years. <u>Child Develop</u>. 42(6):1673-1683.

Rousseau, J.J. 1762. <u>Emile</u>. Barbara Foxley (Transl.) 1916.
    Everyman's Library, New York.

Salama, A.A., and Hunt, J.McV. 1964. "Fixation" in the Rat as a
    Function of Infantile Shocking, Handling, and Gentling. <u>J.
    Genet. Psychol</u>. 105:131-162.

Sears, R.R., Maccoby, E.E., and Levin, H. 1957. <u>Patterns of Child
    Rearing</u>. Row, Peterson, & Co., Evanston, Ill.

Skeels, H.M. 1966. Adult Status of Children with Contrasting Early
    Life Experiences. Monogr. Soc. Res. Child Develop. 31(3),
    Serial No. 105, 1-65.

Skeels, H.M., and Dye, H.B. 1939. A Study of the Effects of Differ-
    ential Stimulation of Mentally Retarded Children. Proc. Amer.
    Assoc. Ment. Defic. 44:114-136.

Skeels, H.M., Updegraff, R., Wellman, B.L., and Williams, H.M.
    1938. A Study of Environmental Stimulation: An Orphanage
    Preschool Project. University of Iowa Study of Child Welfare
    15(4):1-191.

Skinner, B.F. 1938. The Behavior of Organisms: An Experimental
    Analysis. Appleton-Century-Crofts, New York.

Skinner, B.F. 1950. Are Theories of Learning Necessary? Psych.
    Rev. 57:193-216.

Sokolov, E.N. 1963. Higher Nervous Functions: The Orienting
    Reflex. Annual Review of Physiology 25:545-580.

Stern, W. 1912. The Psychological Methods of Testing Intelligence.
    G.M. Whipple (Transl.) 1914. Warwick and York, Baltimore.

Stoddard, G.D. 1939. The IQ: Its Ups and Downs. Educ. Rec.,
    Suppl. 20:44-57.

Stone, L.J. 1954. A Critique of Studies of Infant Isolation.
    Child Develop. 25:9-20.

Terman, L.M., and Merrill, M.A. 1960. Measuring Intelligence.
    Houghton and Mifflin, Boston.

Thompson, W.R., and Heron, W. 1954. The Effects of Restricting
    Early Experience on the Problem-Solving Capacity of Dogs.
    Canad. J. Psychol. 8:17-31.

Thompson, W.R., and Melzack, R. 1956. Early Environment. Sci.
    Amer. 114:38-42.

Thorndike, E.L. 1898. Animal Intelligence. Psych. Rev., Monogr.
    Suppl. 2:1-109.

Thorndike, E.L. 1913a. Educational Psychology. The Original
    Nature of Man, Vol. 1. Columbia University, Teachers College,
    New York.

Thorndike, E.L. 1913b. Educational Psychology. The Learning
    Process, Vol. 2. Columbia University, Teachers College, New

York.

Thorndike, R.L. 1933. The Effect of the Interval Between Test and
    Retest on the Constancy of the IQ. J. Educ. Psychol. 24:543-
    549.

Thorndike, R.L. 1940. "Constancy" of the IQ. Psych. Bull. 37:
    167-186.

Uzgiris, I.C., and Hunt, J.McV. 1966. An Instrument for Assessing
    Infant Psychological Development. University of Illinois,
    Psychological Development Laboratory. (Mimeographed.)

Uzgiris, I.C., and Hunt, J.McV. 1975. Assessment in Infancy:
    Ordinal Scales of Psychological Development. University of
    Illinois Press, Urbana, Ill.

Valverde, R., and Esteban, M.E. 1968. Peristriate Cortex of Mouse:
    Location and the Effects of Enucleation on the Number of
    Dendritic Spines. Brain Res. 9:145-148.

Volkmar, F.R., and Greenough, W.T. 1972. Rearing Complexity
    Affects Branching of Dendrites in the Visual Cortex of the
    Rat. Science 176:1445-1447.

Wachs, T.D., Uzgiris, I.C., and Hunt, J.McV. 1971. Cognitive
    Development in Infants of Different Age Levels and From
    Different Environmental Backgrounds: An Exploratory Investiga-
    tion. Merr. Palm. Quart. 17:283-317.

Watson, J.B. 1916. The Place of the Conditioned-Reflex in Psycho-
    logy. Psych. Rev. 23:89-117.

Watson, J.B. 1917. An Attempted Formulation of the Scope of
    Behavior Psychology. Psych. Rev. 24:329-352.

Watson, J.B. 1926. Behaviorism: A Psychology Based on Reflex
    Action. Arch. Neurol. Psychiat. 15:185-204.

Wechsler, D. 1958. The Measurement and Appraisal of Adult Inte-
    lligence (4th ed.) Williams and Wilkins, New York.

Weikart, D.P. 1972. Relationship of Curriculum, Teaching, and
    Learning in Preschool Education. In J.C. Stanley (ed.).
    Preschool Programs for the Disadvantaged: Five Experimental
    Approaches to Early Childhood Education. Johns Hopkins Press,
    Baltimore.

Weikart, D.P. 1975. Development of Effective Preschool Programs:
    A Report on the Results of the High/Scope Ypsilanti Preschool

Projects. High/Scope Educational Research Foundation, Ypsilanti, Mich.

Weizmann, F., Cohen, L.B., and Pratt, R.J. 1971. Novelty, Familiarity, and the Development of Infant Attention. Develop. Psychol. 4:149-154.

Wetherford, M., and Cohen, L.B. 1973. Developmental Changes in Infant Visual Preferences for Novelty and Familiarity. Child Develop. 44:416-424.

White, B.L. 1967. An Experimental Approach to the Effects of Experience on Early Human Behavior, pp. 201-227. In J.P. Hill (ed.). Minnesota Symposium on Child Psychology. University of Minnesota Press, Minneapolis.

White, B.L. 1974. Child-Rearing Practices and the Development of Competence. Harvard Preschool Project, Graduate School of Education, Harvard University, Cambridge, Mass.

White, B.L. 1975. Critical Influences in the Origins of Competence. Merr. Palm. Quart. (in press).

White, B.L., and Watts, J.C. 1973. Experience and Environment: Major Influences on the Development of the Young Child. Prentice-Hall, Englewood Cliffs, New Jersey.

White, S. 1970. The Learning Theory Approach, Chap. 8. In P.H Mussen (ed.). Carmichael's Manual of Child Psychology. Wiley, New York.

Wiesel, T.N., and Hubel, D.H. 1963. Effects of Visual Deprivation on Morphology and Physiology of Cells in the Cat's Lateral Geniculate Body. J. Neurophysiol. 26:978-993.

Woolley, H.T. 1925. The Validity of Standards of Mental Measurement in Young Childhood. School and Sociology 21:476-482.

Yarrow, L.J. 1961. Maternal Deprivation: Toward an Empirical and Conceptual Re-evaluation. Psych. Bull. 58:459-490.

Yarrow, L.J., Rubenstein, J.L., and Pedersen, F.A. 1974. Infant and Environment: Early Cognitive and Motivational Development. Hemisphere-Halsted, Wiley, Washington, D.C.

THE INFLUENCE OF SEVERE MALNUTRITION IN INFANCY ON THE INTELLIGENCE

OF CHILDREN AT SCHOOL AGE: AN ECOLOGICAL PERSPECTIVE

Stephen A. Richardson

Department of Pediatrics
Albert Einstein College of Medicine
1300 Morris Park Avenue
Bronx, New York 10461

The rationale for including a chapter on malnutrition in a book dealing with brain dysfunction is that severe malnutrition in infancy may cause central nervous system damage which leads to permanent intellectual impairment. The insertion of the word "may" in the preceding sentence is necessary because widely different interpretations have been made of the results of malnutrition studies. Two summaries by reviewers illustrate these differences.

> There is overwhelming evidence that severe malnutrition during the early years of life, especially the first two years, leads to retarded brain growth, permanent reduction in brain size, and defective intellectual development. Malnutrition has, therefore, been rightly blamed as one of the main causes of mental retardation. (Crane and Stern, 1967, cited in Manocha, 1972, p. 123)

> Our review of knowledge about the effects of postnatal nutrition in later development suggests to us that such effects do exist but that they are not large or easily detected. There are many areas of ambiguity. There is as yet no evidence to support the hypothesis that nutritional deprivation not only retards development but that its effects persist into adulthood and prevents the full realization of potential mental competence. (Stein et al., 1975, p. 32)

To understand what has led to such different conclusions it is necessary to review the design of studies of the long range consequences of severe malnutrition, the results, and how they have been interpreted. No attempt will be made here to review independent studies because a number of recent reviews are available (Pan

American Health Organization, 1972; Cravioto et al., 1967; Frisch, 1970; Warren, 1973; Stein et al., 1975; Hertzig, et al., 1972; Scrimshaw and Gordon, 1968; Riccuiti, 1973; Manocha, 1972). Studies of malnutrition in both animals and humans have shown in general that subjects severely malnourished in infancy later perform less well on various tests of learning and intelligence than do "controls" who were not severely malnourished. Authors have used various degrees of caution in suggesting that the malnutrition led to mental retardation or impairment.

Such interpretations of results have become increasingly questioned following close scrutiny of the extent to which the animals and human subjects used as "controls" in the studies met the requirements of experiment controls. That is, everything about the experimental and control cases is matched except for the independent variable of severe malnutrition. In animal experiments the opportunity for manipulating variables is greater than in studies of man. In order to produce malnutrition in animals investigators have disturbed the normal mother-child interactions during early rearing so that the results can be a function of disturbances in early rearing, malnutrition, or some interaction effect (see the chapter by Levine and Wiener, this volume). In human studies, using infants hospitalized for severe malnutrition as subjects, the "controls" were selected matching on a limited number of variables such as age, sex, social class and neighborhood (Champakan et al., 1968; Cabak and Najdanvic, 1965; Chase and Martin, 1970; Pollitt and Granoff, 1967; Stoch and Smythe, 1963, 1967; Birch et al., 1971; Hertzig et al., 1972). Such matching variables are hardly adequate to control on all factors in the children's life experience which may influence intellectual development. In fact there is some evidence in a number of the studies that the "controls" have social and biological histories which are generally considered more advantageous for intellectual development. Increasingly, the question has been raised as to whether severe malnutrition in infancy is an indicator of a more generally disadvantageous set of social and biological conditions which collectively may be sufficient to account for the later differences in intellect found between experimental and control subjects without invoking the additional variable of malnutrition. Stated in this manner the issue has to be examined as a biosocial problem rather than as a problem of brain lesions and their effects.

The use of the term "control" has been partly responsible for diverting attention from the alternative interpretations which have just been discussed. Once the label "control" was attached to the subjects who were not severely malnourished, it was easy for the investigators who introduced the label to begin thinking of the "controls" as though they possessed the ideal experimental requirements, and then to interpret the results as though an ideal experimental design had been employed.

A few studies of humans have employed a research design using siblings as controls for the children who were hospitalized for severe malnutrition (Birch et al., 1971; Hansen et al., 1971; Evans et al., 1971; Hertzig et al., 1972). The rationale for use of siblings is that their background experiences should closely approximate those of the malnourished children. The results of these studies vary. Some show differences in the expected direction of the siblings doing better on intelligence tests, while others show no differences. Again there are problems in the interpretation of findings both of no differences and differences. No difference can be interpreted to mean that severe malnutrition does not lead to later intellectual impairment. Alternatively it may be argued that in a household where there was a severely malnourished child, the other children were also likely to be poorly nourished, and that there was little difference in the level of nutrition that caused the experimental subject to be hospitalized and the sibling control not to be. In both cases impairment of intellect would result from poor nutrition.

The studies which show that the children hospitalized for malnutrition have lower intelligence than their siblings may be interpreted to mean that severe malnutrition was responsible for the difference. However, the presence or absence of hospitalization may suggest that malnutrition is an indicator of a more generally disadvantageous set of life experiences which impair intellectual development. There are further difficulties in the interpretation of findings using siblings as "controls". The study design requirements of having siblings who were not hospitalized for severe malnutrition and matching on variables such as sex and age within three-four years of the hospitalized child restricts the number of cases of hospitalized children who can be studied. For example, in one study of 71 hospitalized children there were only 38 siblings who met the study design requirements (Hertzig, 1972; Richardson et al., 1972, 1973, 1975). Some siblings were not included because they had been hospitalized. Their omission removes from the study families where the problem of malnutrition may be most serious. The absence of a sibling who can be used as a "control" also excludes broken families where siblings have not been living together. In summary, sibling "control" studies introduce selective factors into the identification of "experimental" and "control" subjects which are only partially known and may restrict the findings only to particular sets of family conditions.

In all studies of malnutrition which use the criterion of hospitalization for severe malnutrition, there are four factors which may have long term consequences for intellectual development but have been omitted from research reports. The first is the severity of the malnutrition when the infant is admitted. The second is the quality of the medical care the infant receives during the acute phase in the hospital. These are difficult to

measure. The third factor is the convalescent period following
the acute episode. There is good evidence that during convalescence,
if the caloric intake is sufficiently high, children grow at rates
which are four to six times as great as those of normal infants of
a similar weight or height (Ashworth et al., 1968; Ashworth, 1969;
Suckling and Campbell, 1957; McWilliam and Dean, 1965). If nutrition
is poor during this convalescent period it is possible that this may
have long term detrimental consequences for intellectual impairment.
It may therefore be important to take into account nutrition during
convalescence. The fourth factor omitted from research reports is
the overall growth of the child up to the point of follow-up.
Physical growth at later ages in part reflects the level of nutrition
of the child over his life span. The acute episode as measured by
hospitalization may have differing consequences for intellectual
development depending on the level of nutrition the child receives
during the remainder of his life.

Some studies have inferred malnutrition from the height of
older children and used a study design comparing the tallest and
shortest among a selected set of children (Cravioto et al., 1966;
Cravioto and De Licardie, 1968). These studies have used children
from poor areas where it is thought that severe malnutrition in
infancy is common. These studies generally show the small children
have lower intelligence than the large children. There is no direct
evidence the children had an acute episode of severe malnutrition in
infancy and the studies have not systematically examined the social
and biological background histories of the study subjects to determine whether the small children have had more disadvantageous general
circumstances for intellectual development.

This review suggests that it may be useful to consider changes
in the way the problem of malnutrition has been looked at and then
consider changes in the nature of study design, data collection,
and analysis. Because it is known that a variety of factors influence intellectual development, it is useful to consider some of
these factors when examining the potential role of severe malnutrition in impairment of intellect. Instead of asking, "Does
severe malnutrition in infancy cause later mental retardation or
impairment?", the question might well be changed to, "Under what
circumstances and conditions in the life history of children does
severe malnutrition in infancy contribute to later mental impairment?" To answer the latter question requires some changes from
and addition to the study designs that have been used in the past.

A major change relates to the kinds of data gathering required
for the children hospitalized for severe malnutrition and for the
nonhospitalized children used for comparisons. It is reasonable to
select the comparisons matching on a limited number of variables
such as age, sex, and neighborhood. Instead however, of calling
these comparisons "controls" and assuming that they share the same

kinds of social and biological backgrounds as the hospitalized
children, data collection should include a life history of each
malnourished and comparison child in order to take into account
variations in the background histories which may effect later
intelligence. This more ecological approach requires a selection
of those background factors which research has shown or suggested
to influence the intellectual development of children. This is a
formidable task both to review the literature of research results,
concepts, and theories from which the background factors must be
selected and then to translate the variable selected into data
gathering procedures. Figure 1 illustrates the kinds of variables
which have been derived from a review of previous work in social
and human deprivation, child development, pediatrics, and obstetrics.

     Because the medical care during the acute phase in hospital
and convalescence after an acute episode of severe malnutrition
may be a critical period related to the child's later intellectual
development, studies should report at least on the medical care and
on the kind of feeding received during convalescence and possibly
also the kind and extent of intellectual stimulation and social
experiences during this period.

     In order to obtain some indication of the life time history
of malnutrition, as well as the limited period at the time of the
severe episode of malnutrition in infancy, size of the child at
follow-up should be looked at in relation to IQ. In the past, these
two indicators of child growth have been looked at separately.

I. A STUDY OF SCHOOL CHILDREN SEVERELY MALNOURISHED IN INFANCY

     To illustrate an attempt to approximate the suggested research
approach, a study will be reported of Jamaican children (Richardson,
1975d). (For a fuller set of reports see Hertzig et al., 1972;
Richardson et al., 1972; Richardson et al., 1973; Richardson, 1975a;
Richardson et al., 1975; Richardson, 1975b.) Seventy-four severely
malnourished boys (hereafter referred to as index cases) were selected who had been treated in a hospital for severe malnutrition during
their first two years of life. The malnutrition was reflected
variously in syndromes of marasmus, kwashiorkor, or marasmic-
kwashiorkor. Marasmus is characterized by wrinkled, loose hanging
skin, absence of subcutaneous fat, muscle atrophy, and prominent
bones and joints. The abdomen is usually scaphoid but may be dis-
tended. Temperature and blood pressure are often subnormal.
Physical activity is almost nil. In kwashiorkor there is reduced
physical activity, weakness, apathy, and irritability. Edema may
be gross and generalized, or slight and localized. Changes in pig-
mentation of the skin and hair are often present. When severe loss
of fat and muscle atrophy are also present, the diagnosis of

Child's Biologic Mother
    Reproductive history
    Health history
Mother's or Caretaker's Capabilities and Activities
    Verbal ability
    Values
    Exposure to ideas
    Activities and affiliations
    Human resources
    Training and upbringing of the child
    Aspirations for the child
    Mother as teacher of the child
Father or Adult Male
    Presence of adult male role model in the household
    Existence of affectionate ongoing relationship with the child
    Joint activities of husband and wife with the child
    Degree of conflict or cooperation between husband and wife in
        childrearing
Family
    Composition
    Stability
    Extended family
    Social relations between family, friends and neighbors
    Alternative caretakers available for the child
Physical and Economic Resources of the Family
    Income in cash and kind
    Type and size of dwelling
    Water supply
    Availability of electricity
    Appliances
    Type of fuel used
    Transportation
Area of Residence
    Spectrum ranging from isolated rural location to large urban
        center
Child's Background History
    Pregnancy number and ordinal position
    Birth weight and general health history (other than malnutrition)
    Feeding during the first two years of life
    Continuity in prime caretaker
    Continuity in composition of family
    Relationships with adults
    Relationships with other children
    Exposure to ideas and language
    Activities and experiences outside the home
    School history

Fig. 1. Ecological factors related to intellectual development[*]

---

[*](Richardson, 1972)

marasmic-kwashiorkor is usually made (Barnett and Einhorn, 1972, pp. 171-173). Evidence of the malnutrition was obtained from the detailed clinical and metabolic hospital records. These children received an average eight weeks of inpatient care with good medical care and feeding of good quality and quantity. Afterwards follow-up visits were made by nurses to the boys' homes for two years following discharge. These boys were later traced and at the time of follow-up ranged in age from six through ten years. These ages were selected so as to be far enough removed from the time of acute illness to eliminate the effects of immediate sequelae and for the boys to be at an age when intelligence testing has predictive value.

A classmate or neighbor comparison was selected for each index case. For index boys attending school a classmate nearest in age and of the same sex was chosen. Eleven of the 74 index boys were not attending school because of lack of school facilities. For these 11 cases a comparison was chosen by finding the nearest neighboring child who was not a relative, was of the same sex and within six months of age of the index case. It was determined that none of the comparisons had ever been hospitalized for severe malnutrition. This method of selection obtained matched pairs of index and comparison cases who lived in the same general neighborhood. This made it unlikely that index and comparison matched cases would come from widely differing socioeconomic classes, but provided for variability of life experiences among the study subjects within the same neighborhood.

Each child's intellectual level was individually evaluated by means of the WISC. Clearly the IQs obtained for Jamaican children are not directly comparable with those of children in the cultures where the test was standardized. However as Vernon (1969) has pointed out, comparisons of children within a culture on a test standardized in another setting is appropriate provided the test discriminates between the individuals tested. Experienced testers were used who did not know whether a subject was an index or comparison case.

To obtain background histories of the study subjects which included variables hypothesized to be associated with intellectual development, a detailed home interview and set of observations was developed and data were collected at the child's home from the mother or principal guardian of the child. (Hereafter the term 'guardian' will be used to cover both parents and guardians.) From the questions and answers, and from the observational data, a series of quantified variables were derived, each variable based on combining a number of indicators of that variable (for details of the measures see Richardson, 1975b). For each social, economic, or biological variable it was predicted that the index boys would be more at a disadvantage, and that for each variable, those boys with the hypothesized disadvantageous scores would have lower IQs than those with advantageous scores. The list of variables selected is shown in Fig. 2.

To obtain a single composite measure of the boys' background histories, one variable was selected from each of the general categories: a variable concerning the guardian; an economic and housing variable; and an educational and social variable. The variables selected are shown in Table 1, together with the indicators used in obtaining a score for each variable. On each variable, the index boys are found to be significantly more disadvantaged. For each variable, there is a significant correlation in the predicted direction between higher IQs and a more advantageous score on the variable. Each of these variables was given equal weight, and the scores on the three variables were added to give a composite score of the child's background history.

At the time of the follow-up study, the height of each study subject was obtained. To make the heights comparable across the age range of the subjects, standard scores were obtained based on standards developed for Jamaican primary school boys seven years and older (Ashcroft and Lovell, 1966) and for rural Jamaican boys under seven (Ashcroft et al., 1965).

```
Guardian Variables
      Guardian's upbringing and education
      Mother's general reproductive history
      Mother's pregnancy with study child
      Guardian's level of capacity
      Guardian's contact with media
      Guardian's human resources
Mortality Variable
      Mortality among siblings
Economic and Housing Variables
      Structure and condition of the house
      Home furnishings and appliances
      Amount of crowding in the house
Educational and Social Variables (pertaining to child)
      Extent and diversity of child's social relationships
      Intellectual stimulation
      Caretaker's child rearing practices
      Amount of schooling
```

Fig. 2. Variables used in the study of the background histories of Jamaican index and comparison boys[*]

---

[*](Richardson, 1975b)

TABLE 1.   Variables Selected for A Composite Background History
           Score*

		Differences Between Index and Comparison Boys	
	χ^2	Significance Level of the Difference	Correlation with I.Q.
Caretaker's Level of Capacity	13.79	$p < 0.01$	0.43
Use of free time			
Degree of literacy			
Use of caretaker by others as a source of help or advice			
State of neatness & organization of house			
Caretaker's comprehension, language & level of intelligence			
Home Furnishings & Appliances	5.34	$p < 0.025$	0.53
Use of electricity & refrigerator			
Number of electrical appliances			
Fuel used for cooking			
Person:bed ratio			
Presence of sewing machine			
Presence of transistor radio			
Intellectual Stimulation	7.27	$p < 0.05$	0.46
Toys given to child			
Child has books or magazines			
Child listens to radio			
Frequency of child's TV watching			
Frequency of trips child taken on			
Stories told or read to child			

*Adapted from Richardson, 1975c.

II.   RESULTS

The first step was to determine whether the index boys were
smaller in stature at follow-up and whether they experienced more
disadvantageous background histories. The index boys were found to
be significantly smaller in height at school age (Richardson, 1975a).

The index boys were also found to have significantly more disadvantageous background histories (Richardson, 1975b).

The second step was to determine the associations between each of the three variables of malnutrition, height and background history, and the measure of I.Q. The index boys were found to have significantly lower IQs than the comparisons (Hertzig et al., 1972). To examine the relations between height, background history and IQ, the index and comparison cases were combined. The taller boys were found to have significantly higher IQs than the smaller boys (Table 2). The boys with the lowest or more disadvantageous background history composite scores were found to have significantly lower IQs than boys with the highest or more advantageous background history scores (Table 3).

Having shown that malnutrition in infancy, height at follow-up, and the background history measure are each associated with I.Q. in the expected direction, the next step was to determine the relative contribution of each of the three variables to I.Q. To do this, a multiple correlation coefficient was obtained. The overall coefficient is 0.674, which indicates that 46% of the variance is accounted for. When the overall variance is broken down into the three components, the largest contributor is the background history measure, which provides 0.294 of the variance. Hospitalization in infancy for severe malnutrition is the smallest contributor with 0.049 of the variance, and height provides an intermediate variance of 0.112 (Table 4).

TABLE 2. Index and Comparison Boys Combined by I.Q. and Height[*]

Height	Full Scale I.Q.		
	≤ 55	56–65	≥ 66
> 1/2 S.D. below mean[†]	26	12	9
1/2 S.D. below mean to 1/2 S.D. above mean	20	15	13
> 1/2 S.D. above mean	10	14	26

$\chi^2 = 16.88$ $p < 0.01$

[*](Richardson, 1976)

[†]Mean heights for age taken from Ashcroft & Lovell, 1966; Ashcroft et al., 1965.

TABLE 3.   Index and Comparison Boys Combined by I.Q. and
           Background History Scores[*]

Background History Score	Full Scale I.Q.		
	≤ 55	55-65	≥ 66
Lowest 3 Deciles	31	9	5
Middle 4 Deciles	20	22	14
Highest 3 Deciles	5	10	29

χ^2 = 45.2   p < 0.0005

[*](Richardson, 1976)

TABLE 4.   Relative Contributions of Background History Score,
           Malnutrition and Height to I.Q. Variance Estimates[*]

	Background History Score	Malnutrition	Height	
Multiple Correlation Coefficient	= R^2 = 0.294	+ 0.049	+ 0.112	= 0.455

R = 0.674   [*](Richardson, 1976)

TABLE 5.   I.Q. Scores for Two Extreme Groups of Index and
           Comparison Boys[*]

Subset 1 (n = 14)
    Index
    Height > 1/2 S.D. below mean
    Background History Score in lowest 4 deciles

Subset 2 (n = 19)
    Comparison
    Height > 1/2 S.D. above mean
    Background History Score in top 4 deciles

Subset 1 I.Q. Scores:

46,46,46,46,46,46,46,47,48,51, | 53,54,54,   62, |

Subset 2 I.Q. Scores: | 53,   59, | 63,64,67,68,68,69,
                               | | 69,69,72,72,76,79,
                               | | 86,86,89,101,113

[*](Richardson, 1976)

A somewhat different perspective of the results is obtained by examining the IQs of boys with different combinations of acute malnutrition in infancy, height at follow-up, and background history. First, we examined the I.Q. scores of the two extreme subsets of study subjects. Subset 1 consisted of boys who were hospitalized (index), whose height was more than half a standard deviation below the Jamaican standards (Ashcroft and Lovell, 1966; Ashcroft et al., 1965), and whose composite background history score was in the lowest four deciles. Subset 2 consisted of boys not hospitalized, with heights more than half a standard deviation above the Jamaican standards, and whose background history score was in the top four deciles. The IQs of these two subsets are strikingly different (Table 5). Half of the cases in Subset 1 have IQs on the floor of the test; only two of Subset 2 overlap in I.Q. scores with Subset 1.

The mean and median IQs of index and comparison boys who have different heights and background history scores are shown in Table 6. It shows that under certain conditions the index boys have higher IQs than the comparisons. For example, index boys who are tall and have an advantageous background history have an average I.Q. score 11 points higher than comparison boys who are short in stature and have a disadvantageous background history. Table 6 also provides an opportunity to examine whether the difference in I.Q. between index and comparison boys varies under different conditions of height and background history when these are held constant for both groups. Under the most favorable conditions of being tall and having an advantageous background history, the average I.Q. of the index boys is only two points lower than the comparisons. Under the most unfavorable conditions of short stature and disadvantageous background histories, the average I.Q. of the index boys is 9 points lower than comparisons. The combinations of advantageous background histories and short stature, and of disadvantageous background history and tall stature, show I.Q. differences between index and comparison cases of 3 and 7 points respectively. These differences are summarized in Fig. 3.

The results suggest that an acute episode of severe malnutrition in the first two years of life has differing consequences for intellectual impairment, depending on the background history and characteristics of the child's guardian, the economic conditions of the household, and the kind of social experience the child has had. Further, the consequences are influenced by the life history of the child which is reflected in his stature at time of follow-up. Height provides some indication of the child's nutritional history, and possibly something of his overall health, in addition to having a genetic component. If severe malnutrition in infancy occurs in a context of a life history which is generally favorable for intellectual development, the early malnutrition appears to have a negligible effect on intellectual functioning. If early malnutrition occurs in

TABLE 6. I.Q. Means and Medians of Index and Comparison Boys by Height and Background History Scores*

BACKGROUND HISTORY SCORE[†]

	Lowest 4 Deciles			Middle 2 Deciles			7th,8th,9th Deciles		
	N	I.Q. Mean	I.Q. Median	N	I.Q. Mean	I.Q. Median	N	I.Q. Mean	I.Q. Median
I N D E X Height									
> 1/2 S.D. below mean[†]	14	49	47	9	54	54	8	62	57
1/2 S.D. above and below mean	11	52	51	6	58	62	7	67	66
> 1/2 S.D. above mean	8	55	55	4	66	67	6	69	73
C O M P A R I S O N S Height									
> 1/2 S.D. below mean[†]	7	58	58	1	¶	--	4	65	65
1/2 S.D. above and below mean	14	55	53	1	--	--	6	69	67
> 1/2 S.D. above mean	6	62	62	7	67	65	13	71	69

*(Richardson, 1976).

[†]10th Decile scores not included because 1 index & 12 comparison boys were in this decile. Disparate proportion of boys in 10th decile reduces extent to which more advantageous background history category can be held constant for index & comparison boys.

[†]Mean heights for age taken from Ashcroft & Lovell, 1966; Ashcroft et al., 1965.

¶Indicates lack of sufficient cases.

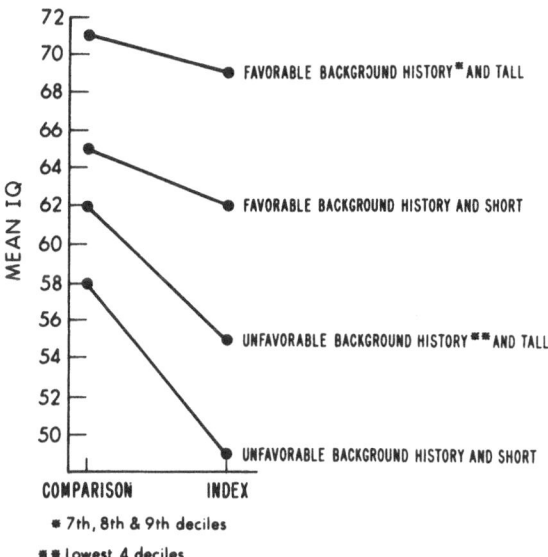

Fig. 3. Mean IQ's of index and comparison boys when background history score and height are held constant (Richardson, 1976).

an unfavorable general ecology for intellectual development, the severe episode of malnutrition has a clear relation to later intellectual impairment. This type of interactional effect of several deleterious variables on intellectual function is similar to that reported by Beckwith for premature infants and by Davenport for hormonal imbalance in this volume.

A similar example of the effect of a potential early insult to a child's intellectual development is the differential consequences of low birth weight and gestational age depending on the socioeconomic conditions of the family into which the child is born. A study which dealt with the obstetrical histories of school children in Scotland reports:

The purpose was to examine the association between combinations of birth weight and gestational age, and later intellectual functioning of the children. Further, we wished to see whether low birth weight and gestational age would have different associations with the child's intelligence at age 7. We therefore looked at the associations for each social-class category separately. In order to avoid the effects of obstetrical and neonatal compli-

cations, any cases with such complications were removed and analyzed separately...(The analysis was
also restricted to children who had not been adminis-
tratively classified as mentally subnormal. We had
found separately that low birth weight...and low gestational age were more frequent for mentally subnormal
children than for children who were not mentally subnormal.)

(Figure 4 of the present paper) shows the average I.Q.
of children with different birth weights and gestational ages within each social class category. For
each social class, children with birth weights of less
than 37 weeks have lower I.Q. scores than the I.Q. for
all children within the same social classes. With the
exception of the upper social class I-IIIa, when children have experienced both low birth weight and low
gestational age, they have lower average intelligence
scores than when low gestational age was present, but
not low birth weight. The size of difference in average
I.Q. between all children in a social class and the
children with low birth weight and gestational age is
larger in the lower than in the upper social classes.
This suggests that there is a bio-social interaction,
with children of lower social class families at greater
risk of intellectual impairment from low birth weight
and gestational age than children from upper class
families (Richardson, 1974).

If all mentally subnormal children had been included in this
analysis, the differences by social class of the relationship between birth weight and gestational age, and I.Q. at age seven would
have been even more marked.

It appears clear that the concept that severe malnutrition in
infancy causes central nervous system damage which then, in turn,
causes mental retardation or impairment is too simple. A more complex conceptualization is needed which accounts for biological and
social variables that may influence the child's intellectual functioning and development over his life span, including the period of
fetal growth and the neonatal period. The Jamaican study reported
only makes a start in this direction and will require the addition
of further background history variables using a broad ecological
perspective. It will also require the use of multivariate forms of
analysis which take into account the interactions between variables.
The only functional outcome or dependent variable reported here was
I.Q. A broader conceptualization is needed which provides some
functional profile of the child which would include social, emotional
and motor functioning. This is necessary to expand our understanding

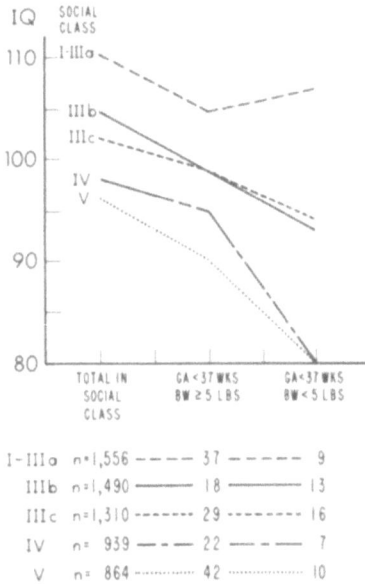

Fig. 4. I.Q. test scores and social class of seven year old children with different gestational age (GA) and birth weight (BW) in Aberdeen, Scotland, 1962 (Richardson, 1972, 1974).

of the long-range consequences of early malnutrition for child development. It should be emphasized that the Jamaican study applies to boys at ages six through ten who have had high standards of medical care during the acute phase of malnutrition after hospitalization and good nutrition during the period of convalescence following the severe malnutrition. Further, the severe malnutrition occurred for our study subjects during the first two years of life. We have examined whether the consequences of severe malnutrition for later I.Q. varied depending on the age at hospitalization within the first two years and found no differences by age. Whether different results would have been obtained using girls, different ages at follow-up, and poor conditions of medical care and nutrition during the acute episode and convalescence are open questions which other studies must answer.

The finding that, under disadvantageous circumstances for intellectual development, the index boys have lower IQs than the comparisons does not tell us what it was about the episode of severe malnutrition that caused the lower IQs. The hospitalization may have been associated with other factors which we have not identified, but which contribute toward later intellectual impairment.

In closing it may be useful to consider the content of this
chapter from the viewpoint of the title, Environments As Therapy
For Brain Dysfunction. The only forms of therapeutic intervention
were medical and nutritional during hospitalization and convalescence. The major focus in this chapter has been the variations
that naturally occur in the ecology of Jamaican life and how these
relate to the intellectual development of children. The study suggests that, when the problem of malnutrition is posed, therapy
should not be restricted to consideration of how to provide more
food for children, but should take into account the more complex
array of factors which have been considered. Further, therapy should
not be restricted to one approach, but needs a variety of approaches
if it is to have any chance of success. By examining the ecology of
those children who live in the same neighborhoods as children who
have experienced early acute malnutrition, but who are found to be
functioning well above the average, we can begin to learn about the
conditions of socialization these children have experienced, and
how those responsible for their upbringing have used local resources,
customs, and practices. What is learned from such studies may suggest forms of intervention and therapy which will benefit the overall
development of children and be more acceptable than therapy developed
in other settings which may not be either acceptable or effective in
the particular setting. There is always political appeal in simple
approaches to complex problems. Ecological multivariate studies of
child development will hopefully yield results which will provide a
basis for more complex forms of therapeutic intervention which will
be beneficial to children.

REFERENCES

Ashcroft, M. T., and Lovell, H. G. 1966. Heights and Weights of
    Jamaican Primary School Children. J. Trop Ped. 12:37-43.

Ashcroft, M. T., Lovell, H. G., and Williams, A. 1965. Heights
    and Weights of Infants and Children in a Rural Community of
    Jamaica. J. Trop Ped. 11:56-68.

Ashworth, A. 1969. Growth Rates in Children Recovering From
    Protein-Calorie Malnutrition. Br. J. Nutr. 23:835-845.

Ashworth, A., Bell, R., James, W. P. T., and Waterlow, J. C. 1968.
    Calorie Requirements of Children Recovering From Protein-
    Carolie Malnutrition. Lancet 2:600.

Barnett, H. L., and Einhorn, A. H. (eds.). 1972. Pediatrics (15th
    ed.). Appleton-Century-Crofts, New York.

Birth, H. G., Piñeiro, C., Alcade, E., Toca, T., and Cravioto, J.

1971. Relation of Kwashiorkor in Early Childhood and Intelligence at School Age. Pediat. Res. 5:579-585.

Cabak, V., and Najdanvic, R. 1965. Effect of Under Nutrition in Early Life on Physical and Mental Development. Arch. Dis. Child. 40:532-534.

Champakam, S., Srikantia, S. G., and Gopalan, C. 1968. Kwashiorkor and Mental Development. Amer. J. Clin. Nutr. 21:844-852.

Chase, H. P., and Martin, H. P. 1970. Undernutrition and Child Development. N. Engl. J. Med. 282:933-939.

Crane, L. C., and Stern, J. 1967. Pathology of Mental Retardation. Churchill, London.

Cravioto, J., and De Licardie, E. R. 1968. Intersensory Development of School-Age Children, pp. 252-268. In N. S. Scrimshaw and J. E. Gordon (eds.). Malnutrition, Learning, and Behavior. MIT Press, Cambridge, Massachusetts.

Cravioto, J., Birch, H. G., De Licardie, E. R., and Rosales, L. 1967. The Ecology of Infant Weight Gain in a Pre-Industrial Society. Acta Paediat. Scand. 56:71-84.

Cravioto, J., De Licardie, E. R., and Birch, H. G. 1966. Nutrition, Growth, and Neurointegrative Development: An Experimental and Ecologic Study. Pediatrics Suppl. 38:319.

Evans, D. E., Moodie, A. D., and Hansen, J. D. L. 1971. Kwashiorkor and Intellectual Development. S. Afr. Med. J. 45:1413-1426.

Frisch, R. E. 1970. Present Status of the Supposition that Malnutrition Causes Permanent Mental Retardation. Am. J. Clin. Nutr. 23:189-195.

Hansen, J. D. L., Freesemann, C., Moodie, A. D., and Evans, D. E. 1971. What Does Nutritional Growth Retardation Really Imply? Pediatrics 47:299.

Hertzig, M. E., Birch, H. G., Richardson, S. A., and Tizard, J. 1972. Intellectual Levels of School Children Severely Malnourished During the First Two Years of Life. Pediatrics 49: 814-824.

Manocha, S. L. 1972. Malnutrition and Retarded Human Development. Charles C. Thomas, Springfield, Illinois.

McWilliam, K. M., and Dean, R. F. A. 1965. The Growth of Malnourished Children After Hospital Treatment. E. Afr. Med. J.

42:297-304.

Nutrition, The Nervous System and Behavior. 1972. Pan American
    Health Organization, Scientific Publication No. 251.

Pollitt, E., and Granoff, D. 1967. Mental and Motor Development
    of Peruvian Children Treated for Severe Malnutrition. Rev.
    Interamer. Psicol. 1:93.

Ricciuti, H. N. 1973. Malnutrition and Psychological Development,
    pp. 63-78. In Biological and Environmental Determinants of
    Early Development. Research publication A. R. N. M. D. 50.

Richardson, S. A. 1976. The Relation of Severe Malnutrition in
    Infancy to the Intelligence of School Children Under Different
    Ecological Conditions. Pediatric Research 10:1.

Richardson, S. A. 1975a. Physical Growth of Jamaican School Child-
    ren Who Were Severely Malnourished Before Two Years of Age.
    J. Biosoc. Sci. 7:445-462.

Richardson, S. A. 1975b. The Background Histories of School Child-
    ren Severely Malnourished in Infancy, pp. 167-195. In
    I. Schulman (ed.). Advances in Pediatrics, Vol. 21. Yearbook
    Publishers, Chicago.

Richardson, S. A. 1975c. The Ecology of Severe Malnutrition and
    Intellectual Development, pp. 528-531. In D. A. A. Primrose
    (ed.). Proceedings of the Third Congress of the I. A. S. S.
    M. D. Polish Medical Publishers, Warsaw, Poland.

Richardson, S. A. 1974. The Reduction of Stress for Persons With
    Handicaps, pp. 426-430. In L. Levi (ed.). Society, Stress and
    Disease: Childhood and Adolescence. Oxford University Press,
    Oxford, England.

Richardson, S. A. 1972. Ecology of Malnutrition: Non-nutritional
    Factors Influencing Intellectual and Behavioral Development.
    In Nutrition, The Nervous System and Behavior. Pan American
    Health Organization, Scientific Publication No. 251.

Richardson, S. A., Birch, H. G., and Ragbeer, C. 1975. The Behavior
    of Children at Home Who Were Severely Malnourished in the First
    Two Years of Life. J. Biosoc. Sci. 7:255-267.

Richardson, S. A., Birch, H. G., and Hertzig, M. E. 1973. School
    Performance of Children Who Were Severely Malnourished in In-
    fancy. J. Mental Def. 77:623-632.

Richardson, S. A., Birch, H. G., Grabie, E., and Yoder, K. 1972. The Behavior of Children in School Who Were Severely Malnourished in the First Two Years of Life. J. Health Soc. Behav. 13:276-284.

Scrimshaw, N. S., and Gordon, J. E. (eds.). 1968. Malnutrition, Learning and Behavior. The M.I.T. Press, Cambridge, Massachusetts.

Stein, Z., Susser, M., Saenger, G., and Marolla, F. 1975. Famine and Human Development. Oxford University Press, New York.

Stoch, M. B., and Smythe, P. A. 1967. The Effect of Undernutrition During Infancy on Subsequent Brain Growth and Intellectual Development. S. Afr. Med. J. 41:1027-1030.

Stoch, M. B., and Smythe, P. M. 1963. Does Undernutrition During Infancy Inhibit Brain Growth and Subsequent Intellectual Development? Arch. Dis. Child. 38:546.

Suckling, P. V., and Campbell, J. A. H. 1957. A Five-Year Follow-Up of Coloured Children With Kwashiorkor in Cape Town. J. Trop. Ped. 2:173-180.

Vernon, P. E. 1969. Intelligence and Cultural Environment. Methuen, London.

Warren, N. 1973. Malnutrition and Mental Development. Psychol. Bull. 80:324-328.

CAREGIVER-INFANT INTERACTION AS A FOCUS FOR

THERAPEUTIC INTERVENTION WITH HUMAN INFANTS

Leila Beckwith

Infant Studies Project
Rehabilitation Institute
23-39 UCLA Campus
Los Angeles, California 90024

I. STATEMENT OF PROBLEM

This chapter will focus upon the effects of the postnatal environment upon behavioral capacity in high risk infants. Specifically it asks: By what process do at-risk infants from favorable environments overcome their deficits? What are the significant dimensions of such environments?

Prenatal and perinatal hazards, such as complications of pregnancy and delivery, prematurity, and abnormal neonatal conditions, may determine not only the probability of survival of the human infant but may also put him/her at greater statistical risk during childhood for a wide range of handicapping conditions. These include sensory, perceptual-motor, cognitive, and/or neurological dysfunctioning (e.g. Caputo and Mandell, 1970; Drillien, 1964; Wiener, 1962), as well as behavior problems (Pasamanick et al., 1956) and even such deviant interpersonal syndromes as autism (Knobloch and Pasamanick, 1962) or schizophrenia (Garmezy and Streitman, 1974). However, such adverse consequences are not inevitable and there is considerable controversy as to which obstetrical conditions are hazardous (Parmelee and Haber, 1973). Many infants show no deleterious effects of prenatal and perinatal problems. In behavior that has been investigated, individual vulnerable infants differ as widely in range of performance as do individual normal infants. Further, many vulnerable infants appear to overcome initial handicaps. Several investigators point to the "wash out" of perinatal effects in later childhood (Drillien, 1964; Werner et al., 1971).

In addition, and most pertinent to this chapter, postnatal

experience may amplify or diminish the probability of deficits (Drillien, 1964; Sameroff and Chandler, 1975; Werner et al., 1971). Variables in social status have been found to be as potent in the development of risk children (Drillien, 1964; Werner et al., 1971) as in normal children (Deutsch, 1973). Lower social status not only seems to increase the incidence of reproductive hazards, but may increase their likelihood of developmental handicaps for affected individuals (Braine et al., 1966; Drillien, 1964; Werner et al., 1971). Furthermore, such factors as family stability (Drillien, 1964; Werner et al., 1971), intellectual stimulation (Werner et al., 1971), and emotional support (Werner et al., 1971) have been found to be as important as social status in modifying the incidence of later difficulties.

II. SIGNIFICANCE OF INFANCY EXPERIENCES

Our inquiry into the empirical findings and theoretical issues will focus on preterm babies without specific severe sensory or motor handicaps. Prematurity has been suggested to be a model problem for assessing effects of the continuum of reproductive casualty (Birch and Gussow, 1970), and is the single most prevalent abnormality associated with birth. The emphasis follows the strategy suggested by Knobloch and Pasamanick.

> Since human development is affected by so many different modes of integration, with the social forces frequently influencing the psychologic behavior by way of the biologic functions, any attempt to unravel them must involve an understanding of the various factors influencing behavior as early in life as they can be studied and analyzed. (1960, p. 210)

More specifically, this chapter adopts a position espoused by Sameroff and Chandler (1975). They ascribe to a complex of mutual influences between the child and his environment which dissipate or amplify the effects of earlier developmental insults. Rather than interpret development as a chain of efficient causes and invariant effects operating on passive organisms, they believe that development proceeds from children regularly restructing themselves and their environments. The suggested analogy is self-righting rather than tabula rasa.

Piaget's work (1952) issues from a parallel emphasis on the organism, on one hand, and its transactions with the environment on the other. Intelligence, as well as social adaptation, derives from the ongoing creative process of an infant and child acting on the environment (see chapter by Hunt, this volume). Piaget's position is supported by, and has contributed to, an explosion in infancy research. From an earlier view of babies as helpless and

incompetent, the power of neonates and young infants to discriminate
among stimuli to show preferences and to evoke selectively, respond
to, maintain, adapt to, and even terminate transactions with their
environment is being increasingly recognized (Stone et al., 1973).
As capacities of neonates are delineated, wide ranges of individual
performances are demonstrated (e.g. Barten, Birns, and Rouch, 1971;
Bell, Weller, and Waldrop, 1971; Birns, 1965; Korner, 1971). The
differences are probably not ephemeral. Some have been shown to be
stable over situations (Osofsky and Danzger, 1974), and over days as
well as several months (Barten and Rouch, 1971; Osofsky, 1975).

The increased understanding of normal neonates has not been
matched in infants who have sustained prenatal and perinatal hazards.
Investigation of individual differences among such risk infants and
comparison with normal infants has been limited, with some notable
exceptions. Investigators seeking to describe innate temperamental
differences, and recognizing the potential impact of prenatal
environmental events and their sequelae, have specifically excluded
babies with deviant obstetrical histories. Such examination could
increase our understanding of the development of risk children. At
least three issues are relevant.

1) In what ways is the development of risk children a direct
consequence of changes in the nervous system? 2) In what ways is
the development of risk children a consequence of changed caregiver-
infant transactions? 3) Can caregiver-infant transactions alleviate
early problems? In regard to the second question, one might speculate that early differences might make the mutual adaptation of the
infant to his environment more difficult, and may contribute to the
increased incidence of gross abuses of caretaking found in one group
of risk children (Sameroff and Chandler, 1975). That is, preterm
infants may show not only deficits in their own development but they
are also subject to an increased incidence of child battering (Klein
and Stern, 1971). In regard to the third question, since an infant
is not a stable complete organism but one that changes by transactions with the environment, greater understanding of the infancy
period offers the hope of prevention rather than more difficult
remediation of crystallized problems.

This chapter will examine the significant dimensions of experience to which a human infant is exposed by transactions with the
caregiver. The evidence is clear that behavior does not unfold by
maturation alone. Different early rearing conditions associated
with the quantity and nature of caregiver-infant interaction are
capable of significantly influencing a wide range of developing
behavior in infants of normal obstetrical histories. The effects
have been seen in the course and timing of basic maturational
sequences such as visually directed reaching (White and Held, 1967),
crawling, and walking (Dennis and Najarian, 1957). The effects have
also been demonstrated in the most significant issues of adulthood,

that is independent work, marriage, and parenthood (Skeels, 1966).

However, as the far-reaching consequences of early experience have been demonstrated, impermanence of effects has also been exposed. Among the more dramatic and perplexing examples are the following: orphanage life in Lebanon or Iran, although retarding in infancy (Dennis, 1960; see chapter by Hunt, this volume) does not appear to produce the gross cognitive deviance in the six-year-old child (Dennis and Najarian, 1957) that might be expected from certain kinds of orphanage life in western countries (Goldfarb, 1943; Skeels, 1966). Similarly, the lack of face-to-face vocalization with the caregiver does not appear to retard Guatemalan children from functioning in their culture (Kagan and Klein, 1973), whereas such a deficiency is thought to contribute to lower IQ scores in lower social status children in our culture (Kagan, 1968; Kagan and Tulkin, 1971; Tulkin and Kagan, 1972).

An explanation which might be posited illustrates two elements to be considered in unraveling the effects of early experience. One is the nature of the behaviors influenced by early experience. The other points to the importance of the post-infancy environment in sustaining behaviors shaped during infancy (Wachs and Cucinotta, 1971; Yarrow, 1964). A point of view that is supported by animal research (Denenberg, 1969; Levine, 1969) suggests that motivational factors are affected more than skills (Lewis and Goldberg, 1969; Provence and Lipton, 1962; Tulkin, 1972). If that is so, then motivational factors such as risk-taking and achievement striving would become manifest in our culture and effect differences in cognitive performance. In other cultures, although the underlying processes would be the same, differential performances post-infancy would not be evident. In any case, as the malleability of the human ensures the impact of early experience, the plasticity allows for changes to be wrought by post-infancy experiences. Capacities change. The environment itself may change. No simple assumptions can be made about consistency of the caregivers' behavior, the constitution of the family, or changes in role expectations in society. In addition, the subsequent environment may change in its reinforcement of given characteristics dependent on sex and age as well as situation (Kagan and Moss, 1962; Yarrow, 1964). The ontogeny of cognitive abilities (Bayley and Schaefer, 1964; Hunt and Kirk, 1971; McCall et al., 1972) as well as social behaviors (Bronson, 1971; Macfarlane, 1964; Rheingold, 1973; White and Watts, 1973) is just beginning to be investigated (see Hunt, this volume).

The intricacies inherent in the preceding discussion necessitate further empirical investigations. We reason that the complexities will be no different in substance from those in other life periods, since we adopt the point of view that the individual develops and changes throughout the life span dependent on the sustaining environment.

In sum, prenatal and perinatal hazards may lead to deficits depending on the occurrence of conditions in a child's life. The total cognitive and affective adaptation of the infant to the environment is what matters. With the exception of gross mental retardation and life-threatening incapacities, even sensory deficits and neurological dysfunctioning do not necessarily predict the course of child and adult life. The transactions with the caregiver in reaction to the problems may make them more or less pathological by limiting or expanding opportunities for other avenues of cognitive growth and other modes of affective expression (Parmelee et al., 1975). This chapter then, does not deal with single cases and individual therapy. It does not examine modes of remediation for identified disabilities. Rather, it relates selected aspects of empirical findings on the nature and significance of normal infant-caregiver transactions to infants who have been exposed to prenatal and perinatal hazards.

III. MEDIATING PROCESSES BETWEEN PERINATAL EVENTS AND LATER DEFICITS

A. Brain Dysfunctioning

Pasamanick and Knobloch and their associates (e.g. Knobloch and Pasamanick, 1960; Weiner et al., 1968) have been most prominent in stating and investigating empirically the following set of propositions: Since complications of pregnancy and delivery, including prematurity, are associated with brain injury resulting in fetal and neonatal death, there ought to remain a residue of children who are not killed by their traumatic experiences but survive to develop various sequelae of brain injury. A continuum of reproductive casualty exists with a lethal component of cerebral damage giving rise to fetal or neonatal death and a sublethal component resulting in various degrees of disability.

An association of cerebral palsy with certain obstetrical hazards, including prematurity, had already been recognized by Lilienfeld and Parkhurst (1951). Further reasoning suggested that epilepsy, mental deficiency, and even some behavior disorders and reading disabilities might be determined by brain injury and thereby linked to prenatal events. In an extensive series of carefully controlled retrospective studies, they did find that those disorders were significantly associated with some obstetrical complications, including prematurity (Kawi and Pasamanick, 1958; Lilienfeld and Pasamanick, 1956; Pasamanick and Lilienfeld, 1955; Pasamanick et al., 1956). Furthermore, premature infants also suffered other physical sequelae since their mean heights and weights remained less than those of full-term controls (Knobloch et al., 1959).

Cerebral palsy, epilepsy, and gross mental retardation are

manifest syndromes of brain dysfunctioning whereas behavior and
reading problems may represent inferred syndromes of "minimal"
brain dysfunctioning. Other disabilities associated with the syndrome of "minimal" brain dysfunctioning were also related to prematurity. In a carefully controlled prospective study, general
motor incoordination, perceptual-motor difficulties, and poor
Bender-Gestalt performance were found to characterize more premature infants than full-term infants of similar social status
(Wiener et al., 1965; Wiener et al., 1968). Further evidence was
adduced to show that brain injury mediated the behavioral deficits
found (Harper et al., 1959). A composite index of neurological
status was derived from neonatal indicators and a neurological
examination conducted at approximately 40 weeks of age. Most of
the variance in psychological performance which could be attributed
to obstetrical complications was explained by the composite neurological index (Wiener et al., 1965).

Other investigators have provided additional evidence that
attentional defects suggestive of "minimal" brain dysfunctioning
are more likely in infants of poorer birth condition. Honzik,
Hutchings, and Burnip (1965) found that those infants whose prenatal and perinatal conditions were judged most suspect for neurological involvement were more likely to be judged during infant test
examination at eight months to have a shorter span of attention, to
be markedly more distractible, to be hypo- or hyperactive. Lilienfeld et al. (1955) also found premature children to be judged to be
more distractible and hyperactive than normals. Judgments of
deviant attention are supported by objective measurements. Term
infants of poorer birth condition, as measured by a newborn neurological examination, showed less total visual fixation at birth
(Sigman et al., 1973). At four months post-term, preterms, as compared to full-terms, manifested less total visual fixation to a
novel stimulus as well as a slower rate of habituation (Sigman and
Parmelee, 1974). Similarly, at a later age, nine and 13 months post-
term, in a different sample, and using lower Apgar scores to measure
birth condition, less total visual fixation as well as a slower
degree of habituation were again noted (Lewis et al., 1967).

Although the evidence for neurological deficit is suggestive,
the equivocal indirect nature of the evidence has generated controversy. From my point of view, two main issues can be raised.
As Birch (1964) cogently stated, "minimal" brain dysfunctioning is
an enigmatic entity, difficult to demonstrate. It is an inferred
organic substrate for an array of symptoms. Evidence is limited
that children with the "minimal" brain damage syndrome have brain
damage. Alternatively, there is evidence that individuals with
brain damage do not always exhibit the syndrome. Thus, to assume
that similarity of symptoms in infants and children has been
effected by an inferred "minimal" brain dysfunctioning is question-
able. On the other hand, the coincidence of symptoms lends support

to the existence of such an entity.

Nevertheless, a relationship between prenatal hazards and
"minimal" brain damage syndrome can be questioned on other grounds.
As Caputo and Mandell (1970) judged from their review of then
existing studies, the evidence was not clear that preterms of birthweights between 2000-2500 g manifested any sequelae. The evidence
was clear that very low birthweight (1500 g or less) individuals
did. Investigations more recent than their review now indicate
that changes in postnatal nursery procedures not only have decreased
mortality for very low birthweight infants, but have markedly decreased their later neurological, sensory, and psychological
deficits.

Since neonatal hospital care is continually changing, the
extent of the improved prognosis reflects those changes in nursery
procedures which were specific to the year and hospital of birth.
In contrast to the incidence of neurological abnormalities reported
by Lubchenco et al. (32%, 1963) and Drillien (28%, 1964) in children
born prior to 1960 of less than 1500 g, Fitzhardinge and Ramsey
(1973) found a 6% incidence in low birthweight individuals born in
the years 1960-1966. In contrast to Drillien (9%, 1964) and Lubchenco et al. (25%, 1963), Fitzhardinge and Ramsey (1973) found 40%
of their subjects to perform at an IQ level equal to or greater than
100. Other studies of that period report similar progress with
fewer gross neurological or sensory disabilities, fewer severely
retarded, and more individuals with IQ scores above 100 (Francis-
Williams and Davies, 1974). The outcome for low birthweight babies
was improved but could still be considered discouraging. Two points
should be noted. The low birthweight individuals were not compared
to term infants of similar social circumstances. Therefore, social
status effects were confounded with the sequelae of low birthweight,
since lower social status is associated with a higher incidence of
preterm births and also acts to lower IQ scores. The extent of the
contribution of lower social status rather than low birthweight
cannot be determined. That lower social status is a major factor
is suggested by Stewart and Reynolds (1974). On one hand, only 43%
of the low birthweight children in their study obtained IQs above
100. On the other hand, the distribution of values obtained in the
children was no different from that of their parents. Second, even
more recent studies are reporting increasingly more salutary outcomes. Hunt et al. (1974) estimated that those infants in their
study who weighed 1500 g or less and were born in the years 1969-
1972 would evidence at least a 50% decrease in incidence of retardation in comparison to the low birthweight subjects born in 1965-
1968. A caution is still presented. All investigators have recognized that very low birthweight individuals may still be vulnerable
to more subtle handicaps, as in reading deficits.

As Drillien stated (1972, p. 563), the improved prognosis for

infants of very low birthweight implies that much of the handicap
previously reported and attributed to prenatal brain damage "was
postnatally determined and potentially preventable." All studies,
therefore, which were conducted in the 50's and 60's, and which
had a high percentage of very low birthweight individuals (e.g.
Braine et al., 1966; Drillien, 1964; Wiener, 1970) have to be
reconsidered as to the evidence for brain damage and to the severity and extensiveness of deficits associated with presumed prenatal
hazards.

B. Other Mediating Processes

     Although one source of brain dysfunctioning as well as
behavioral deficits in preterm infants may now be diminished, other
sources of hazardous postnatal experiences remain. At least two
other mediating processes have been suggested which might augment
behavioral deficits (Sameroff and Chandler, 1975; Wiener, 1962).
One stresses the disrupting effect of the deviant birth on the
family and primary caregiver. This view suggests that there may be
disruption in the attachment of the caregiver to the infant effected
by the imposed separation from the baby, the delay in carrying out
natural caregiving functions, and the increased emotional stress of
an abnormal birth and pregnancy. The other hypothesis emphasizes
the deviant sensory environment that neonates experience in the
hospital in contrast to intrauterine conditions or extrauterine
family rearing.

     1. Disrupting Effect on Caregiver of Separation from Baby. It
is apparent that parental reaction to the birth of a preterm baby is
an acute emotional crisis (Kaplan and Mason, 1960). The parents must
prepare for possible loss. Then, as the baby continues to exist, the
parents must resume the process of relating to the infant. They must
learn how preterm differ from full-term babies and understand any
special needs. They must do so while dealing with their failure to
deliver a full-term normal infant. Finally, separation from the baby
and from natural caregiving responsibilities may further threaten the
caregiver's attachment to the infant.

     Klaus and Kennell and their associates have suggested that a
"critical" period may exist immediately after delivery for the formation of the mother's attachment to her infant. The impact of
separation on attachment behaviors has been studied using several
strategies. When mothers of preterm infants were compared with
mothers of full-terms as to their style of contact with their infants
in the initial meetings, mothers of preterms were more tentative in
their physical contact and showed less eye-to-eye contact (Klaus et
al., 1970). Augmenting contact immediately after birth even for an
experimental group of women with normal full-term infants was related
one month later to more reluctance to leave the infants with someone
else, to greater soothing behaviors, more en face behavior, and more

fondling (Klaus et al., 1972). The effects persisted one year
after delivery. Experimental mothers soothed more and stayed
closer to their babies during physical examination (Kennell et al.,
1974).

Increasing the opportunity for early contact of mothers with
their preterm infants also changed their caregiving styles. Using
time lapse photography of the first ten minutes of a feeding conducted just before the infant's discharge from the hospital, Klaus
and Kennell (1970) compared the behavior of mothers who had been
separated from their preterm infants for 20 days with that of
mothers who had been permitted close physical contact within the
first five days of life with their preterm infants. The group that
had been allowed early contact showed many more intervals of cuddling
and more en face intervals. These differences persisted and one
month after discharge, during a similar filming of a feeding, early
contact mothers provided more stimulation by changing the babies'
position more, burping them more, and holding them differently.
Leiderman et al. (1973) compared a group of mothers of full-terms
to two groups of mothers of preterms. One of the preterm groups
was encouraged to have more contact and to participate more in caretaking interactions with their infants in the nursery while the
other preterm group was separated in the usual hospital procedure.
Although the greater contact group showed more ventral contact at
one week post-discharge than did the other preterm group, no differences among preterm groups were seen by one month. However, mothers
of full-terms smiled more and had more ventral contact at one month,
although they did not differ from the mothers of preterms in total
attentiveness. At three months, the full-terms scored higher on
the Bayley Scales of Mental Development than did either preterm
group.

To summarize, there are probably subtle differences in the
care given by families to their preterm and full-term infants. It
is apparent that separation is one of the many stressful factors
contained in a preterm infant's birth. Maternal attitudes and
behaviors may be impeded, but the strength, the extensiveness, and
the short and long-term consequences of the effect have not yet been
delineated. Separation may be a phenomenon which has its most significant effect only when other conditions are deleterious and the
effect may then show in gross disruptions of family life, rather
than in moment-to-moment caregiving. Thus Leifer et al. (1972)
reported more frequent occurrence of relinquishment of infants to
foster care, and increased number of divorces, in a late contact
preterm group as compared to an early contact group. Similarly,
Klein and Stern (1971) found an apparent association between low
birthweight and child battering, and suggested that the enforced
separation so commonly practiced in premature units contributes to
an abnormal maternal-child relationship.

2. Early Sensory Experiences in the Hospital. The studies reviewed in this section are noteworthy methodologically as well as theoretically. All studies were experimental-predictive rather than retrospective or even anteorespective. Thus, they have the strength and elegance of experimental design, although the subject numbers have been few, and the designation of a control group has been as difficult and inconclusive at times as many of the retrospective or prospective naturalistic-descriptive studies. The investigations grew out of the conviction that the hospital environment, particularly that of an isolette or incubator, is deviant from the normal intrauterine environment and from the extrauterine environment provided by the family. Investigators have pointed out that the hospital environment is grossly bombarding in excess sound and light stimuli, grossly depriving in patterning of visual, auditory, tactile, and vestibular stimuli, as well as lacking reciprocal stimulus feedback (reafferent) experiences. Each investigator has intervened to change one or more of these aspects for a selected group of preterm infants.

Solkoff et al. (1969) increased the tactile stimulation received by infants of birthweights below 1600 g for their first ten days. The experimental babies regained their birthweight faster than did the control babies. At seven to eight months of age the handled babies were all rated as active and healthy by the pediatrician while half of the nonhandled babies were not. A substantially smaller percentage of experimental babies displayed poor gross and fine motor development. Furthermore, babies who had been handled were found to have more toys and greater mother-infant interaction, possibly because handling modified the baby's characteristics, which then changed the care received, and thus further modified development. This has been suggested by recent research described later in this chapter.

Korner (1973) reported a study by Neal in which preterms were provided complex vestibular stimulation in a swinging cot inside an incubator for 30 minutes three times a day. When compared to control subjects, they achieved significantly greater motor, visual, and auditory development, and weighed more. Korner et al. (1975) provided increased vestibular stimulation for preterms in another way. Preterms residing on water beds and otherwise cared for by usual hospital procedure manifested significantly fewer apnea spells while in the hospital.

Powell (1974) provided extra handling twice a day in the hospital. The experimental group performed significantly higher on Bayley mental and motor scales at four months of age. Scarr-Salapatek and Williams (1973) also provided increased handling to preterm infants during six weeks in the nursery. After discharge, and throughout the first year, the experimental group continued to receive additional help by weekly home visits to improve maternal

care. At one year, the mean IQ for the experimental group was 95,
whereas the control group mean was only 85. However, the effect of
the interventions may have been confounded with effects of parity as
well as maternal IQ. First-borns, whether or not they are preterms,
tend to score higher on infant tests than do later-borns (Bayley,
1965; Cohen, 1975). Not only did the experimental group contain
significantly more first-born infants, but the maternal IQ was also
substantially higher.

Siqueland (1973) has emphasized the lack of response contingent
stimuli in ordinary hospital care. Using a cotwin design, Siqueland
provided for daily ten-minute periods of extra "mothering", handling
in two of the daily feeding sessions, and participation in 11-minute
experimental situations for one member of a series of twins. The
experimental situation supplied stimulation contingent on the neonate's opening his/her eyes. At four months of age, many of the
nonexperimental subjects, in contrast to the experimental subjects,
failed to show evidence of visual reinforcement control of sucking
behavior. Thus, response contingent stimulation influenced either
learning strategies or visual exploratory behavior.

In sum, there appears to be a trend such that increased handling, or more patterned, and/or more contingent stimulation within
the first few weeks of life, does appear to influence physiological
and behavioral functioning at term date, and four to six months
later. Any longer-lasting effects are not yet known. However, the
existing studies, beset by methodological problems, and too few in
number, can not yet offer conclusive evidence of the effect of hospital experiences on the development of the preterm infant. The
appropriate level and kind of stimulation for a preterm infant
remains uncertain.

IV. SIGNIFICANT DIMENSIONS OF CAREGIVER
BEHAVIOR IN THE POSTNEONATAL PERIOD

A. Environmental Influences on Risk Infants' Development

With few exceptions, social status has been the primary environmental dimension investigated in the postneonatal development of
infants exposed to prenatal and perinatal hazards. All studies
indicate that social status has an important effect in modulating
the impact of perinatal factors, although the extent of modification
remains open to question. Therefore, investigations which have as
their goal exposing the sequelae of reproductive hazards must take
postnatal social status into account.

Much of our information comes from several large studies that
have followed children from infancy through school age. In the
Johns Hopkins Study of Premature Infants, approximately 400 low

birthweight and 400 full-term infants were followed from birth to
12-13 years of age. Examinations were conducted at three-five
years (Harper et al., 1959; Wiener et al., 1965), six-seven (Wiener
et al., 1965), eight-ten (Wiener, 1970; Wiener et al., 1968), and
12-13 years of age (Wiener, 1968). The investigations have sub-
stantiated the association of preterm birth with increased cognitive,
perceptual-motor, and learning problems as discussed elsewhere in
this review. Nevertheless, despite the investigators' emphasis on
the effects of preterm birth, social class was found to provide the
largest correlation with IQ scores.

Werner et al. (1971) followed longitudinally from the prenatal
period to age ten all births on the island of Kauai in the year
1955. Infants were initially scored on a four-point scale for
severity of perinatal complications. The scores were then related
to cognitive and social development at age two and at age ten. At
age two the effects were seen in three ways. Children growing up
in the most favorable environments who had experienced the most
severe perinatal complications had mean IQ scores almost comparable
to children with no perinatal stress who were living in the least
favorable environments. Thus, although some difference still
remained in favor of the child without adverse perinatal circum-
stance, social status clearly contributed. Second, the most retarded children were those who had both experienced the most severe
perinatal complications and who were also living in the least
favorable environments. Note that the effects of perinatal and
postnatal environments interacted to produce the largest deficit
for the least advantaged children. This parallels the malnutrition
findings discussed by Richardson in this volume. Third, social
status differences provided for a greater difference in mean IQ
scores (37 points) for children with severe perinatal stress than
did perinatal experiences for children living in favorable environments (seven IQ points). By age ten, postnatal environmental
influences were even more patent. Children with and without severe
perinatal stress who had grown up in more favorable homes did not
differ. Both groups achieved mean IQ scores well above the average.
On the other hand, social status differences contributed to large
differences in IQ of those children who had experienced severe perinatal stress. IQ scores were seriously depressed in children of
low social status, particularly if they had experienced severe perinatal hazards. Werner et al. concluded that any gradient of retarded
intellectual development that had appeared by age two with increased
severity of perinatal complications had been washed out by age ten.
Only a residue remained contributed by the most severely stressed
children who grew up in unfavorable home environments.

Drillien (1964) also investigated the combined effects of social
status and prematurity. At age four, an interactional effect favor-
ing the most advantaged babies was evident. Term babies living in
higher social status homes performed better than preterm babies being

reared under similar social circumstances. That is, those babies
who had not experienced perinatal hazards and who had available to
them the more beneficial postnatal environments performed significantly better than all others. However, very low birthweight
infants (born weighing less than three-and-a-half pounds) were at
less of a disadvantage in higher social status families than very
low birthweight infants living in lower social status families. At
age four, children of very low birthweight living in the highest
social status families showed a mean deficit of 13 developmental
quotient (DQ) points from their term peers whereas children of very
low birthweight living in the lowest social status families showed
a mean deficit of 32 DQ points from their term peers. By the ages
of five to seven, when the children were tested in school, few
children from middle class homes were retarded, except when the
birthweight had been below three-and-a-half pounds, while in poor
homes there was a marked excess of poorly functioning children in
all weight categories.

It is apparent that the significant correlations between social
status and IQ scores found throughout the age range starting from
age three for children who have not experienced adverse perinatal
factors (Kennedy, Van de Riet, and White, 1963) must be equally
true for children who have. Further, the progressive retardation
over the age span in children of lower class environments is as
evident in children who have experienced perinatal hazards as in
those who have not.

As suggested by some of the data previously discussed, infants
exposed to obstetrical complications may be particularly vulnerable
to the effects of an impoverished and deleterious environment.
Willerman et al. (1970) found that the developmental status of term
infants interacted with social status to influence IQ at four years
of age. Retarded infant development predicted disproportionately
poorer intellectual performance for infants of lower social status.
Braine et al. (1966) did not find that more adverse environments,
within a very restricted range of poverty, produced a uniform detrimental effect for the sample of children taken as a whole. But the
more adverse environments were selectively handicapping to children
who had suffered certain kinds of obstetrical complications.
Drillien (1964) suggested that obstetric complications appeared to
have the effect of lowering the resistance level to stressful situations encountered in early childhood. She found that preterms performed disproportionately more poorly when any one of several other
adverse or depriving factors was in force. Thus, preterms with
additional obstetric complications, or very low birthweight preterms who were not the first-born child in the family, or low birthweight infants from the lower social classes, all did disproportionately more poorly. This type of interaction is reminiscent of some
animal studies in which sensory enrichment may compensate, to some
degree, for prior brain damage (see chapters by Greenough et al.,

Davenport, Walsh and Cummins).

The Baltimore studies have found no such interactive effect except one study which pointed to the converse of vulnerability, that is, the facilitating effect of beneficial social status. In Wiener et al. (1963), those subjects whose IQ scores rose rather than declined from age three-five to ages six-seven were preterms of upper social status with good emotional adjustment. In the other studies, however, when preterms were matched on social status indices with term babies, the preterms of lower class did not perform significantly more poorly than any other group. The effects of birthweight were similar in each social class. However, it is possible that the method of matching controls to preterms, which was by census tract place of residence, may have been too gross in that it obscured true social status differences. In addition, as Richardson's work (this volume) indicates, within the same social class, certain psychosocial characteristics of the mother may predispose to delivery of low birthweight infants and other hazardous obstetrical conditions, as well as producing differences in postnatal stimulation and emotional support to the child. The adequate criteria for defining a control group is a particularly difficult problem in research with preterm infants. A comparison group of equal social status is essential for an evaluation of social status effects. On the other hand, matching by nominal social status membership probably highlights certain psychological-social differences that exist within a social status group and which, in turn, mediate postnatal events as well as prenatal conditions. Assessment of those psychosocial dimensions within and across comparison groups would be useful.

On a broader level, as Sameroff and Chandler (1975) point out, the various longitudinal studies of prenatal and perinatal complications have yet to produce a predictive variable more powerful than familial and social status characteristics of the caretaking environment. Nevertheless, the processes involved in the impact of social status on a child's development are poorly understood and are open for investigation. Moreover, social status cannot be used to understand individual differences within a group. Such differences exist and may supersede the social status groupings.

The question of how social status shapes individuals is particularly pertinent within the infancy period, since most studies find no relationship between social status and mental test performance in that period (Bayley, 1965; Golden and Birns, 1968). Social status is not a unitary variable but an aggregate (Deutsch, 1973). The behaviors and attitudes referred to are not specific nor probably even stable over time. Furthermore, social status, although it may index some significant dimensions of caregiver-infant interaction, may not differentiate others equally pertinent to the development of high risk infants. Initially, a deprivation model arising from

investigations of orphanages had been generalized to lower status
membership. Then an increasing number of studies using naturalistic observations (e.g. Tulkin, 1972; Wachs et al., 1971) indicated
that poverty was not analogous to stimulus deprivation nor to differences in affective variables, nor even to the lack of responsiveness
often associated with orphanage rearing. Infants in lower social
status families do not differ from those of higher social situations
in the amount of physical contact received through holding, soothing,
or affection (Lewis and Wilson, 1972; Tulkin and Kagan, 1972). Nor
do infants in upper social status families necessarily receive more
verbal input (Lewis and Wilson, 1972; Tulkin and Kagan, 1972). The
differences have been found in style and timing. Infants in upper
social status families are exposed to more face-to-face vocalization
and to more reciprocal vocal exchanges (Cohen and Beckwith, 1975;
Lewis and Wilson, 1972; Tulkin and Kagan, 1972). Lower social status
may restrict the opportunities for exploration of the inanimate
environment through fewer available toys. But more important,
crowded living conditions provide a superfluity of auditory and
visual input (see chapter by Hunt, this volume). It now appears as
though a difference model would be more accurate with excessive
stimulation rather than deprivation as one of the components.

The three longitudinal investigations of risk infants that
were summarized in the preceding pages used clinical ratings in
addition to social status to characterize their subjects' postnatal
environments. Drillien (1964) found father's occupation alone provided too narrow a range of social status grades. She therefore
included in her stratification considerations of the standards of
care and management of health, food, and money, as well as the
intellectual ambitiousness of the family. Thus, the social status
influences reflected psychological differences within nominal social
status groups.

The Johns Hopkins Study of Premature Infants used a modification
of Schaefer and Bell's Parental Attitude Research Inventory (Schaefer
and Bell, 1958). Rated were the mother's tendency to ignore the
child, her emotional involvement with the child, her use of fear in
controlling the child, her intellectual interests and achievement
strivings, and the degree of positive relation between mother and
child. Although social class was found to provide the largest component to IQ, maternal attitudes also contributed and with more
influence than birthweight at ages 12-13 (Wiener, 1968). Werner
et al. (1971) as well as Drillien (1964) assessed family stability
during their subjects' preschool years by ratings which took into
account the legitimacy of the child, the presence of a father,
marital discord, long-term separation of the child from the mother
without adequate substitute caretakers, and alcoholism in either of
the parents. By school age, at six to seven years, teachers rated
children of all birthweights who had been subjected to severe preschool familial stress as exhibiting more adverse behavior. The

effect was most marked with the low birthweight individuals (Drillien, 1964). When the subjects of the study of Werner et al. (1971) were age ten, their families were characterized as to the degree of educational stimulation and emotional support provided. By age ten, educational stimulation ratings of the home were found to correlate more closely with children's IQ and achievement than did measures of parental socioeconomic status. Educational stimulation ratings, as well as social status, were more effective in influencing IQ scores than was emotional support, although it too contributed.

It is most likely that environmental variables interact complexly. They may act to heighten, suppress, or compensate for deficits in experiences received through another dimension. Clusters, or combined deficits rather than single factors, may be necessary to produce an observable effect (Yarrow et al., 1972). Such interactions, and the relative weights of each factor have not yet been identified. Social status grading, and judges' ratings of family stability, educational stimulation, or emotional support -- as have been used in studies with risk children -- operate to cluster factors. But they obscure specificity and thereby the understanding of process.

In contrast to the gross clusters measured by judges' ratings, which defined environmental influences in the development of risk infants, specific dimensions of caregiver-infant interaction have been objectively examined through naturalistic observations and experimental manipulations in term infants born without obstetrical complications. These dimensions have been found to be significant in affecting a wide variety of cognitive and social behaviors not only in grossly deprived environments such as institutions but even within the narrower range of family rearing. The dimensions and processes are thoughtfully discussed by Hunt, this volume, and are summarized briefly in the following section. I suggest that an examination of these dimensions would prove useful in understanding the development of infants who have been exposed to prenatal and perinatal stress.

V. SIGNIFICANT DIMENSIONS OF EXPERIENCE WITH AVERAGE INFANT

There is a growing body of evidence that the human infant may be biologically programmed to be specifically responsive to perceptual features of the human caregiver. It is not only that the caregiver provides gratification and reduces tension through meeting the infant's physiological needs. The infant within the first few months of life is specifically interested in the human voice (Eisenberg, 1965), speech sounds (Eimas et al., 1971), and face, particularly the eyes (Fantz and Nevis, 1967; Haaf and Bell, 1967; Kagan et al., 1966). The human caregiver is the perceptual stimulus

within the baby's environment that is the most salient, the most
complex, as well as the most contingent to the baby's behavior
(Rheingold, 1967). It is both the most familiar and yet is ever
changing, thereby producing novelty necessary to suppress habituation. Moreover, the caregiver not only provides stimulation and
reinforcement herself but mediates stimulation from the inanimate
environment.

The evidence we have for the impact has been conceptualized
in various terms, not necessarily mutually exclusive (see Hunt,
this volume, for more extensive theoretical discussion and report
of research evidence). The caregiver provides stimulation. In so
doing she provides opportunities for observational learning, for
differentiation and integration of skilled goal-directed acts
(Bruner, 1973), as well as for the build-up of expectancies of
forthcoming events (Kagan, 1970). The caregiver also provides
variety. Thus, she functions as an arouser (Hebb, 1946) and on the
other hand, acts to decrease emotional reaction to novelty, to
reduce fear of novelty (Denenberg, 1964), and to increase the level
of adaptation to change (Helson, 1959). The total amount of interaction the primary caregiver has with the infant, regardless of
mode and supplementary to physical care, has been variously labeled
as attentiveness (Rubenstein, 1967) or intensity and level of social
stimulation (Yarrow et al., 1972) and has been shown to influence IQ
scores, whether they are concurrently measured in infancy (Clarke-
Stewart, 1973; Yarrow et al., 1972) or later at age ten (Yarrow et
al. 1973). Attentiveness also has been associated with an infant's
greater exploration of the novel (Rubenstein, 1967; Yarrow et al.,
1972). The dimension does not reflect the overall quantity of time
that the mother is at home with her baby, since time at home may not
necessarily correspond to number or intensity of contacts (Schaffer
and Emerson, 1964).

The caregiver's contact with the infant is important not only
as it provides exposure to perceptual stimuli but as the timing and
appropriateness provide stimulus feedback experiences and schedules
of reinforcement. Such experiences are important in operant learning
theory in shaping infant's behavior, important for increasing the
potency of the caregiver as a generalized secondary reinforcer
(Gewirtz, 1961) and important in affecting a generalized sense of
mastery and the motivation to use capabilities (Lewis and Goldberg,
1969; Provence and Lipton, 1962). In addition, response-contingent
stimulation may operate to determine an harmonious and secure attachment, thus influencing the ability to be active in initiating a
social contact as well as in avoiding or warding off unpleasant
stimuli (Ainsworth, 1973). Secure attachment may also facilitate
detachment and active exploration of the environment (Ainsworth,
1973; Rheingold, 1969a,b; Rheingold and Eckerman, 1970). The dimension has variously been conceptualized as the caregiver's responsiveness to the child's cues (Yarrow et al., 1973), sensitivity to

infant signals (Ainsworth and Bell, 1975), individualization
(Yarrow, 1963), or more narrowly -- contingency to distress (Yarrow
et al., 1972). The dimension influences IQ scores in infancy, and
rate of development of both object and person permanence (Bell,
1970). Further, the dimension has been found to enhance social
effectiveness in boys ten years later (Yarrow et al., 1973). On
the other hand, adverse responsiveness that acts to suppress the
infant's behavior, that is, intrusion, criticism, direction, or
punishment, slows the acquisition of language (Nelson, 1973), and
depresses performance on infant scales (Ainsworth and Bell, 1975)
as well as on intelligence tests later in life (Bayley and Schaefer,
1964). The dimension reflects crudely the fact that social interchanges involve reciprocal and precise temporal organization
(Richards, 1974). The mutual phasing and serial ordering of interactions is just beginning to be investigated (David and Appell,
1969; Brazelton et al., 1974; Richards, 1974; Stern, 1974). The
rhythm of interchange has been found to influence the infant's early
biological rhythms (Sander, 1969). The precise phasing of behaviors
also underlies the development of communication skills (Brazelton
et al., 1974; Richards, 1974; Stern, 1974), verbal and nonverbal.

In addition to participating in social transactions, the caregiver mediates the infant's interaction with the inanimate environment by providing objects and places for exploration. In general,
the more varied the opportunities for inanimate exploration which
are available at the infant's initiation, the more skillful the
infant (e.g. Ainsworth and Bell, 1975; Beckwith, 1971b; Yarrow et
al., 1972). On the other hand, the amount of background stimulus
bombardment out of the infant's control has been shown to slow
language acquisition (Nelson, 1973) and to slow sensory-motor development (Wachs, 1973; Wachs et al., 1971). (See Hunt, this volume, for
a more extensive discussion.)

The purpose of our own research has been to detail through
naturalistic home observations some significant dimensions of interaction between preterm infants and their caregivers and to relate
these dimensions to the infants' development in the first year of
life (Beckwith and Cohen, 1975). The preliminary findings are consistent with research with healthy term infants. Specific environmental encounters, occurring between caregivers and infants as early
as one month of age, were found to influence infant sensorimotor
performance and Gesell DQ at nine months of age. Further, the interactions operated differentially in influencing the discrete skills
measured by each test. Reciprocal social transactions, that is,
transactions which occurred contingent to the infant's signals,
either simultaneously as in mutual gazing, or successively as in
response to fuss-cries and response to nondistress vocalizations,
were associated with infants' faster acquisition of the stages of
object permanence at nine months. On the other hand, less physical
restraint and more experience in practicing independent locomotor

skills were correlated with higher Gesell DQ scores at nine months.
The implications for the babies' further development and for their
relationships with their families await further analysis.

VI. THE CONTRIBUTION OF THE INFANT

The preceding discussion and the research on which it is based
emphasize the caregiver's influence on the infant and ignore the
infant's contribution to his own experience (Bell, 1971; Bruner,
1969a,b; Korner, 1971, 1974). From the earliest weeks of life the
infant effectively promotes many of the interactions. The infant,
through his discriminative crying, looking, and smiling, facilitates
and maintains interaction (Bell, 1974). His influence is not only
immediate but shows long-term effects on the caregiver (Rheingold,
1969a,b). Furthermore, infants actively seek out stimulation,
attend selectively, and show strong preferences among stimuli and
for certain levels of stimulus change. Along with all the capacities that have been demonstrated in infants, significant individual
differences have also been noted.

Do risk infants differ in initial behaviors from infants who
have not experienced hazardous perinatal conditions? If so, how
do differences in infants affect the caregiver? Or how do differences among infants modify the effects of the same experience?
Although some investigations have detailed differences between
risk infants and controls, their focus has been in the main on
behaviors associated with "minimal brain dysfunctioning", that is
on control of attention and activity (Honzik et al., 1965; Sigman
et al., 1973), rather than on eliciting and maintaining qualities
for transactions with the caregiver. That is not to say that
attentional phenomena may not modify the nature and the influence
of transactions with the caregiver. Further, it is likely that
specific transactions with the caregiver could increase attentional
control, even for infants who are more distractible and less flexible in their scanning (Bruner, 1969a,b).

In the early months, an infant's fusses and cries are a potent
initiator of interactions. Moss and Robson (1968) found that one-
month-old-term healthy infants initiated roughly four out of five
of the interactions that occurred with the caregiver and they did
so through fussing and crying. One might speculate that there would
exist within the group of infants who have suffered perinatal complications an increased number of infants who cry less and those
who cry more than term healthy infants. Those infants would change
the number of social interactions to which they were exposed.
Furthermore, the ease of soothing the infant must also be considered.
Moss (1967) found that mothers tended to interact less with more
irritable male babies at three months, whereas they interacted more
with more irritable girls. Moss speculated that mothers might have

been negatively reinforced for responding to the boys but tended
to be positively reinforced for responses toward the girls. That
is, the more irritable boys might have been more difficult to soothe
than the more irritable girls. Prechtl (1963) has described a
"hyperexcitability" syndrome, associated with prenatal and perinatal
complications and manifest on neonatal neurologic examination. The
babies of that group cried more than normal babies, showed sudden
changes of state from being drowsy and difficult to arouse to being
wide awake, crying and difficult to pacify. These infants, when
compared to a control group, elicited much greater anxiety and
rejection from their mothers in the first year of life.

Another dimension holds promise for describing differences
among infants which will in turn influence caregiver behaviors.
Osofsky and Danzger (1974) found that among term infants, those
judged on the Brazelton Neonatal Behavioral Assessment Scale
(Brazelton, 1972) to be more responsive to visual, auditory, and
tactile stimuli had more attentive and stimulating mothers. Moreover, the interrelationship of responsive babies and stimulating,
sensitive mothers persisted over the first year of life (Osofsky,
1975). Powell (1974) has described preterm infants on the same
scales and found that individual differences in responsiveness were
stable through six months, as assessed by Bayley behavior records.

Individual differences among infants may gain importance if one
considers that the stability of the effects of early experience may
be mediated by characteristics of the infant. One factor involved
may be the extent to which the infant's characteristics evoke experiences beyond infancy which consolidate the effects begun during
infancy. For example, Siqueland (1973) found that interventions
with preterm infants in the first few weeks of life so changed the
babies that they evoked more responsive interaction from the mother
later. Alternatively, Ucko (1965) found that perinatal complications
increased the incidence of a syndrome of "difficulty in handling".
The syndrome consisted of a high degree of sensitivity, intense
reactions, and a disequilibrium to change. The syndrome is suggestive of that pointed to by Thomas et al. (1968). In a longitudinal
project of infants born without obstetrical complications, it was
shown that babies who were irritable, intense in their reactions,
and negative or withdrawing from new situations elicited dis-
harmonious relationships with their families and were referred in
the largest proportion for child guidance help. Not all such children had the same outcome. Parents who could maintain emotional
support and promote new experiences helped their infants become
competent children. Note that the syndrome has been found in infants
who have not experienced perinatal complications as well as in
infants who have. Further note that the reaction of the family can
modify outcome. This example may illustrate the complexities en-
tailed in describing effects of perinatal hazards. Incidence rates
may be different, but the range of possible outcomes is similar.

VII.   CONCLUSIONS AND IMPLICATIONS FOR RESEARCH AND PRACTICE

An increased incidence of cognitive, perceptual, and social
problems have been found by some investigators to be associated
with exposure to prenatal and perinatal hazards. Other investigators have found that postnatal experiences so modify the effects
that they are no longer apparent. The environment then can be said
to have been therapeutic, or alternatively, that certain conditions,
triggering factors, must exist for deficits to be manifest. The
evidence suggests that conditions which exist coincident with low
social status, or family instability, or lack of educational stimulation are such triggering factors. How they produce deficits,
whether they do so in ways specific to this group of children, or
more likely, in ways detrimental to all children, or in what ways
high social status acts to suppress deficits is not known. Such
gross clustering of environmental factors acts to obscure process
as well as to obscure the child's contributions. What is clear is
that postnatal experiences are as significant to the development of
risk infants as of normal infants -- if not more so, as risk infants
may be particularly vulnerable to adverse conditions.

Families of risk infants may themselves be particularly vulnerable to adverse conditions. Since prenatal and perinatal complications occur at a higher incidence in unwed women, women without
medical care, and women of lower social status at the time of the
birth and as far back as their own childhood, it would be anticipated that many such mothers and their families would have fewer
resources with which to meet the increased stress which may occur
in the birth and postnatal course of their children. Supportive
services, including family counseling and parent groups, must be
considered necessary for the children's development, as suggested
by Lodge, this volume.

In order to make professional intervention, either in counseling to the families or in direct provision of supplemental experiences to the infants, more meaningful, research should focus on
detailing the daily transactions that occur naturally between caregivers and infants at successive ages. Since it is known that wide
individual differences exist in normal infants (born at term without
obstetrical complications) in their eliciting qualities and responsiveness to experiences, it would be important to detail individual
differences within risk infants, as well as comparing risk infants
to infants who have suffered no prenatal or perinatal complications.
We reason that deviance in some infants may impede opportunities
normally used for salutary environmental encounters, and make the
families' adaptation to their babies more difficult.

The successive patterns of transactions with the environment
should then be examined emphasizing objective, specific dimensions
of experience and their impact on discrete aspects of cognitive and

affective development. While that information is essential, it must also be recognized that caregivers differ widely in styles of interaction even with normal infants. Since it is most likely that environmental variables interact, combined deficits rather than single factors may be necessary to produce an observable effect, and reduced experience in one area may be adequately compensated by experiences received through another dimension. Caregiving, then, could be expected to be successful in encouraging a child's competence through a variety of mediating experiences.

There are some leads which appear promising for further research. An increasing number of studies demonstrate that infants who have experienced hazardous obstetrical events may show deviant organization of states of arousal, and deviant attentional patterns in less total fixation to a novel stimulus and a slower rate of habituation to a redundant stimulus. The association of these deviations as precursors to later attentional defects included in the minimal brain dysfunctioning syndrome needs further investigation. Yet there is hope that environmental encounters can ameliorate these deviations so that they do not become consolidated in pathology. Interactions which have been found to occur naturally between caregiver and infant are relevant. Research with normal infants has shown that proprioceptive-vestibular stimulation associated with picking up and moving in space is significant in increasing visual attentiveness (Korner and Thoman, 1970), in mediating changes in arousal level (Korner and Thoman, 1972), and in increasing visual response decrement to a familiar stimulus (Lewis et al., 1969). Mutual gazing also may increase visual attentiveness (Moss and Robson, 1970), and we have observed that social transactions, specifically, mutual gazing, may mediate the organization of arousal states. Holding and mutual gazing are prominent in normal caregiving in the early months; moving in space occurs in utero. As they are the experiences which are most diminished for the preterm infant in the hospital, their link with later deviant behavior provokes speculation, although the studies are too few and the evidence inconclusive. In any case, the provision of such experiences at a high level during home care should be beneficial.

While some experiences may be particularly significant in modifying deviant behaviors, some forms of experience are essential in facilitating development in normal infants as well as in risk infants. Reciprocal social transactions which are contingent to the infant's signals have been found to be one. Opportunity to explore the inanimate environment at the infant's own rate and initiative is another. For some stressed infants, such as those whose emitted behaviors are diminished, contingent reactions by the caregiver may have to be supplemented by an imposed higher level of social interaction. Self-directed exploration may also have to be specifically encouraged in hypoactive infants or infants who with-

draw from novelty. In essence, self-directed activity in a varied
and responsive environment is beneficial to all infants, and
undoubtedly will modify and ameliorate some, but not all, prenatal
and perinatal hazards.

REFERENCES

Ainsworth, M.D.S. 1973. The Development of Infant-Mother Attach-
    ment, pp. 1-94. In B.M. Caldwell and H.N. Riccuiti (eds.).
    Review of Child Development Research, Vol. 3. University of
    Chicago Press, Chicago.

Ainsworth, M.D.S., and Bell, S.M. 1975. Mother-Infant Interaction
    and the Development of Competence, pp. 97-118. In K.J. Connolly
    and J. Bruner (eds.). The Growth of Competence. Academic
    Press, New York.

Barten, S., and Rouch, J. 1971. Continuity in the Development of
    Visual Behavior in Young Infants. Child Develop. 42:1566-1571.

Barten, S., Birns, B., and Rouch, J. 1971. Individual Differences
    in the Visual Pursuit Behavior of Neonates. Child Develop. 42:
    313-319.

Bayley, N. 1965. Comparisons of Mental and Motor Test Scores for
    Ages 1-15 Months by Sex, Birth Order, Race, Geographical
    Location and Education of Parents. Child Develop. 36:379-411.

Bayley, N., and Schaefer, E.S. 1964. Correlations of Maternal and
    Child Behaviors with the Development of Mental Abilities: Data
    from the Berkeley Growth Study. Monogr. Soc. Res. Child
    Develop. 29(6),Serial No. 97, pp. 1-80.

Beckwith, L. 1971a. Relationships Between Infants' Vocalizations
    and their Mothers' Behaviors. Merr. Palm. Quart. 17:211-266.

Beckwith, L. 1971b. Relationships Between Attributes of Mothers
    and their Infants' IQ Scores. Child Develop. 42:1083-1097.

Beckwith, L., and Cohen, S.E. 1975. Early Cognitive Development of
    Full-Term and Premature Infants: Infant Studies Project Home
    Data. Paper presented at Meeting of Society for Research in
    Child Development, April, Denver, Colorado.

Bell, R.Q. 1971. Stimulus Control of Parent or Caretaker Behavior
    by Offspring. Develop. Psychol. 4:63-72.

Bell, R.Q. 1974. Contributions of Human Infants to Caregiving and
    Social Interaction, pp. 1-20. In M. Lewis and L.A. Rosenblum

(eds.). The Effect of the Infant on its Caregiver. Wiley, New York.

Bell, R.Q., Weller, G.M., and Waldrop, M.F. 1971. Newborn and Preschooler: Organization of Behavior and Relations Between Periods. Monogr. Soc. Res. Child Develop. 36(1-2),Serial No. 142, pp. 1-145.

Bell, S.M. 1970. The Development of the Concept of Objects as Related to Infant-Mother Attachment. Child Develop. 41:291-311.

Bell, S.M., and Ainsworth, M.D.S. 1972. Infant Crying and Maternal Responsiveness. Child Develop. 43:1171-1190.

Birch, H.G. 1964. The Problem of "Brain Damage" in Children, pp. 3-12. In H.G. Birch (ed.). Brain Damage in Children: The Biological and Social Aspects. Williams and Wilkins, Baltimore.

Birch, H.G., and Gussow, C.D. 1970. Disadvantaged Children. Grune and Stratton, New York. 322 pp.

Birns, B. 1965. Individual Differences in Human Neonates' Responses to Stimulation. Child Develop. 36:249-256.

Braine, M., Heimer, C., Wortis, H., and Freedman, A. 1966. Factors Associated with Impairment of the Early Development of Prematures. Monogr. Soc. Res. Child Develop. 31(4),Serial No. 106, pp. 1-92.

Brazelton, T.B. 1972. Neonatal Behavioral Assessment Scale. Unpublished manuscript. Harvard University, Cambridge, Mass.

Brazelton, T.B., Koslowski, B., and Main, M. 1974. The Origins of Reciprocity: The Early Mother-Infant Interaction, pp. 49-76. In M. Lewis and L. Rosenblum (eds.). The Effect of the Infant on its Caregiver, Vol. 1. The Origins of Behavior Series. Wiley, New York.

Bronson, W.C. 1971. The Growth of Competence: Issues of Conceptualization and Measurement, pp. 269-277. In H.R. Schaffer (ed.). The Origins of Human Social Relations. Academic Press, New York.

Bruner, J.S. 1969a. Process of Growth in Infancy, pp. 205-228. In A. Ambrose (ed.). Stimulation in Early Infancy. Academic Press, New York.

Bruner, J.S. 1969b. Phenotypic and Genotypic Variation, Early Stimulation and Cognitive Development: General Discussion,

pp. 261-267. In A. Ambrose (ed.). Stimulation in Early
Infancy. Academic Press, New York.

Bruner, J.S. 1973. Nature and Uses of Immaturity, pp. 11-48. In
K. Connolly and J. Bruner (eds.). The Growth of Competence.
Academic Press, New York.

Caputo, D.V., and Mandell, W. 1970. Consequences of Low Birthweight.
Develop. Psychol. 3:363-384.

Clarke-Stewart, K.A. 1973. Interactions Between Mothers and their
Young Children: Characteristics and Consequences. Monogr. Soc.
Res. Child Develop. 38(6-7),Serial No. 153, pp. 1-109.

Cohen, S.E. 1975. Caregiving Behaviors and Early Cognitive Develop-
ment as Related to Ordinal Position in Premature Infants.
Paper presented at Meeting of Society for Research in Child
Development, April, Denver, Colorado.

Cohen, S.E., and Beckwith, L. 1975. Maternal Language Input in
Infancy. Paper presented at American Psychological Association
Meeting, September, Chicago, Illinois.

David, M., and Appell, G. 1969. Mother-Child Interaction and its
Impact on the Child, pp. 171-190. In A. Ambrose (ed.).
Stimulation in Early Infancy. Academic Press, New York.

Denenberg, V.H. 1964. Critical Periods, Stimulus Input, and
Emotional Reactivity: A Theory of Infantile Stimulation.
Psych. Rev. 71:335-351.

Denenberg, V.H. 1969. Experimental Programming of Life Histories
in the Rat, pp. 21-34. In A. Ambrose (ed.). Stimulation in
Early Infancy. Academic Press, New York.

Denenberg, V.H., and Whimbey, A.E. 1963. Behavior of Adult Rats
is Modified by the Experience Their Mothers Had as Infants.
Science. 142:1192-1193.

Dennis, W. 1960. Causes of Retardation Among Institutional Children:
Iran. J. Genet. Psychol. 96:47-59.

Dennis, W., and Najarian, P. 1957. Infant Development Under Environmental Handicap. Psychol. Monogr. 71(7):1-13.

Deutsch, C.P. 1973. Social Class and Child Development, pp. 233-
282. In B.M. Caldwell and H.N. Ricciuti (eds.). Review of
Child Development Research, Vol. 3. The University of
Chicago Press, Chicago.

Drillien, C.M. 1964. The Growth and Development of the Prematurely
     Born Infant. Williams and Wilkins, Baltimore. 376 pp.

Drillien, C.M. 1972. Aetiology and Outcome in Low Birthweight
     Infants. Develop. Med. Child Neurol. 14:563-584.

Eimas, P.D., Siqueland, E.R., Jusczyk, P., and Vigorito, J. 1971.
     Speech Perception in Infants. Science. 171:303-306.

Eisenberg, R.B. 1965. Auditory Behavior in the Human Neonate: I.
     Methodologic Problems and the Logical Design of Research
     Procedures. J. Audit. Res. 5:159-177.

Fantz, R.L. and Nevis, S. 1967. Pattern Preferences and Perceptual-
     Cognitive Development in Early Infancy. Merr. Palm. Quart.
     13:77-108.

Fitzhardinge, P.M. and Ramsay, M. 1973. The Improving Outlook for
     the Small Prematurely Born Infant. Develop. Med. Child Neurol.
     15:447-459.

Francis-Williams, J. and Davies, P.A. 1974. Very Low Birthweight
     and Later Intelligence. Develop. Med. Child Neurol. 16:709-
     728.

Garmezy, N. and Streitman, S. 1974. Children at Risk: The Search
     for the Antecedents of Schizophrenia. Part 1. Conceptual Models
     and Research Methods. Schizophrenia Bull. 8:14-90.

Gewirtz, J.L. 1961. A Learning Analysis of the Effects of Normal
     Stimulation, Privation and Deprivation on the Acquisition of
     Social Motivation and Attachment, pp. 213-290. In B.M. Foss
     (ed.). Determinants of Infant Behavior. Wiley, New York.

Golden, M. and Birns, B. 1968. Social Class and Cognitive Develop-
     ment in Infancy. Merr. Palm. Quart. 14:139-149.

Goldfarb, W. 1943. The Effects of Early Institutional Care on
     Adolescent Personality. J. Exp. Educ. 12:106-129.

Haaf, R.A., and Bell, R.Q. 1967. A Facial Dimension in Visual
     Discrimination by Human Infants. Child Develop. 38:893-899.

Harper, P.A., Fischer, L.K., and Rider, R.V. 1959. Neurological
     and Intellectual Status of Prematures at Three to Five Years
     of Age. J. Pediat. 55:679-690.

Hebb, D.O. 1946. On the Nature of Fear. Psych. Rev. 53:259-276.

Helson, H. 1959. Adaptation Level Theory, pp. 565-621. In S. Koch (ed.). Psychology: A Study of a Science. Sensory, Perceptual, and Psychological Formulations, Vol. 1. McGraw Hill, New York.

Honzik, M.P., Hutchings, J.J., and Burnip, S.R. 1965. Birth Record Assessments and Test Performance at Eight Months. Amer. J. Dis. Childr. 109:416-426.

Hunt, J.McV., and Kirk, G.E. 1971. Social Aspects of Intelligence: Evidence and Issues, pp. 262-306. In R. Cancro (ed.). Intelligence, Genetic and Environmental Influences. Grune and Stratton, New York.

Hunt, J.V., Harvin, D., Kennedy, D., and Tooley, W.H. 1974. Mental Development of Children with Birthweights ≤ 1500 g. Paper presented at the Meeting of the Western Society for Pediatric Research, February, Carmel, California.

Kagan, J. 1968. On Cultural Deprivation, pp. 211-257. In D.C. Glass (ed.). Environmental Influences. Proceedings of a Conference under the auspices of Russell Sage and Rockefeller University. Rockefeller University and Russell Sage, New York.

Kagan, J. 1970. The Determinants of Attention in the Infant. Amer. Scientist 58:298-306.

Kagan, J., and Klein, R.E. 1973. Cross-Cultural Perspectives on Early Development. Amer. Psychol. 28:947-961.

Kagan, J., and Moss, H.A. 1962. Birth to Maturity: A Study in Psychological Development. Wiley, New York. 381 pp.

Kagan, J., and Tulkin, S.R. 1971. Social Class Differences in Child Rearing During the First Year, pp. 165-183. In H.R. Schaffer (ed.). The Origins of Human Social Relations. Academic Press, New York.

Kagan, J., Henker, B.A., Hen-tov, A., Levine, J., and Lewis, M. 1966. Infants' Differential Reactions to Familiar and Distorted Faces. Child Develop. 37:519-532.

Kaplan, D., and Mason, E. 1960. Maternal Reactions to Premature Birth Viewed as an Acute Emotional Disorder. Amer. J. Orthopsych. 30:539.

Kawi, A., and Pasamanick, B. 1958. Association of Factors of Pregnancy with Reading Disorders in Childhood. J. Amer. Med. Assoc. 166:1420-1423.

Kennedy, W.A., Van de Riet, V., and White, J.C. 1963. A Normative

Sample of Intelligence and Achievement of Negro Elementary Children in the Southeastern United States. Monogr. Soc. Res. Child Develop. 28(6),Serial No. 90, pp. 1-112.

Kennell, J.A., Jerauld, R., Wolfe, H., Chesler, D., Kreger, N.C., McAlpine, W., Steffa, M., and Klaus, M.H. 1974. Maternal Behavior One Year After Early and Extended Postpartum Contact. Develop. Med. Child Neurol. 16:172-179.

Klaus, M.H., and Kennell, J.H. 1970. Mothers Separated From Their Newborn Infants. Pediatr. Clin. N. Amer. 17:1015-1037.

Klaus, M.H., Kennell, J.H., Plumb, N., and Zwehlke, S. 1970. Human Maternal Behavior at the First Contact With Her Young. Pediatrics 46:187-192.

Klaus, M.H., Jerauld, R., Kreger, N.C., McAlpine, W., Steffa, M., and Kennell, J.H. 1972. Maternal Attachment: Importance of the First Postpartum Days. N. Engl. J. Med. 286:460-463.

Klein, M., and Stern, L. 1971. Low Birthweight and the Battered Child Syndrome. Amer. J. Dis. Childr. 122:15-18.

Knobloch, H., and Pasamanick, B. 1960. Environmental Factors Affecting Human Development Before and After Birth. Pediatrics 26:210-218.

Knobloch, H. and Pasamanick, B. 1962. Developmental and Behavioral Approach to Neurologic Examination in Infancy. Child Develop. 33:181-198.

Knobloch, H., Pasamanick, B., Harper, P., and Rider, R. 1959. The Effect of Prematurity on Health and Growth. Amer. J. Publ. Hlth. 49:1164-1173.

Korner, A.F. 1971. Individual Differences at Birth: Implications for Early Experience and Later Development. Amer. J. Orthopsych. 41:608-619.

Korner, A.F. 1973. Early Stimulation and Maternal Care as Related to Infant Capabilities and Individual Differences. Early Child Develop. Care 2:307-327.

Korner, A.F. 1974. The Effect of the Infant's State, Level of Arousal, Sex, and Ontogenetic Stage on the Caregiver, pp. 105-122. In M. Lewis and L.A. Rosenblum (eds.). The Effect of the Infant on its Caregiver. Wiley, New York.

Korner, A.F., and Thoman, E.B. 1970. Visual Alertness in Neonates as Evoked by Maternal Care. J. Exper. Child Psychol. 10:67-78.

Korner, A.F., and Thoman, E.B. 1972. The Relative Efficacy of
    Contact and Vestibular-Proprioceptive Stimulation in Soothing
    Neonates. Child Develop. 43:443-453.

Korner, A.F., Kraemer, H.C., Haffner, M.E., and Cosper, L.M. 1975.
    Effects of Waterbed Flotation on Premature Infants: A Pilot
    Study. Pediatrics. (in press).

Leiderman, P.H., Leifer, A.D., Seashore, M.J., Barnett, C.R., and
    Grobstein, R. 1973. Mother-Infant Interaction: Effects of
    Early Deprivation, Prior Experience and Sex of Infant, pp. 154-
    175. In J.I. Nurnberger (ed.). Biological and Environmental
    Determinants of Early Development. Williams and Wilkins,
    Baltimore.

Leifer, A.D., Leiderman, P.H., Barnett, C.R., and Williams, J.A.
    1972. Effects of Mother-Infant Separation on Maternal Attach-
    ment Behavior. Child Develop. 43:1203-1218.

Levine, S. 1969. Infantile Stimulation: A Perspective, pp. 3-8.
    In A. Ambrose (ed.). Stimulation in Early Infancy. Academic
    Press, New York.

Lewis, M., and Goldberg, S. 1969. Perceptual-Cognitive Development
    in Infancy: A Generalized Expectancy Model as a Function of
    the Mother-Infant Interaction. Merr. Palm. Quart. 15:81-100.

Lewis, M., and Wilson, C.D. 1972. Infant Development in Lower-Class
    American Families. Human Develop. 15:112-127.

Lewis, M., Bartels, B., Campbell, H., and Goldberg, S. 1967.
    Individual Differences in Attention: The Relation Between
    Infants' Condition at Birth and Attention Distribution Within
    the First Year. Amer. J. Dis. Childr. 113:461-465.

Lewis, M., Goldberg, S., and Campbell, H. 1969. A Developmental
    Study of Information Processing Within the First Three Years
    of Life: Response Decrement to a Redundant Signal. Monogr.
    Soc. Res. Child Develop. 34(9),Serial No. 133, pp. 1-41.

Lilienfeld, A.M., and Parkhurst, E. 1951. A Study of the Associa-
    tion of Factors of Pregnancy and Parturition With the Develop-
    ment of Cerebral Palsy. Amer. J. Hyg. 53:262-282.

Lilienfeld, A.M., Pasamanick, B., and Rogers, M. 1955. Relationship
    Between Pregnancy Experience and the Development of Certain
    Neuropsychiatric Disorders in Childhood. Amer. J. Publ. Hlth.
    45:637-643.

Lilienfeld, A.M., and Pasamanick, B. 1956. The Association of

Maternal and Fetal Factors with the Development of Mental Deficiency. II. Relationship to Maternal Age, Birth Order, Previous Reproductive Loss, and Degree of Mental Deficiency. Amer. J. Ment. Def. 60:557-569.

Lubchenco, L.O., Horner, F.A., Reed, L.H., Hix, I.E., Metcalf, D., Cohig, R., Elliot, H.C., and Bourg, M. 1963. Sequelae of Premature Birth: Evaluation of Premature Infants of Low Birth-weights at Ten Years of Age. Amer. J. Dis. Childr. 106:101-115.

Macfarlane, J. 1964. Perspectives on Personality Consistency and Change From the Guidance Study. Vita Humana 7: 115-126.

McCall, R.B., Hagarty, P.S., and Hurlburt, N. 1972. Transitions in Infant Sensorimotor Development and the Prediction of Childhood IQ. Amer. Psychol. 27:728-748.

Moss, H.A. 1967. Sex, Age, and State as Determinants of Mother-Infant Interaction. Merr. Palm. Quart. 13:19-36.

Moss, H.A., and Robson, K.S. 1968. The Role of Protest Behavior in the Development of the Mother-Infant Attachment. Paper presented at the Meeting of the American Psychological Association, September, San Francisco, California.

Moss, H.A., and Robson, K.S. 1970. The Relation Between the Amount of Time Infants Spend at Various States and the Development of Visual Behavior. Child Develop. 41:509-517.

Nelson, K. 1973. Structure and Strategy in Learning to Talk. Monogr. Soc. Res. Child Develop. 38(1-2),Serial No. 149, pp. 1-135.

Osofsky, J.D. 1975. Neonatal Characteristics and Directional Effects in Mother-Infant Interaction. Symposium on Direction of Effects in Studies of Early Parent-Infant Interaction presented at the Society for Research in Child Development, April, Denver, Colorado.

Osofsky, J.D., and Danzger, B. 1974. Relationships Between Neo-natal Characteristics and Mother-Infant Interaction. Develop. Psychol. 10:124-130.

Parmelee, A.H., and Haber, A. 1973. Who is the "Risk Infant"?, pp. 376-387. In H.J. Osofsky (ed.). Clinical Obstetrics and Gynecology. Harper and Row, New York.

Parmelee, A.H., Kopp, C.B., and Sigman, M. 1975. Selection of Developmental Assessment Techniques for Infant at Risk. Paper presented at Merrill-Palmer Institute Conference on Research and Teaching of Infant Development, February, Detroit, Michigan.

Pasamanick, B., and Lilienfeld, A.M. 1955. Association of Maternal
    and Fetal Factors with the Development of Mental Deficiency:
    I. Abnormalities in the Prenatal and Paranatal Periods. J.
    Amer. Med. Assoc. 159:155-160.

Pasamanick, B., Rogers, M.E., and Lilienfeld, A.M. 1956. Pregnancy
    Experience and the Development of Behavior Disorder in Children.
    Amer. J. Psychiat. 112:613-618.

Piaget, J. 1952. The Origins of Intelligence in Children. Inter-
    national Universities Press, New York. 419 pp.

Powell, L.F. 1974. The Effect of Extra Stimulation and Maternal
    Involvement on the Development of Low Birthweight Infants and
    on Maternal Behavior. Child Develop. 45:106-113.

Prechtl, H.F.R. 1963. The Mother-Child Interaction in Babies with
    Minimal Brain Damage, pp. 53-59. In B.M. Foss (ed.). Deter-
    minants of Infant Behavior, Vol. 2. Wiley, New York.

Provence, S., and Lipton, R.C. 1962. Infants in Institutions: A
    Comparison of Their Development with Family-Reared Infants
    During the First Year of Life. International Universities
    Press, New York. 191 pp.

Rheingold, H.L. 1967. A Comparative Psychology of Development,
    pp. 279-293. In H.W. Stevenson, E.H. Hess, and H.L. Rheingold
    (eds.). Early Behavior: Comparative and Developmental
    Approaches. Wiley, New York.

Rheingold, H.L. 1969a. The Social and Socializing Infant, pp.
    779-790. In D.A. Goslin (ed.). Handbook of Socialization
    Theory and Research. Rand McNally, Chicago.

Rheingold, H.L. 1969b. The Effect of a Strange Environment on the
    Behavior of Infants, pp. 137-168. In B.M. Foss (ed.). Deter-
    minants of Infant Behavior, Vol. 4. Wiley, New York.

Rheingold, H.L. 1973. Independent Behavior of the Human Infant,
    pp. 178-203. In A.D. Pick (ed.). Minnesota Symposia on Child
    Psychology, Vol. 7. University of Minnesota Press, Minneapolis,
    Minnesota.

Rheingold, H.L., and Eckerman, C.D. 1970. The Infant Separates
    Himself From His Mother. Science 168:78-83.

Richards, M.P.M. 1974. The Development of Psychological Communica-
    tion in the First Year of Life, pp. 119-132. In K. Connolly

and J. Bruner (eds.). The Growth of Competence. Academic Press, New York.

Rubenstein, J. 1967. Maternal Attentiveness and Subsequent Exploratory Behavior in the Infant. Child Develop. 38: 1089-1100.

Sameroff, A., and Chandler, M. 1975. Reproductive Risk and the Continuum of Caretaking Casualty, pp. 187-244. In F. D. Horowitz, E.M. Hetherington, M. Siegel, and S. Scarr-Salapatek (eds.). Review of Child Development Research, Vol. 4. University of Chicago Press, Chicago, Illinois. (in press).

Sander, L.W. 1969. Regulation and Organization in the Early Infant-Caretaker System, pp. 311-333. In R.J. Robinson (ed.). Brain and Early Behaviour. Academic Press, New York.

Scarr-Salapatek, S., and Williams, M.L. 1973. The Effects of Early Stimulation on Low Birthweight Infants. Child Develop. 44: 94-102.

Schaefer, E.S., and Bell, R.Q. 1958. Development of a Parental Attitude Research Instrument. Child Develop. 29:339-361.

Schaffer, H.R., and Emerson, P.E. 1964. The Development of Social Attachments in Infancy. Monogr. Soc. Res. Child Develop. 29(3), Serial No. 94, pp. 1-77.

Sigman, M., Kopp, C.B., Parmelee, A.H., and Jeffrey, W.E. 1973. Visual Attention and Neurological Organization in Neonates. Child Develop. 44:461-466.

Sigman, M., and Parmelee, A.H. 1974. Visual Preferences of Four-Month-Old Premature and Full-Term Infants. Child Develop. 45:959-965.

Siqueland, E.R. 1973. Biological and Experimental Determinants of Exploration in Infancy, pp. 822-823. In L.J. Stone, H.T. Smith, and L.B. Murphy (eds.). The Competent Infant. Basic Books, New York.

Skeels, H. 1966. Adult Status of Children With Contrasting Early Life Experiences. Monogr. Soc. Res. Child Develop. 31(3), Serial No. 105, pp. 1-65.

Solkoff, N., Yaffe, S., Weintraub, D., and Blase, B. 1969. Effects of Handling on the Subsequent Development of Premature Infants. Develop. Psychol. 1:765-768.

Stern, D.N. 1974. Mother and Infant at Play: The Dyadic Interaction

Involving Facial, Vocal, and Gaze Behaviors, pp. 187-213.
In M. Lewis and L. Rosenblum (eds.). The Effect of the Infant
on its Caregivers. The Origin of Behavior Series, Vol. 1,
Wiley, New York.

Stewart, A.L., and Reynolds, E.O.R. 1974. Improved Prognosis for
    Infants of Very Low Birthweight. Pediatrics 54:724-735.

Stone, J., Smith, J., and Murphy, L. 1973. The Competent Infant.
    Basic Books, New York. 1314 pp.

Thomas, A., Chess, S., and Birch, H. 1968. Temperament and Behavior
    Disorders in Children. New York University Press, New York.
    309 pp.

Tulkin, S.R. 1972. An Analysis of the Concept of Cultural Depriva-
    tion. Develop. Psychol. 6:326-339.

Tulkin, S.R., and Kagan, J. 1972. Mother-Child Interaction in the
    First Year of Life. Child Develop. 43:31-41.

Ucko, L.E. 1965. A Comparative Study of Asphyxiated and Nonasphyx-
    iated Boys From Birth to Five Years. Develop. Med. Child
    Neurol. 7:643-657.

Wachs, T.D. 1973. Utilization of a Piagetian Approach in Investiga-
    tion of Early Experience Effects: A Research Strategy and Some
    Illustrative Data. Paper presented at the Meeting of the
    American Psychological Association, August, Montreal, Canada.

Wachs, T.D., and Cucinotta, P. 1971. The Effects of Enriched Neo-
    natal Experiences Upon Later Cognitive Functioning. Paper
    presented at the Meeting of the Society for Research in Child
    Development, April, Minneapolis, Minnesota.

Wachs, T.D., Uzgiris, I.C., and Hunt, J.McV. 1971. Cognitive Devel-
    opment in Infants of Different Age Levels and From Different
    Environmental Backgrounds: An Explanatory Investigation. Merr.
    Palm. Quart. 17:283-317.

Werner, E.E., Bierman, J.M., and French, F.E. 1971. The Children
    of Kauai. A Longitudinal Study from the Prenatal Period to Age
    Ten. University of Hawaii Press, Honolulu. 199 pp.

White, B.L., and Held, R. 1967. Plasticity of Sensorimotor Devel-
    opment in the Human Infant, pp. 291-313. In J. Hellmuth (ed.).
    Exceptional Infant. The Normal Infant, Vol. 1. Brunner-Mazel,
    New York.

White, B.L., and Watts, J.C. 1973. Experience and Environment.

Prentice-Hall, Englewood Cliffs, New Jersey. 552 pp.

Wiener, G. 1962. Psychologic Correlates of Premature Birth: A Review. J. Nerv. Mental Dis. 134:129-135.

Wiener, G. 1968. Scholastic Achievement at Age 12-13 of Prematurely Born Infants. J. Spec. Educ. 2:237.

Wiener, G. 1970. The Relationship of Birthweight and Length of Gestation to Intellectual Development at Ages 8 to 10 Years. J. Pediat. 76:694-699.

Wiener, G., Rider, R.V., and Oppel, W. 1963. Some Correlates of IQ Changes in Children. Child Develop. 34:61-67.

Wiener, G., Rider, R.V., Oppel, W., Fischer, L.K., and Harper, P.A. 1965. Correlates of Low Birthweight: Psychological Status of 6-7 Years of Age. Pediatrics 35:434-444.

Wiener, G., Rider, R.V., Oppel, W., and Harper, P.A. 1968. Correlates of Low Birthweight. Psychological Status at 8 to 10 Years of Age. Pediatr. Rev. 2:110-118.

Willerman, L., Broman, S.H., and Fiedler, M. 1970. Infant Development, Preschool IQ, and Social Class. Child Develop. 41: 69-79.

Yarrow, L.J. 1963. Research in Dimensions of Early Maternal Child Care. Merr. Palm. Quart. 9:101-114.

Yarrow, L.J. 1964. Personality Consistency and Change: An Overview of Some Conceptual and Methodological Issues. Vita Humana 7:67-72.

Yarrow, L.J., Rubenstein, J.L., Pederson, F.A., and Jankowski, J.J. 1972. Dimensions of Early Stimulation and Their Differential Effects on Infant Development. Merr. Palm. Quart. 18:205-218.

Yarrow, L.J., Goodwin, M.S., Manheimer, H., and Milowe, I.D. 1973. Infancy Experiences and Cognitive and Personality Development at Ten Years, pp. 1274-1281. In L.J. Stone, H.T. Smith, and L.B. Murphy (eds.). The Competent Infant: Research and Commentary. Basic Books, New York.

DETERMINATION AND PREVENTION OF INFANT BRAIN DYSFUNCTION:

SENSORY AND NONSENSORY ASPECTS

Ann Lodge

Department of Pediatrics
Children's Hospital of San Francisco
3801 Sacramento Street
San Francisco, California 94119

I. STATUS OF THE PROBLEM

There is accumulating evidence that environmental conditions
during the prenatal and perinatal periods and the early years of
life have a determining impact upon the intellectual and emotional
development of the human infant. This has special relevance for
environmental planning for the increasing numbers of infants born
at-risk for central nervous system dysfunction associated with such
conditions as malnutrition, drug effects, prematurity, infection,
respiratory distress, and hyperbilirubinemia. A 68% improvement in
survival rate between the years of 1962 and 1971 was found for premature infants born in New York City with birthweights under 1000 g,
according to a recent report (Culliton, 1975). Approximately 150,000
infants per year, or one of every 20 babies born in the United States,
are placed in neonatal intensive care units for observation and
treatment (Steinmann, 1975). Evidence suggests that 20% to 30% of
these infants may develop handicaps including sensory and perceptual
deficits, learning disabilities, and various behavioral problems
(Drillien, 1964, 1965; Knobloch and Pasamanick, 1960; Rogers, 1968).
Nevertheless, considerable variability is seen in developmental outcome which cannot be satisfactorily accounted for in terms of prenatal risk factors, birth distress, or neonatal status. Newer treatment methods appear to offer hope of significantly reducing the
developmental hazards associated with high-risk birth; however, their
long-range impact still requires intensive investigation. This
emphasizes the urgent need for more precise identification of both
the sensory and nonsensory factors which affect infant neurodevelopmental processes and the nature of their susceptibility to environmental influences. Such knowledge could provide an improved basis
for formulating diagnostic, preventive and therapeutic measures.

This chapter discusses available assessment procedures and some
therapeutic approaches which appear to be effective.

II. ENVIRONMENTAL INFLUENCES UPON DEVELOPMENT

A. Prenatal Environment

Wilson (1973) has defined environment as all influences from
outside the skin of the developing organism. These may initially
include amniotic fluid and placenta, the state of the mother's
body and other physical and chemical influences transmitted through
the mother, as well as the more subtle impact of all the mother's
life experiences and stresses.

While mankind has a long history of both intuitive and ritual-
ized practices for safeguarding the mother and unborn child,
specialized medical care of the pregnant woman and concern with
the prenatal health of the child are a relatively recent emphasis
of our culture. This trend may reflect a growing atmosphere of
humanistic commitment to improving the quality of life, an acceptance
of both the possibility and the responsibility for ensuring this,
and an increased awareness of the dire implications of its neglect.

There are a number of chromosomal, metabolic and other abnormalities associated with retardation which may be detected
prenatally through amniocentesis. These include Down's syndrome,
Tay-Sachs disease, Hunter's and Hurler's syndromes, galactosemia
(Butler, 1972). Two metabolic disorders, galactosemia and phenyl-
ketonuria (detectable only after birth), show significant response
to therapy with early diagnosis and dietary treatment. Hypothyroidism, the only endocrinopathy known to be associated with
mental retardation, and hydrocephalus are also identifiable and
treatable from the time of birth.

Less specific than the identifiable cytogenic, metabolic, or
gross structural abnormalities are intrauterine factors such as
malnutrition and drug exposure which may affect brain development.
There is much conflicting evidence concerning the impact and even
the definition of malnutrition (see chapter by Levine and Wiener;
and Richardson, this volume), while effects of extrauterine agents
vary. Despite the protective filtering influence of the placenta,
the rapidly developing fetal brain is subject to exposure to hormones, viruses, maternal blood, drugs, and chemicals at various
stages of gestation, with known and unknown implications for development. For example, with no maternal immunity the fetus is particularly susceptible to viruses such as rubella during the first
trimester, which can produce multiple defects. The congenital
rubella epidemic of 1964-65 afflicted large numbers of infants in
the United States with a wide range of symptoms including both

peripheral and central nervous system damage and systemic involvement (Dudgeon, 1968; Barnet and Lodge, 1966).

The profound fetal organ damage and malfunction which may
result from drugs taken by the mother during pregnancy gained even
wider recognition following the thalidomide tragedy of 1964 (Bowes
et al., 1970).

Drug and alcohol abuse have become major world problems with
serious neurodevelopmental implications. Both heroin and methadone
may cross the placental barrier, with unknown consequences for the
developing brain of the fetus (e.g., Fabro, 1973). Symptoms of the
neonatal withdrawal syndrome may include hypertonicity, tremulous-
ness, gastrointestinal distress, hyperacousis, depressed visual
attention, inadequate sucking, and seizures, which indicate both
autonomic and central nervous system involvement (e.g., Kron et al.,
1973; Lodge et al., 1975; Soule et al., 1973; Zelson et al., 1971).
Evidence also indicates that heroin may serve as an enzyme inducer,
which appears to be associated with a lower incidence of jaundice
and possibly other effects (Stern, 1973, p. 41; Zelson et al.,
1971). A neonatal alcohol syndrome with distinct physical characteristics has also been described, and it may be associated with retardation (Jones, 1974). Commonly prescribed analgesic medications
administered during pregnancy and delivery can depress newborn
alertness, visual attention, sucking, and mother-infant interaction
(e.g., Brazelton, 1970; Kron, 1966; Stechler, 1964). Excess vitamin
A during pregnancy has been implicated in deficits of later discrimination learning (Hutchings and Gibbon, 1971). The scope of
pre-natal drug risk is indicated by a survey of drug use in pregnant
women in Scotland; 82% of the women received medically prescribed
drugs and 65% took drugs on their own initiative (Forfar, 1973).

Any major handicap or the interaction of minor ones may predispose to further disadvantaging situations and experiences so as
to produce cumulative deficits. Lourie (1971) has suggested that
during prenatal formative stages a functional organ system may
develop a pattern of reaction to stress which may predispose it to
subsequent developmental distortion. Prescott (1971) has hypothesized that the relative immaturity of the cerebellum at birth is
associated with particular vulnerability to such early insults as
premature birth and neonatal anoxia. These effects may be compounded
by inappropriate sensory environments such as lack of maternal/social
contact. In addition to the relatively localized impact of environmental trauma upon various developing organ systems, the overall
question of nonspecific stress (Selye, 1956), or just "how sick the
baby is" and for how long, may be of overriding importance.

B. Postnatal Environment

At birth, the baby loses the protective insulation of the

mother's body and becomes abruptly and more directly exposed to a
wide range of environmental influences. He is thrust into reliance
upon his own untested coping mechanisms and upon the support of
those around him. Now sensory impairment in any modality will dis-
tort the baby's capacity for adequate information processing and
learning of adaptive responses. A central, nonspecific disturbance
such as the irritability and inconsolability of a baby undergoing
drug withdrawal seriously interferes with his ability to deal adapt-
ively with the surrounding environment; furthermore, it is apt to
have a negative effect upon the reaction of other persons upon whom
he is dependent. Neurological involvement which is associated with
diminished visual attention and eye-contact may also have a deleterious effect upon mother-infant interaction (see Beckwith, this
volume).

There is increasing suspicion that Western civilization may
have gone too far in the direction of treating birth in the manner
of a medical illness, and that current hospital practices may
frequently subject mother, baby, and father to more trauma and disruption of living conditions than are normally necessary. The
notion that birth may be a traumatic experience was emphasized by
Rank (1929); more recently, Leboyer (1975) has argued that the newborn be recognized as a person exquisitely sensitive to pain and
therefore deserving of a more gradual and kindly introduction to
the world. He recommends such practices as placing the newborn on
its mother's belly and welcoming it with gentle massage, and the
postponement of the severing of the umbilicus, with its protective function as a back-up source of oxygen, until the infant's
breathing is established. However, there is evidence that early
clamping of the cord of normal newborns is associated with a higher
percentage of time spent in a quiet awake state, while late-clamped
infants display more quiet sleep and increased blood volume (Theorell
et al., 1973). The authors suggest that late clamping may further
stress the infant, while early clamping may be more conducive to a
positive mother-infant relationship.

When the prenatally-at-risk infant is born, or an infant is
placed at-risk as a result of complications related to the birth
process, he then becomes exposed to another set of distorting
environmental conditions through days, weeks, or even months spent
in a hospital nursery intensive care unit. At this point, iatro-
genic and environmental factors in developmental damage cannot be
overlooked, although they may unavoidably accompany the decision to
save the child's life. The infant, monitored by numerous electrodes,
fed through tubes, often repeatedly subjected to injections and surgery, may come to associate human approach with pain. In addition
he is typically exposed to a chaotic and unsympathetic visual and
auditory environment with isolette noise levels frequently in
excess of a deafening 80 to 90 db (League et al., 1972). The result may be a temporary deafness, as evidenced by diminished audit-

ory responsiveness and the lack of a vertex evoked EEG response to
click stimulation (Marcus, M.M., unpublished data). Damage to the
auditory system of the fetus or newborn has also been suspected to be
among the possible side effects associated with prolonged exposure
to certain forms of antibiotic therapy administered to the mother
(Bowes et al., 1970).

Retrolental fibroplasia, or retinal damage associated with
excessive oxygen administration, has been identified and has been
less significant as a cause of blindness than in previous years.
Treatment of hyperbilirubinemia frequently involves phototherapy
which necessitates blindfolding the baby within the isolette for
relatively long periods of time in order to prevent retinal damage.
Both animal and human studies suggest this could have deleterious
effects, at least for full-term infants. The visual system of a
number of animals including cats and infant monkeys is highly
susceptible to damage as a result of eye closure during the early
weeks of life (e.g., Hubel and Wiesel, 1963; Von Noorden et al.,
1970; see Walsh and Cummins, this volume). Children whose eyes
were occluded for surgery for short periods of time during the
first year of life displayed diminished visual acuity in later
years (Awaya et al., 1973). Earlier age of occlusion tended to be
associated with a greater incidence of abnormal visual evoked responses and greater resistence of the condition to treatment. The
results indicate stimulus deprivation amblyopia involving central
visual pathways, since the electroetinograms of all patients
were normal (Awaya et al., 1973).

The somatosensory environment which surrounds the high-risk
infant is equally unsympathetic: a plexiglass box with a relatively
unyielding mattress upon which the head, of necessity, flops to
one side or the other -- a condition which may be related to the
narrow, somewhat egg-shaped head characteristic of prematurity
(Baum and Searls, 1971). The possible long-range effects of the
manner in which the premature baby is typically positioned in the
isolette and the way in which he is clothed are not sufficiently
well understood; however, there is an obvious lack of the tactile,
proprioceptive, and kinesthetic stimulations that are experienced
both in utero and after birth by normally-born infants. Dreyfus-
Brisac has noted that "the presence of a circadian rhythm differ-
entiates intrauterine from extrauterine life" (Dreyfus-Brisac, 1974,
p. 136). There is evidence that temperature, lighting, and other
factors affect the development of sleep patterns in prematures,
who often experience later sleep disturbances (Dreyfus-Brisac, 1970,
1974; Parmelee et al., 1962; Sander et al., 1972).

C. Mother-Infant Interaction

In addition to the phenomena above, with most risk births the
crucial mother-infant interaction is severely disrupted and the

family typically experiences extreme emotional distress. Pierre
Budin (1907), who pioneered the medical specialty of neonatology,
recognized the importance of avoiding separation of mother and
infant and encouraged the mother's sharing in the care of her baby
to the extent possible to prevent the loss of her interest and
involvement in the child. Nevertheless, subsequent nursery practices have led, until recently, to increased separation rather than
the rooming-in and participation prevalent in earlier days (Klaus
and Fanaroff, 1973). The impact of the usually unanticipated
failure to have produced a normal baby, combined with abrupt separation and often alarming treatment procedures, would tax the
emotional resources of the best-adjusted family. The maternal
reaction in some instances may be comparable to traumatic neurosis
(Kaplan and Mason, 1960).

There is evidence that deprivation of contact with the infant
in the nursery may have a profound effect upon self-confidence as
a mother and commitment to the baby, as well as upon skill in caregiving and developmental stimulation (Barnett et al., 1970). A
disproportionate incidence of child abuse and failure to thrive
has also been reported associated with a history of high-risk birth
(Fanaroff et al., 1972). This appears congruent with observations
based on animal studies which indicate that early mother-infant
separation alters subsequent maternal attachment and quality of
infant care, especially in terms of timing and duration of contact,
sensory modalities of interaction, and caretaking nature of interaction (Barnett et al., 1970).

Maternal perception of the neonate as differing from average,
a factor built into the high-risk birth situation, has also been
found, in a study based upon normal infants, to show a significant
relationship to subsequent psychopathology in the child (Broussard
and Hartner, 1970). Maternal visiting patterns were also found to
provide an informative index concerning the quality of mothering
received by low birthweight infants (Fanaroff et al., 1972).

These considerations have led to some attempts to ameliorate
the sources of stress for parents of high-risk infants. It was
demonstrated that mothers could be permitted greater contact with
their babies shortly after birth without clinical hazard, although
some staff adjustment was necessary (Barnett et al., 1970). Increased communication, both formal and informal, between parents
and hospital staff has been beneficial (e.g., DuHamel et al., 1974).
Beckwith (this volume) discusses these issues in greater detail.

D. Need for Clarification of Environmental Variables

At every stage of development, different hazards are encountered and different opportunities arise for appropriate intervention.
The complexities of assessment of infant status has led to the

concept of "cumulative risk" (Parmelee et al., 1974), while Prechtl
(1968) has found optimality, or absence of significant complications,
a more useful approach to identification of babies at-risk for brain
dysfunction.

Part of the confusion in assessing the source of deprivation
effects would appear to arise from the difficulty in achieving clear
differentiation of the environmental variables involved. Yarrow et
al. (1971) have tackled this problem by employing time-sampling
observations and other ratings of the availability, stimulus value,
and responsiveness of both caregiver behavior and inanimate objects.
By so doing they have introduced greater precision into the definition and measurement of the infant's natural environment as it
affects development. Papoušek and Papoušek (1975) have demonstrated
that both social and nonsocial environmental events may be usefully
viewed in the context of their contingency relationships with the
infant's behavior.

Another difficulty arises from the lack of a satisfactory
definition of developmental retardation itself and of the role of
differing rates of development in different areas. Kagan (1973)
has pointed out that restricted early experience may appear to be
associated with a lack of certain culturally arbitrary skills, such
as reading ability, which constitutes retardation relative to a given
reference group at a certain point in time. He cites his study of
Guatemalan Indian children who experienced close physical contact
with their mothers but were otherwise isolated inside their homes
during the earliest years of their lives and appeared developmentally
retarded at 18 months, yet by the age of 11 appeared to function
with normal capability in all areas. He concludes that "an abnormal
experience in the first two years of life in no way affects basic
intellectual processes or the ability to be affectively normal -- to
experience gaiety and sadness, guilt and shame". A third difficulty
in definitive assessment of the impact of early environmental restrictions upon subsequent development (the lack of sufficient knowledge concerning the relative plasticity of human central nervous
system function) concerns the possibility of normalization of development (through appropriately timed and sequenced interventions).
An example is furnished by Richardson's findings (this volume) of
normalization of intellectual functions in malnourished infants from
stimulating home environments.

A disproportionate incidence of developmental retardation with
respect to culturally prevalent standards of intellectual functioning is found among socioeconomically disadvantaged children.
Characteristics such as lack of verbal facility, low self-esteem,
inability to form abstract concepts, low frustration tolerance, and
lack of intellectual curiosity or motivation for achieving success
through sustained constructive effort have variously been ascribed
to this group. The issue of values involved in criterion measures

of development and resultant implications for intervention through
environmental modification is a difficult one, especially during
this era of heightened sensitivity to the imposition of the values
of a dominant cultural group upon minorities.

Assessment of the impact of differing environmental conditions
upon developing brain function is further complicated by the necessity of understanding the role of a particular response within the
total organizational framework of an individual infant's behavioral
repertoire. It is to be hoped that greater understanding and appreciation of both genetically and culturally determined individual differences, as well as sources of preventable deficits, will provide
a broader basis for informed and humanitarian decisions in this
area.

III. APPROACHES TO ASSESSMENT OF SENSORY FUNCTION
AND NEURODEVELOPMENTAL STATUS

In view of the evidence for environmental sources of potential
damage, there is reason to expect that some aspects of developmental
dysfunction may be averted through preventive or rehabilitative
intervention. Much appropriate intervention may be undertaken on
an intuitive basis; however, for effective planning for environments as therapy for prevention of brain dysfunction, a necessary
first step is the earliest possible precise and comprehensive diagnosis of the individual child's physical status and psychological
characteristics, along with an evaluation of the therapeutic potential of his family situation.

A. The Problem of Infant "Intelligence"

Few topics are more perplexing than the mind of the developing child, and there is as yet no agreed-upon definition or measure
of infant intelligence. The developmental model which has emerged
from pediatric neurology has revealed a great deal about the reflexive status and sensorimotor abilities of infants, while traditional
psychological developmental assessment has further explored motoric,
language, social, and problem-solving skills during the early developmental period. Gesell and Amatruda (1945) introduced the notion
of embryology of behavior and pioneered an approach to "developmental diagnosis" based on the age of emergence of typical observable and readily recordable infant behaviors (see Knobloch and
Pasamanick, 1974). Some approaches have continued or further elab-
orated Gesell and Amatruda's division into four traditional developmental areas: motor, adaptive, personal-social, and language.
Another approach, represented by Cattell (1947) and Bayley (1969),
has been to concentrate on the overall developmental picture in
terms of age equivalents and developmental quotients or indices,
divided in the case of the more recent Bayley Infant Scales into

mental and motor areas (Bayley, 1965, 1969).

The Bayley Scales have the advantage of extensive standard-
ization using a more representative population sample, thereby
providing more adequate behavioral norms than have previously been
available (Bayley, 1965, 1969). In addition to permitting the
derivation of overall age equivalents for both mental and motor
areas, each test item has been assigned a developmental age equivalent based upon the average age at which it was passed by the stand-
ardization sample. On this basis the items have since been grouped
into nine subscales which yield a descriptive behavioral profile
for the following areas considered to be of clinical and theoretical
significance: sensory responsiveness and orientation, gross motor,
fine motor, exploratory drive, competence motivation, social re-
latedness, imitation, perceptuo-cognitive development, and language
(Lodge, 1973). Preliminary studies suggest that this approach may
be more useful in pinpointing specific areas of deficit than are the
overall developmental indices. Characteristic developmental patterns with respect to these areas may aid in identifying and differ-
entiating among causes of developmental handicaps (Lodge, 1968, 1973;
Lodge and Kleinfeld, 1973; Lodge et al., 1970). For example, the
gross motor subscale is concerned with large muscle control and coordination and is largely dependent upon maturation. However, this
area is also found to be particularly susceptible to the effects
of maternal deprivation and constricting environmental conditions
(Lodge, 1968). Neurochemical and electrophysiological abnormalities
which may disrupt the overall organization of behavior also appear
to be reflected in gross motor function (Lodge and Kleinfeld, 1973).
Imitative learning, which is often highly developed in home-reared
Down's syndrome infants, is generally conspicuously lacking in
institution-reared infants who were considered normal at birth
(Lodge, 1968). The relative contribution of the different developmental areas to determination of the Bayley Infant Scale Mental
Developmental Index varies at different ages (Lodge et al., 1970;
Lodge, 1973). Initially it is largely determined by sensory responsiveness but with maturation the major determinants become unskilled
exploration (six months), fine motor skills and imitation (12
months), with language predominant by 24 months.

The value of developmental testing has been most clearly demonstrated in terms of assessment of current status and identification of specific problem areas, rather than predictive value with
regard to subsequent intelligence measures such as the Stanford-
Binet (Terman and Merrill, 1960). This has led to questioning the
value of the more general infant behavioral tests (e.g., Lewis and
McGurk, 1972) and has spurred the development of tests directed at
more specifically cognitive aspects of infant functioning, usually
on the basis of Piaget's (1952) theory of the role of sensorimotor
development (see Hunt, this volume).

Perhaps instead of too severely criticizing the early developmental test for its generality and further constricting our picture of the infant to a search for variables that will reflect later intellectual and academic prowess, we should consider broadening our emphasis at later ages to include a more comprehensive picture of development than is reflected in prevalent IQ tests. While of undisputed importance, they should not be the only basis, for instance, for evaluating the effects of intervention programs. Surely, social intelligence and nonverbal communication skills, athletic ability, craftsmanship, and creativity, as well as vitality, purpose, and overall integration constitute a significant part of the total developmental picture at any age.

B. Other Approaches to Assessment of Developmental Status and Sensory Function

1. Behavioral Methods. An innovative and qualitatively different emphasis in developmental assessment is represented by Brazelton's (1973) Neonatal Assessment Scale. Here the primary emphasis is upon the infant's capacity to interact with both animate (human) and inanimate features of the surrounding environment. State variables, defined according to observable behavioral criteria developed by Prechtl and Beintema (1964), are also taken into account and it is intended to bring the baby through the whole spectrum of states during the course of the examination. By sampling hitherto largely unrealized capabilities for differential discrimination in the newborn, such as head turning to the coaxing of a human voice as compared with orienting to inanimate auditory stimuli, it offers a sensitive descriptive assessment for a wide range of behaviors. Neonatal ethnic differences in such areas as temperament, state organization, and social attentiveness have been obtained with Oriental, Zambian, and Mexican Indian populations as compared with Caucasian norms (Brazelton et al., 1969; Freedman and Freedman, 1969; Tronick et al., 1973). This scale, which appears to have value in assessing status and anticipating adjustment problems for both high-risk and normal infants, is being further modified for use with premature infants.

The clinical approach, while often the most sensitive and relevant to the real life situation and needs of the individual infant, has proved difficult to quantify. The application of systematic laboratory methods to the areas of both classical and instrumental learning and perceptuocognitive development is a valuable supplement to clinical observation but has as yet received relatively little application to clinical problems. Behaviors such as sucking and head turning have been demonstrated to respond to operant as well as classical conditioning procedures from the neonatal period and can provide sensitive measures of abnormal behavior in this area (e.g., Papoušek, 1959; Lipsitt and Kaye, 1964; Kron, 1966; Siqueland and Lipsitt, 1966). Kron's studies have identified a variety of mater-

nal and neonatal drug conditions associated with depressed sucking
patterns which appear to possess some unique diagnostic and prog-
nostic features (Kron, 1966; Kron et al., 1973).

Attempts to condition the blink response have revealed wide
individual differences which may reflect different levels of central
nervous system maturity or qualitative differences in the organization of neural functions (Papoušek, 1965). While neonatal conditioning is possible, responses such as the eyeblink which may be quickly
conditioned to a variety of stimuli at 2 or 3 months of age may be
conditioned only slowly and with great difficulty in younger infants.
The detailed developmental analysis of the course of learning specific adaptive behaviors such as sucking and blinking has important
implications for both diagnosis and therapeutic intervention.

Fantz's (1958, 1963) method for recording preferential attention in infants by means of differential fixation times (observed
by corneal reflection) to a variety of stimuli and charting of the
developmental course of pattern preferences paved the way for the
study of a wide range of parameters involved in perceptual development. The effect of stimulus characteristics such as color, form
(including pattern and contour), depth, as well as more subtle
dimensions such as the role of novelty, complexity, and meaning
have been studied in detail. (For reviews of the now extensive
literature in this field, see Hershenson, 1967; Stone et al., 1973).
The establishment of normative data in these areas also has important bearing for assessing, monitoring, and intervening in the perceptual development of the potentially developmentally handicapped
infant. For example, Fantz and Nevis (1967) found relative acceleration of perceptual development in home-reared versus institution-
reared infants.

Certain aspects of intelligent adaptive behavior may be importantly related to sensorimotor skills. Many significant aspects of
perceptuocognitive function may be predominantly mediated through
visual, auditory, and other sensory systems in interaction with
central organizational processes. The actions of the eyes, which
have received little attention in Piaget's theoretical formulation
of the importance of the sensorimotor period for cognitive development, are now being intensively studied in infants, utilizing a
variety of photographic and electronic recording techniques (e.g.
Haith et al., 1969; Hershenson, 1967).

2. Electrophysiological Methods. An inevitable shortcoming
of tests based upon observable behavior is that they may not adequately reflect underlying sensory, perceptual, or cognitive
functioning. We are forced to rely on inference, sometimes on the
basis of very little observable behavioral information. A baby may
see and even recognize a visual configuration or hear a sound or
comprehend speech but give little or no sign of such information

processing. This is where recent developments in electrophysiological recording may provide an important supplementary and sometimes sole source of information, as for example, in the case of
an unresponsive or comatose infant or one lacking means of expression or communication. In addition to eye movement photography and
the electro-oculogram (EOG), other indicators of the infant's
responses are the electroencephalogram (EEG) and averaged evoked
potentials, electrocardiogram (EKG), respiration, psychogalvanic
skin resistance (PGR), electroretinogram (ERG), and electromyogram
(EMG).

Until recently, clinical evaluation of the infant's hearing
ability had often been based upon observation of such reflexes
as the startle (Moro) or blink to sound, changes in activity level
(quieting, perhaps followed by increased movement), or directional
search as revealed by turning of head and eyes toward the source
of sound. These responses, however, tend to be variable, subtle,
and elusive in their manifestation and their observation provides
only cursory examination of auditory function in the young infant.
The technique of averaging of brain waves or electroencephalographic
(EEG) responses recorded from scalp electrodes in response to visual
and auditory stimulation has revealed that the brain of even the
newborn infant responds selectively to differences in intensity
and other characteristics of both light and sound stimulation.
Repetitive stimulation leads to habituation or decreased responsiveness in normal infants, but not in Down's syndrome infants
(Barnet et al., 1971). Autonomic response measures which have
yielded significant information about sensory responsiveness and
perceptual functioning of the infant include heart rate, respiration, and galvanic skin response. Suppression of sucking behavior
(measured through a special electronically-monitored bottle) has
also proved to be a sensitive indicator of perception and learning
in the infant. Findings indicative of a broad range of auditory
discrimination capabilities in infants, based upon such variables
as band-width, duration, repetition rate, interstimulus interval,
frequency, sound pressure level, dimensionality, as well as more
complex dimensions including tone pattern, are emerging in the area
of auditory perception (reviewed in Eisenberg, 1970). Issues of
the stress of testing itself, of when such special studies are
justified, are important and difficult decisions, involving both
the evaluation of possible risks and the possible contribution of
such studies to the patients' welfare.

While traditional neurological examinations and clinical EEG
tracings obtained during the neonatal period and subsequently
during the first year do not appear to predict future status of the
child except in the case of gross abnormalities, there is evidence
that cortical evoked responses may serve as an early indicator of
later perceptual and cognitive dysfunction. A large body of normative data concerning these response characteristics permits

precise assessment of their relative maturity. In general, this
increasing accuracy of measurement and comparison of the characteristics of different response systems has revealed a greater degree
of development of sensory responsiveness and perceptual capacity
in early infancy than has been traditionally assumed on the basis
of anatomic data and/or observable behavioral responses to auditory
and visual stimulation.

Evoked EEG potentials obtained to auditory, visual, and somatosensory stimuli are prominent at birth and provide one of the
most direct indices of cortical function during the perceptual
process (Ellingson, 1964). In fact, responses to light stimulation
have been recorded as early as 28-29 weeks gestational age (Ellingson, 1964; Engel and Butler, 1963). A substantial amount of systematic information now exists concerning longitudinal change in
development of the wave form components of the auditory evoked
potential (AEP) from the premature period into early childhood
(e.g., Weitzman and Graziani, 1968; Ellingson et al., 1974; Barnet
et al., 1975).

Barnet and her research group (1966, 1967, 1971), Rapin and
Graziani (1967), and others have explored the diagnostic value of
auditory evoked response audiometry in normal and brain-injured
infants. Sleep stage has been found to play an important role in
vertex derived recordings particularly, and Schulman's (1969)
report of disturbed sleep patterns in heroin-addicted infants,
which include a predominance of disorganized REM periods and
absence of normal periods of quiet sleep, suggests the probable
importance of predominant state variables in other conditions.

Evidence for hemispheric specialization in EEG of six-month-
old infants has been reported (Gardiner and Walter, 1973) in terms
of a power shift in the frequency range of the alpha precursor (4
hz) in response to verbal as compared with nonverbal (musical)
stimuli. Molfese (1975) has reported similar right-left differences
in neonatal evoked potentials. Using sucking rate as the response
measure, three-week-old infants were found to manifest lateral
asymmetry for dichotically presented speech and nonspeech stimuli
(Entus, 1975). These findings would appear to hold promise for
increasing diagnostic specificity in assessing developmental disabilities in information processing.

Low amplitude waves of extremely short latency (less than 10
msec) known as far field potentials, described by Jewett et al.
(1970), are believed to represent early synapses in the auditory
pathway at the level of the brainstem (cochlear nucleus, superior
olivary nucleus, lateral lemniscus, inferior colliculus). While
averages from many repeated stimuli are required to detect these
responses, they have proved extremely stable and apparently unaffected by anesthesia or state variables. They have been recorded

in infants between three weeks and three years of age by Hecox and Galambos (1974) and the results suggest that this technique has promise for increasing the efficacy of evoked response analysis of auditory dysfunction in infants and may eventually lead to specific identification of various levels of subcortical dysfunction.

The neonatal visual evoked response, while less mature and more variable and state-dependent than the auditory response, is also complex at birth. In contrast to the auditory evoked response, which is most prominent at the vertex, the visual response (VEP) is maximal in the occipital region. The vertex potential evoked by auditory stimuli appears to represent a nonspecific response system related to arousal, while the visual evoked potential is considered to arise more directly from a specific sensory system, although it may contain nonspecific components as well. Vertex responses evoked by visual stimulation tend to be more affected by behavioral and attentional factors and less dependent upon stimulus characteristics than is the occipital response. Nevertheless, both types of response are found to vary from earliest infancy as a function of both stimulus characteristics and behavioral state.

Despite differences in amplitude and latency, the electrophysiological responses to visual stimulation in the neonate, as measured by the ERG and VEP, were found to be relatively well-differentiated and generally comparable in wave form to those found with adults. It was concluded from these studies that the photopic and scotopic systems develop together at both the retinal and cortical levels and appear consistent with some capacity to perceive color, form and pattern (Barnet et al., 1965; Lodge et al., 1969; Oster, 1975).

Electroencephalographic and evoked response characteristics of premature and low birthweight infants have been described and found useful in the assessment of CNS maturity (e.g., Dreyfus-Brisac, 1964; Engel and Benson, 1968; Hrbek and Mareš, 1964; Weitzman and Graziani, 1968). Watanabe et al. (1972) found the wave form of the visual evoked response to be of aid in distinguishing true preterm from small-for-date infants. Work by Marcus (1971, 1975) has indicated that evoked responses to checkerboard patterns are more reliable than those obtained with simple flashes and, furthermore, that the latency of these responses is significantly correlated with the five-minute Apgar rating. Maturational characteristics of these wave forms appear to be of value in monitoring the CNS development of high-risk infants (Marcus, 1976).

Butler and Engel (1969) have reported a significant correlation between the latency characteristics of the visual evoked response at birth and Bayley developmental scores obtained at eight months of age. Rhodes et al. (1969b) found the later occipital components of dull children to be smaller than those of bright children. A tentative interpretation is that enhancement of these early components in dull or retarded infants may reflect some kind of dominance of the response by simpler primary processes or more sensory aspects of the stimulus, while elaboration of later components may represent the operation of more highly developed secondary processes which may characterize a higher level of development.

The electrophysiology of other sensory systems has received much less attention in developmental research. Some developmental patterns have been reported for somatosensory and chemical response measures which suggest potential for assessment (Desmedt and Manil, 1970; Barnet and Lodge, 1966; Barnet et al., 1975).

Thus, both amplitude and latency attributes of various components of evoked responses as well as the overall wave form have been demonstrated to be significantly associated not only with severe mental retardation but with behavioral indicators of minimal developmental dysfunction during the first year of life. These early indications of possible CNS impairment and associated perceptual deficit may or may not be reflected in the immediate growth pattern of the child, but may be precursors of later cognitive impairments including dyslexia and behavioral disturbances such as hyperactivity.

C. Nonsensory Processes

While considerable insight has been gained into the infant's sensory processes, much less is understood about nonsensory central regulating and integrative aspects of information processing and the organization of behavior. Prechtl has suggested that the concept of states be taken beyond descriptive categorization and be seen not as a continuum of arousal but as "finite and discrete vectors representing distinct and qualitatively different conditions, each of them considered as particular modes of nervous activity" (Prechtl, 1974, p. 185). While normal infants tend to have clearly defined state cycles with closely linked physiological parameters, abnormal infants may be more variable and not display this close coupling. For example, Prechtl et al. (1969) have reported that in both apathetic and hyperexcitable babies the normally positive correlation found between respiration and heart rate may become a negative one. The organization of states in the high-risk infant is particularly in need of further investigation as data from normals may have little relevance for their functioning.

The neurologically damaged infant tends to display abnormal sleep states. These are usually characterized by lack of normal periods of the quiet sleep which represents capacity for cortical control and has been suggested by Parmelee et al. (1975) to be neurologically related to visual attention, a capability which has also been found significantly lowered in such infants (Sigman et al., 1973). Early developmental patterns of infants born at-risk for central nervous system damage show some similarities to Goldstein's (1942) findings with brain-injured adults. Important disturbances appear to occur in such central regulating processes as the capacity for appropriate initiation and regulation of behavior, response decrement to repeated stimulation, organization of sleep/wake cycles, activity level, attentional characteristics, and flexibility of adaptation to new experience (Lodge, 1975). The evaluation of habituation to sensory stimulation in normal and abnormal newborns, using both behavioral and electrophysiological methods, appears to hold promise as an early diagnostic technique for assessment of CNS integrity and maturity (Barnet et al., 1971; Brazelton, 1973; Martinius and Papoušek, 1970).

By now the urgent need for bringing together the various approaches to infant assessment to form the basis for a more comprehensive and precise multilevel "developmental diagnosis" is becoming apparent (see chapter by Senf, this volume). Several investigators are beginning to examine the interaction of multiple measures to avoid the danger of being misled by a single category of responses, as Prechtl et al. have cautioned (1969). Leavitt et al. (1973) found a heart rate deceleration or orienting response in six-week-old infants to computer-simulated auditory characteristics of the human voice, while acceleration has generally been obtained to a click. Such information could be compared with a behavioral description of responsiveness to voice, as is afforded by the Brazelton scale, to constitute a multifaceted assessment procedure. The comparison of responses to stimuli varied along a number of dimensions, such as complexity, meaningfulness, or novelty, may be used both diagnostically and to monitor the CNS impact of therapeutic intervention. For example, deficits in linguistic information processing at a cortical level were suggested by the findings of Barnet et al. (1974) that marasmic Mexican infants between the ages of five and 12 months failed to show the normal increased amplitude of the AEP obtained from the left side in response to their own names. Both normal and drug-dependent neonates exhibit a significant positive correlation between the latency of the most prominent positive component of the auditory evoked potential and auditory orienting measured by the Brazelton scale (Lodge et al., 1974). This further supports the value of tapping both behavioral and electrophysiological response systems in order to clarify the mechanisms involved in brain/behavior relationships in infancy.

The increasing range and precision of response measures has generally revealed more complex sensory information processing capabilities than inferred previously on the basis of a more limited behavioral response repertoire. By then increasing the complexity of stimuli utilized along qualitatively different stimulus dimensions and using multiple response measures it becomes possible to assess the organization of response systems in infants and the level at which deficits in information processing may occur.

IV. PREVENTIVE AND THERAPEUTIC INTERVENTION IN INFANCY

A. Basis for Intervention

Because retardation is neither a uniform nor a consistently-defined condition, precise multilevel and continuing diagnosis is a prerequisite to adequate planning for intervention. Such assessment should begin as soon after birth as possible and be carried out at regular intervals during the early years in order to identify the individual child's unique pattern of strengths and vulnerabilities in terms of both rate and adequacy of developmental trends. The knowledge obtained can provide the basis for specific intervention procedures to be initiated during the period of optimal capacity for language learning, perceptual-motor skills, and perceptuo-cognitive development. Intervention may additionally aid in the prevention of secondary emotional and personality disturbances. Blind children, for example, often display a limited repertoire of social communication skills and exploratory and motor delays which can be significantly modified by intervention directed towards normalizing mother-infant interactions and sensorimotor experiences (Fraiberg, 1974).

However, for intervention to be consistently effective it must be individualized to the requirements of each situation. The popularized concept of "stimulation" in itself can be misleading and even dangerous in this regard, and even the notion of a strict "developmental prescription" is over-simplified if misused. Any such recommendations must be based upon overall neurodevelopmental status, and additionally must remain flexible and modifiable in relation to the reactions of the child. For example, physical therapists, who have been pioneers in this field along with occupational therapists and nurses, have long been aware of the possible negative effects of certain exercises and play equipment which in a hypertonic child may increase spasticity and reinforce poor habits such as tiptoeing or teeth-clenching (see Bobath, 1967). It is also important to separate sensory from nonsensory aspects of the infant's problems in order to determine an effective treatment approach. The existence and level of sensory deficit must be determined for each modality. Similarly, the nature of the deficit in central processes must be assessed and appropriate interventions devised. It is possible to encourage age-appropriate stages in concept formation development, such as for object constancy, through teaching simple problem-solving tasks as searching for a hidden toy (e.g., Gordon, 1971). The goals of the activities should be suited to the capabilities of the child and they should be encouraged in a playful, spontaneous manner, so that frustration is minimal and the child experiences the delight and sense of mastery which accompany achievement (see Hunt, this volume). The provision of adult or older child guidance in such educational play is crucial for, while some experience of free creative play is important, too much time alone with complex play materials may lead to repetitiously simple play patterns, prolonged periods of disorganized activity, and wasted learning potential in vulnerable children.

B. Experiments in Intervention

Since Skeels' (1966) dramatic demonstration that provision of more sufficient mothering to institutionalized infants could effectively encourage greater adequacy in intellectual, social, personal, and occupational adjustment, there have been a number of studies concerned with the role of various aspects of caregiving upon infant development. The extensive area of the impact of differing conditions of early rearing and the role of different modes of caregiver-infant interaction is reviewed and evaluated by Beckwith and Hunt elsewhere in this volume. This chapter focuses more on the effects of differential rearing on infants already disadvantaged by either sensory or nonsensory impairments.

An intensive program of language stimulation and reading training with a group of young, severely retarded mongoloids who had been institutionalized from early infancy was carried out by the Special Projects Unit of Sonoma State Hospital (Rhodes et al., 1969a; Bayley et al., 1971). This highly structured program emphasized language-related activities, immediacy and relevance of stimulus materials, and use of a sequenced approach, built-in feedback, and reinforcement. It took place in a unit which provided a somewhat higher level of environmental stimulation than did the usual institutional environment. The children, age six to ten, enjoyed the activities involved and came to be described as happier and more normal in looks and actions than the usual institutionalized Down's children. Before beginning training at age six, the experimental group scored significantly lower in IQ, with a mean of 29, when compared with matched home-reared Down's syndrome controls who had a mean IQ of 45. By age ten, after experiencing the enrichment program, the two groups were approximately equal in IQ and those in the enriched group were able to communicate verbally and read with comprehension at approximately the second grade level. Most of the trained group were subsequently able to function outside the institution in foster family care and attend special education classes in the community. Modification of evoked response characteristics in the trained group was also reported and they showed less deviation from the template of the typical Down's syndrome response (Marcus and Schafer, 1973). The performance of the trained institutionalized Down's syndrome children was compared with that of matched untrained institutionalized Down's syndrome children, and with untrained institutionalized non-Down's syndrome retardates, on a variety of perceptuo-cognitive and learning tasks. The trained children performed

significantly better than the untrained groups on 75% of the
measures. On the Illinois Test of Psycholinguistic Abilities
(ITPA), the trained Down's syndrome children performed significantly better than the other two groups on all but two tasks (auditory reception and object discrimination) (Marcus and Mallory, 1973).

There is evidence that some of the deficits which appear to
be associated with high-risk birth may be modified by caregiving
experience and environmental surroundings. Lewis et al. (1975)
studied a group of infants of adolescent mothers who during their
first two years received regular day-care in a program specially
designed to foster their optimal development. Both normal and high-
risk birth infants were assigned individual ratings of "environmental risk" based upon information obtained concerning the quality
of their home environments and family life. Among the normal-birth
babies, no relationship was found to exist between either mental or
motor development and the risk factor of their home environment.
However, for the high-risk birth infant group a significant correlation was found between mental development, as measured by the
Bayley Scales, and relative degree of freedom from environmental
risk, beginning at the age of 18 months and continuing through two
years of age. No such correlation was found for psychomotor development and environmental risk rating.

Scarr-Salapatek and Williams (1973) have reported the results
of a supplementary program of visual, tactile and kinesthetic stimulation during their first six weeks in the nursery with low birthweight infants (less than 1800 g) born to disadvantaged mothers.
This program, aimed at encouraging sensorimotor development, was
further implemented by weekly home visits to enhance the quality of
maternal care. The stimulated infants showed significantly greater
weight gain and developmental improvement in several areas during
the first four weeks when compared with matched controls. At one
year of age the experimental group maintained their developmental
advantage over controls who had not received home intervention,
with mean developmental quotients averaging ten points higher.
Maternal play stimulation was related to developmental status within
the experimental group.

The developmental impact of a program of vestibular stimulation
upon small prematures with gestational ages between 28 and 32 weeks
was examined in an innovative study by Neal (1968). Beginning on
the fifth day of life, the babies received 30 minutes of supplementary swinging within a small motorized hammock suspended inside
the isolette. When compared with age-matched controls, the experimental infants demonstrated significantly better-developed responses
in motor, auditory, visual, and muscle tension tests, as well as
superior weight gain. At the University of Washington, Barnard
(1973) developed a program of stimulation for premature infants
based on results of a controlled study concerned with provision of

regulated auditory and kinesthetic stimulation to infants at 33
and 34 weeks gestational age as important and appropriate supplements to extrauterine experience. Kinesthetic stimulation was
provided by a rocker bed, while the recording of a heart beat constituted the auditory stimulation. Experimental subjects gained
significantly more weight than controls and received higher estimates of gestational age according to the Dubowitz procedure at a
35-week assessment. Experimental subjects also showed a significantly greater gain in quiet sleep, while controls showed a decline.
Korner et al. (1975) present evidence suggesting that apneic epi-
sodes, which have been implicated in sudden infant death syndrome,
occur with less frequency when infants are provided with stimulation
from a warm oscillating waterbed.

     Casler (1965) and Hasselmeyer (1964) have examined the com-
bined effects of handling and stroking upon infant behavior and
development. Casler (1965) found that short periods of added
tactile stimulation over a ten-week period resulted in significantly higher levels of developmental test performance of institutionalized but otherwise normal infants in a number of areas
(language, adaptive, personal-social) measured by the Gesell
Developmental Schedule when compared with institutionalized controls. Ourth and Brown (1961) found an inverse relationship between
tactile stimulation and crying, while Hopper and Pinneau (1957)
reported lessened regurgitation as a function of added tactile
stimulation. Knudtson (1975) is currently completing a study
designed to examine both short and longer range effects of extra
tactile stimulation upon social aspects of the development of high-
risk premature infants. Preliminary findings appear to suggest
that stroking per se is not associated with increased weight gain,
as has been predominantly found in vestibular stimulation studies,
but that stroking may have at least temporary effects upon social
as well as both gross and fine motor development. Knudtson (1975)
is also examining a physiologic measure not previously investigated
in human infant studies, the amount of hydrocortisol present during
pre- and post-crying sessions as an index of ability to cope with
stress in the stroked as compared with control infants.

C. Planning for Effective Intervention

     While there are genetic and maturational bases for individual
differences in both rate and pattern of behavioral development,
there is accumulating evidence that the high-risk infant may be
unusually susceptible to the impact of surrounding environmental
conditions (e.g., Bayley et al., 1971; Lewis et al., 1975). Within
certain general limits, the environment must make available the
right type of stimulation at the right time for full development of
the nervous system and its learning potential. The rapidly developing sensorimotor repertoire of the young infant constitutes his
primary means of contact, communication, and adjustment to the

world around him. On the receptive or input side, he is dependent
upon his sensory apparatus to transmit impinging stimulation.
These afferent signals are of primary importance both in stimulating the development and organization of his cortical activity and
in the initiation and guidance of motor responses. Any condition
or process which interrupts the reciprocal interaction of this
continuous learning sequence, such as congenital deafness, blindness, or loss of a limb, prevents or distorts the sensory and motor
feedback necessary to appropriate learning. Early intervention to
restore or initiate such feedback and to bring them into the fullest
possible contact with their environment is required to maximize the
developmental potential of such infants. If partial or complete
correction of the condition is impossible, early provision of alternative modes of stimulus reception or motor responding (e.g. by
means of hearing aids, corrective lenses, or prosthetic or sensory-
substitution devices) is desirable.

Excellent programs for dealing with the more obvious sensorimotor handicaps, such as are involved in cerebral palsy, are frequently available in infancy in this country. However, it is with
regard to the more elusive deficits involving perceptuocognitive
function and central integrative attentional and organizational
processes, which usually only gradually become apparent, that an
appropriate therapeutic environment has rarely been made available
and that years of remediation may be necessary.

Improvement appears to be vitally needed in several areas to
facilitate the delivery of more comprehensive and continuous health
care, including programs designed to prevent early developmental
disabilities. First, greater emphasis should be placed upon education at basic training levels, for physicians and other health professionals, concerning the impact of early environment upon infant
and child development. There is also need for a developmentally-
oriented restructuring of the priorities involved in infant care
practices in institutions entrusted with the care and upbringing
of infants. The education-oriented day-care movement which has
become widespread in recent years has much to offer in terms of
methods which can be adapted for use in such infant programs.

More community facilities are needed to provide a variety of
supportive services for families with high-risk infants, including
family counseling, infant education centers, home-based tutoring
and parent groups and educational programs. The establishment of
follow-up clinics and other longitudinal programs for the provision
of continuous care, both during the course of pregnancy and throughout the early formative years, appears desirable. Perhaps the function of existing community and regional centers could be expanded
to provide a framework for effective coordination of the preventive
efforts of physicians, psychologists, public health nurses, and
infant education specialists and their respective agencies.

There are indications of the evolution of an interdisciplinary professional specialty of infant and child development within the fields of psychology and medicine, and the parallel development of subspecialties within nursing, occupational and physical therapy, and teaching may be a natural outgrowth of this trend. Support for longitudinal interdisciplinary research directed towards refinement of diagnostic procedures and exploration of intervention techniques continues to be essential. Some of the more traditionally academic and research oriented approaches, such as experimental psychology and psychophysiology, might be brought into more clinical settings to encourage a more unified endeavor in this area.

A number of unanswered questions remain, both theoretical and practical, concerning environmental modification as an instrument for prevention and therapy in infant brain dysfunction. For example, methodological difficulties arise in the adaptation of experimental procedures to real life situations. There is also the problem of evaluating the long-range effectiveness of early intervention. However, as early neurodevelopmental status becomes increasingly well established as a basic concern within the overall context of the treatment resources available to high-risk infants and their families, prospects hopefully will improve for accomplishment of both the requisite research and the practical implementation of an effective preventive approach.

REFERENCES

Awaya, S., Miyake, Y., Imaizumi, Y., Shiose, Y., Kanda, T., and Komuro, K. 1973. Amblyopia in Man Suggestive of Stimulus Deprivation Amblyopia. Jap. J. Ophthalmol. 17:69-82.

Barnard, K. 1973. A Program of Stimulation for Infants Born Prematurely. (Mimeographed.)

Barnet, A.B., and Lodge, A. 1966. Diagnosis of Deafness in Infants with Use of Computer-Averaged Electroencephalographic Responses to Sound. J. Pediat. 69:753-758.

Barnet, A.B., and Lodge, A. 1967. Click Evoked EEG Responses in Normal and Developmentally Retarded Infants. Nature 214:252-255.

Barnet, A.B., Lodge, A., and Armington, J.C. 1965. Electroretinograms in Newborn Human Infants. Science 148:651-654.

Barnet, A.B., Ohlrich, E.S., and Shanks, B.L. 1971. EEG Evoked Responses to Repetitive Auditory Stimulation in Normal and Down's Syndrome Infants. Develop. Med. Child Neurol. 13:321-329.

Barnet, A.B., Vicentini de Sotillo, M., and Campos S.M. 1974. EEG
    Sensory Evoked Potentials in Early Infancy Malnutrition. Paper
    presented at Society for Neuroscience, October, St. Louis,
    Missouri.

Barnet, A.B., Ohlrich, E.S., Weiss, I.P., and Shanks, B. 1975.
    Auditory Evoked Potentials During Sleep in Normal Children
    From Ten Days to Three Years of Age. Paper presented at the
    Biennial Meeting of the Society for Research in Child Develop-
    ment, April, Denver, Colorado.

Barnett, C.R., Leiderman, P.H., Grobstein, R., and Klaus, M. 1970.
    Neonatal Separation: The Maternal Side of Interactional
    Deprivation. Pediatrics 45:197-204.

Baum, J.D., and Searls, D. 1971. Head Shape and Size of Newborn
    Infants. Develop. Med. Child Neurol. 13:572-581.

Bayley, N. 1965. Comparisons of Mental and Motor Test Scores for
    Ages 1-15 Months by Sex, Birth Order, Race, Geographical
    Location, and Education of Parents. Child Develop. 36:379-411.

Bayley, N. 1969. Manual for the Bayley Scales of Infant Develop-
    ment. The Psychological Corporation, New York.

Bayley, N. Rhodes, L., Gooch, B., and Marcus, N. 1971. Environ-
    mental Factors in the Development of Institutionalized Child-
    ren, pp. 450-472. In J. Hellmuth (ed.). Exceptional Infant:
    Studies in Abnormalities, Vol. 2. Brunner/Mazel, New York.

Bobath, B. 1967. Very Early Treatment of Cerebral Palsy. Develop.
    Med. Child Neurol. 9:373-390.

Bogen, J.E., and Bogen, G.M. 1969. The Other Side of the Brain:
    III. The Corpus Callosum and Creativity. Bull. Los Angeles
    Neurol Soc. 34:191-220.

Bowes, W., Jr., Brackbill, Y., Conway, E., and Steinschneiden, A.
    1970. The Effects of Obstetrical Medication on Fetus and
    Infant. Monogr. Soc. Res. Child Develop. 35(4), Serial No.
    137.

Brazelton, T.B. 1970. Effect of Prenatal Drugs on the Behavior
    of the Neonate. Amer. J. Psychiat. 126:1262-1266.

Brazelton, T.B. 1973. Neonatal Behavioral Assessment Scale.
    Clinics in Developmental Medicine, No. 50. Spastics Inter-
    national Medical Publications. J.B. Lippincott Co.,
    Philadelphia.

Brazelton, T.B., Robey, J.S., and Collier, G.A. 1969. Infant Development in the Zinacanteco Indians of Southern Mexico. Pediatrics 44:274-293.

Broussard, E.R., and Hartner, M.S.S. 1970. Maternal Perception of the Neonate as Related to Development. Child Psychiat. Hum. Develop. 1:16-25.

Bruner, J. 1967. Eye, Hand and Mind. Paper presented at the Meetings of the Society for Research in Child Development. (Mimeographed.)

Budin, P. 1907. The Nurseling. Caxton Publishing Co., London.

Butler, L.J. 1972. Antenatal Detection of Chromosomal and Metabolic Abnormalities, pp. K.S. Holt (eds.). Mental Retardation: Prenatal Diagnosis and Infant Assessment (Symposia 6 and 8). Butterworth & Co., Ltd., London.

Butler, B.V., and Engel, R. 1969. Mental and Motor Scores at 8 Months in Relation to Neonatal Photic Response. Develop. Med. Child Neurol. 11:77-82.

Casler, L. 1965. The Effects of Extratactile Stimulation of a Group of Institutionalized Infants. Genet. Psychol. Monogr. 71:137-175.

Cattell, P. 1947. The Measurement of Intelligence in Infants and Young Children. The Psychological Corporation, New York.

Culliton, B.J. 1975. Intensive Care for Newborns: Are There Times to Pull the Plug? Science 188:133-134.

Desmedt, J.E., and Manil, J. 1970. Somatosensory Evoked Potentials of the Human Neonate in REM Sleep, in Slow Wave Sleep and in Waking. Electroenceph. Clin. Neurophysiol. 29:113-126.

Dreyfus-Brisac, C. 1964. The EEG of the Premature Infant and the Full-Term Newborn, pp. 186-207. In P. Kellaway and I. Peterson (eds.). Neurological and EEG Correlative Studies in Infancy. Grune and Stratton, New York.

Dreyfus-Brisac, C. 1970. Ontogenesis of Sleep in the Human Premature after 32 Weeks of Conceptional Age. Develop. Psychobiol. 3:91-121.

Dreyfus-Brisac, C. 1974. Organization of Sleep in Prematures: Implications for Caregiving, pp. 123-140. In M. Lewis and

A. Rosenblum (eds.). The Effect of the Infant on Its Caregiver. Wiley, New York.

Drillien, C.M. 1964. The Growth and Development of the Prematurely
Born Infant. William and Wilkins, Baltimore.

Drillien, C.M. 1965. The Effect of Obstetrical Hazard on the Later
Development of the Child, pp. 82-109. In D. Gairdner (ed.).
Recent Advances in Paediatrics (3rd Ed.). Little, Brown, Boston.

Dudgeon, J.A. 1968. Breakdown in Maternal Protection: Infections.
Proc. Roy. Soc. Med. 61:1236-1243.

DuHamel, T.R., Liu, S., Skelton, A., and Hantke, C. 1974. Early
Parental Perceptions and the High Risk Neonate: Preliminary
Results of an Early Parent Education Program. Clin. Pediatrics
13: 1052-1056.

Eisenberg, R.B. 1970. The Organization of Auditory Behavior.
J. Speech and Hearing Res. 13:461-464.

Ellingson, R.J. 1964. Cerebral Electrical Responses to Auditory
and Visual Stimuli in the Infant (Human and Subhuman Studies),
pp. 78-116. In P. Kellaway and I. Petersen (eds.). Neurological and Correlative Studies in Infancy. Grune and
Stratton, New York.

Ellingson, R.J., Danahy, T., Bessmark, N., and Lathrop, G.L. 1974.
Variability of Auditory Evoked Potentials in Human Newborns.
EEG Clin. Neurophysiol. 36:155-162.

Engel, R., and Benson, R. 1968. Estimate of Conceptional Age by
Evoked Response Activity. Biol. Neonat. (Basel) 12:201-213.

Engel, R., and Butler, B.V. 1963. Appraisal of Conceptual Age of
Newborn Infants by Electroencephalographic Methods. J.
Pediat. 63:386-393.

Entus, A.K. 1975. Hemispheric Asymmetry in Processing of Dichotically Presented Speech and Nonspeech Sounds by Infants. Paper presented Soc. Res. Child. Devel., April, Denver, Colorado.

Fabro, S. 1973. Passage of Drugs and Other Chemicals into the Ute-
rine Fluids and Preimplantation Blastocyst, pp. 443-461. In
L. Boréus (ed.). Fetal Pharmacology. Raven Press, New York.

Fanaroff, A.A., Kennell, J.H., and Klaus, M.H. 1972. Follow-Up of
Low Birthweight Infants - The Predictive Value of Maternal
Visiting Patterns. J. Pediat. 71:287-290.

Fantz, R.L. 1958. Pattern Vision in Young Infants. Psychol. Rec.
8:43-47.

Fantz, R.L. 1963. Pattern Vision in Newborn Infants. Science 140: 296-297.

Fantz, R.L., and Nevis, S. 1967. The Predictive Value of Changes in Visual Preferences in Early Infancy, pp. 349-413. J. Hellmuth (ed.). Exceptional Infant. The Normal Infant, Vol. 1. Special Child Publications, Seattle, Washington.

Forfar, J. 1973. Symposium on Drugs and the Unborn Child, sponsored by the National Foundation-March of Dimes, March, 1973. Reported in J.L. Marx. Drugs During Pregnancy: Do They Affect the Unborn Child? Science 180:174-175.

Fraiberg, S. 1974. Blind Infants and Their Mothers: An Examination of the Sign System, pp. 215-232. In M. Lewis and A. Rosenblum (eds.). The Effect of the Infant on Its Caregiver. Wiley, New York.

Freedman, D.G., and Freedman, N. 1969. Behavioral Differences Between Chinese-American and European-American Newborns. Nature 224:1227.

Gardiner, M.F., and Walter, D.O. 1973. Evidence of Hemispheric Specialization from Infant EEG. In R. Fischer (ed.). Proceedings of the Conference on Hemispheric Specialization, Fall, Montreal, Canada. (in press).

Gesell, A., and Amatruda, C.S. 1945. The Embryology of Behavior: The Beginnings of the Human Mind. Harper and Brothers, New York.

Goldstein, K. 1942. Aftereffects of Brain Injuries in War. Grune and Stratton, New York.

Gordon, I.J. 1971. Baby Learning Through Baby Play. St. Martin's Press, New York.

Haith, M.M., Collins, D., and Kessen, W. 1969. Response of the Human Infant to Level of Complexity of Intermittent Visual Movement. J. Exp. Child Psychol. 7:52-69.

Hasselmeyer, E. 1964. The Premature Neonate's Response to Handling, pp. 15-22. In Conventional Clinical Session, Expanding Horizons in Knowledge: Implications for Nursing, II. ANA, Atlantic City, New Jersey.

Hecox, K., and Galambos, R. 1974. Brain Stem Auditory Evoked Responses in Human Infants. Arch. Otolaryngol. 99:30-33.

Hershenson, M. 1967. Development of the Perception of Form.

Psychol. Bull. 67:326-336.

Hopper, H.E., and Pinneau, S.R. 1957. Frequency of Regurgitation
in Infancy as Related to the Amount of Stimulation Received
from the Mother. Child Develop. 28:229-235.

Hrbek, A., and Mareš, P. 1964. Cortical and Premature Newborns.
EEG Clin. Neurophysiol. 16:575-581.

Hubel, D.H., and Wiesel, T.N. 1963. Single-Cell Responses in
Striate Cortex of Kittens Deprived of Vision in One Eye. J.
Neurophysiol. 26:1003-1017.

Hutchings, D.E., and Gibbon, J. 1971. Effects of Vitamin A Excess
Administered in Late Pregnancy on Discrimination Learning in
Offspring. Proceedings, 79th Annual Convention, American
Psychological Association 6:211-212.

Jewett, D.L., Romano, M.N., and Williston, J.S. 1970. Human
Auditory Evoked Potentials: Possible Brain Stem Components
Detected on the Scalp. Science 167:1517-1518.

Jones, K. 1974. Outcome of Pregnancy in the Chronic Alcoholic: The
Fetal Alcohol Syndrome. Paper presented at NIDA/Vanderbilt
Perinatal Addiction Research Conf., Sept., Nashville, Tenn.
Addictive Diseases: An International Journal. (in press).

Kagan, J., and Klein, R.E. 1973. Cross-Cultural Perspectives on
Early Development. Amer. Psychologist 28:947-961.

Kaplan, D.M., and Mason, E.A. 1960. Maternal Reactions to Premature Birth Viewed as an Acute Emotional Disorder. Amer. J.
Orthopsych. 30:539-552.

Klaus, M.H., and Fanaroff, A.A. 1973. Care of the High Risk Neonate. W. B. Saunders, Philadelphia.

Knobloch, H., and Pasamanick, B. 1960. Environmental Factors
Affecting Human Development, Before and After Birth.
Pediatrics 26:210-218.

Knobloch, H., and Pasamanick, B. (eds.). 1974. Gesell and Amatruda's
Developmental Diagnosis: The Evaluation and Management of
Normal and Abnormal Neuropsychologic Development in Infancy and
Early Childhood (3rd. ed.) Harper and Row, Hagerstown, Mary-
land.

Knudtson, F. 1975. Effect of Extra Tactile Stimulation on Physical
and Psychological Development in High Risk Premature Infants.
(Mimeographed.)

Korner, A.F., Kraemer, H.C., Haffner, M.E., and Cosper, L.M. 1975.
Effects of Waterbed Flotation on Premature Infants: A Pilot
Study. Pediatrics 56(3):361-367.

Kron, R.E. 1966. Instrumental Conditioning of Nutritive Sucking
Behavior in the Newborn. Rec. Adv. in Biol. Psychiatry 9:
295-300.

Kron, R.E., Litt, M., and Finnegan, L.P. 1973. Behavior of Infants
Born to Narcotic-Addicted Mothers. Pediatric Res. 7:292.

League, R., Parker, J., Robertson, M., Valentine, V., and Powell,
J. 1972. Acoustical Environments in Incubators and Infant
Oxygen Tents. Preventive Med. 1:231-239.

Leavitt, L.A., Morse, P.A., Brown, J.W., and Graham, F.K. 1973.
Cardiac Orienting of Six-Week-Old Infants to Speech and Non-
Speech Stimuli. Pediatric Res. 7(4):419.

Leboyer, F. 1975. Birth Without Violence. Alfred A. Knopf, New
York.

Lewis, J., Latzko, T., Kleinfeld, P., Lyman, P., and Lodge, A. 1975.
Family Developmental Center: A Demonstration Project. Final
report to the Office of Human Development, Department of Health,
Education, Welfare, June. (Grant No. OCD-CB-17).

Lewis, M., and McGurk, H. 1972. Evaluation of Infant Intelligence.
Science 178:1174-1177.

Lipsitt, L.P., and Kaye, H. 1964. Conditioned Sucking in the Human
Newborn. Psychonom. Sci. 1:29-30.

Lodge, A. 1968. Environmental and Biological Aspects of Developmental Retardation in Infancy. Presented at the Round Table
on Social Aspects of Mental Retardation, 12th International
Congress of Pediatrics, December, Mexico City.

Lodge, A. 1973. Innovations in the Assessment of Infant Behavior.
Presented at the symposium on "Innovations in the Electrophysiological and Behavioral Assessment of Mental Retardation",
53rd Annual Convention of the Western Psychological Association,
April, Anaheim, California.

Lodge, A. 1975. Early Developmental Patterns Associated with High
Risk Birth Conditions. Paper presented at First European
Neurosciences Meeting, September, Munich, Germany.

Lodge, A., and Kleinfeld, P.B. 1973. Early Behavioral Development in Down's Syndrome, pp. 61–86. In M. Coleman (ed.). Serotonin in Down's Syndrome. North-Holland Publishers, Amsterdam.

Lodge, A., Armington, J.C., Barnet, A.B., Shanks, B.L., and Newcomb, C. 1969. Newborn Infants' Electroretinograms and Evoked Electroencephalographic Responses to Orange and White Light. Child Develop. 40:267-293.

Lodge, A., Huntington, D.S., Robinson, M.E., and Lewis, J. 1970. Enhancing the Development of Institutionalized Infants. Medical Annals of the District of Columbia 39:628-631.

Lodge, A., Marcus, M.M., and Ramer, C.M. 1975. Neonatal Addiction: A Two-Year Study.: II. Behavioral and Electrophysiological Characteristics of the Addicted Neonate. Addictive Diseases: An International Journal 2(2):235-255.

Lourie, R.S. 1971. The First Three Years of Life: An Overview of a New Frontier of Psychiatry. Amer. J. Psychiat. 127:1457-1463.

Marcus, M.M. 1971. Developmental Change and Age Related Wave Forms in the Visual Evoked Response. Psychophysiol. 8:271.

Marcus, M.M. 1976. VEP's to Flash and Pattern in Normal and High Risk Infants. In J.E. Desmedt (ed.). Evoked Potentials in Man. Oxford University Press, London. (in press).

Marcus, M.M., and Mallory, W.A. 1973. The Development of Learning Tasks for the Assessment of the Mentally Retarded. Presented at the symposium on "Innovations in the Electrophysiological and Behavioral Assessment of Mental Retardation," 53rd Annual Convention of the Western Psychological Association, April, Anaheim, California.

Marcus, M.M., and Schafer, E.W.P. 1973. Evoked Response as a Measure of Development. Presented at the symposium on "Innovations in the Electrophysiological and Behavioral Assessment of Mental Retardation", 53rd Annual Convention of the Western Psychological Association, April, Anaheim, California.

Martinius, J.W., and Papoušek, H. 1970. Responses to Optic and Exteroceptive Stimuli in Relation to State in the Human Newborn: Habituation of the Blink Reflex. Neuropädiatrie 1:452-460.

Molfese, D.L. 1975. The Ontogeny of Cerebral Asymmetry in Man:

Auditory Evoked Potentials to Linguistic and Non-Linguistic Stimuli. Paper presented at the International Symposium on Cerebral Evoked Potentials in Man, April, Brussels. In J.E. Desmedt (ed.). Evoked Potentials in Man. Oxford University Press, London. (in press).

Neal, M. 1968. Vestibular Stimulation and Developmental Behavior of the Small Premature Infant, pp. 1-5. In Nursing Research Report, Vol. 3. American Nurses' Foundation, New York.

Ourth, L., and Brown, K.B. 1961. Inadequate Mothering and Disturbance in the Neonatal Period. Child Develop. 32:287-295.

Oster, H.S. 1975. Color Perception in Ten-Week-Old Infants. Paper presented at the Biennial Meeting of the Society for Research in Child Development, April, Denver, Colorado.

Papoušek, H. 1959. A Method of Studying Conditioned Food Reflexes in Young Children up to the Age of Six Months. Zhurnal Vysshei Nervnoi Deiatelnosti 9:136-140.

Papoušek, H. 1965. The Development of Higher Nervous Activity in Children in the First Half-Year of Life, pp. 102-111. In P.H. Mussen (ed.). European Research in Cognitive Development: Report of the International Conference on Cognitive Development. Monogr. Soc. Res. Child Develop., Vol. 30(2),Serial No. 100.

Papoušek, H., and Papoušek, M. 1975. Concepts and Methods Underlying Our Approach to Social Interactions of Human Infants. Loch Lomond Symposium, University of Strathclyde, September, Scotland.

Parmelee, A.H., Bruck, K., and Bruck, M. 1962. Activity and Inactivity Cycles During the Sleep of Premature Infants Exposed to Neutral Temperatures. Biol. Neonat. 4: 317-339.

Parmelee, A.H., Sigman, M., Kopp, C.B., and Haber, A. 1974. The Concept of a Cumulative Risk Score for Infants. Paper presented at the Symposia on Aberrant Development in Infancy, March, Gatlinberg, Tennessee. In N.R. Ellis (ed.). Aberrant Development in Infancy: Human and Animal Studies. (in press).

Parmelee, A.H., Kopp, C.B., and Sigman, M. 1975. Selection of Developmental Assessment Techniques for Infants at Risk. Paper presented at the Merrill-Palmer Institute Conference on Research and Teaching of Infant Development, February, Detroit, Michigan.

Piaget, J. 1952. The Origins of Intelligence in Children. M. Cook

(Transl.). International Universities Press, New York.

Prechtl, H.F. 1968. Neurological Findings in Newborn Infants After
    Pre- and Paranatal Complications, pp. 303-321. In J.H.P.
    Jonxis, H.K.A. Visser, and J.A. Troelstra (eds.). Aspects of
    Praematurity and Dysmaturity. H.E. Stenfert Kroese N.V., Leiden.

Prechtl, H.F. 1974. The Behavioural States of the Newborn Infant
    (A Review). Brain Res. 76:185-212.

Prechtl, H., and Beintema, D. 1964. The Neurological Examination
    of the Full Term Newborn Infant. Clinics in Developmental
    Medicine No. 12. Spastics International Medical Publications.
    J.B. Lippencott Co., Philadelphia.

Prechtl, H.F., Weinmann, H., and Akiyama, Y. 1969. Organization of
    Physiological Parameters in Normal and Neurologically Abnormal
    Infants. Neuropädiatrie 1:101-128.

Prescott, J.W. 1971. Early Somatosensory Deprivation as an Onto-
    genetic Process in the Abnormal Development of the Brain and
    Behavior, pp. 1-20. In I.E. Goldsmith and J. Moor-Jankowski
    (eds.). Medical Primatology. S. Karger, Basel, New York.

Rank, O. 1929. The Trauma of Birth. Harcourt, Brace and Co., New
    York, and Routledge and Kegan Paul, Ltd., London.

Rapin, I., and Graziani, L. 1967. Auditory-Evoked Responses in
    Normal, Brain-Damaged and Deaf Infants. Neurology 17:881-
    894.

Rhodes, L., Gooch, B., Siegelman, E.Y., Behrns, C.A., and Metzger,
    R. 1969a. A Language Stimulation and Reading Program for
    Severely Retarded Mongoloid Children: A Descriptive Report.
    California Mental Health Research Monograph No. 11, California
    Department of Mental Hygiene.

Rhodes, L.E., Dustman, R.E., and Beck, E.C. 1969b. Visually Evoked
    Potentials of Bright and Dull Children. EEG Clin. Neuro-
    physiol. 27:364-372.

Richardson, S.A., Birch, H.G., and Hertzig, M.E. 1973. School
    Performance of Children Who Were Severely Malnourished in
    Infancy. Amer. J. Ment. Defic. 77:623-632.

Rogers, M.G.H. 1968. Risk Registers and Early Detection of Handi-
    caps. Develop. Med. Child Neurol. 10:651-661.

Sander, L.W., Julia, H.L., Stechler, G., and Burns, P. 1972. Con-
    tinuous 24 Hour Interactional Monitoring in Infants Reared in

Two Caretaking Environments. Psychosom. Med. 3:170-282.

Scarr-Salapatek, S., and Williams, M.L. 1973. The Effects of Early Stimulation on Low-Birthweight Infants. Child Develop. 44:94-101.

Schulman, C.A. 1969. Alterations of the Sleep Cycle in Heroin-Addicted and "Suspect" Newborns. Neuropädiatrie 1:89-100.

Selye, H. 1956. The Stress of Life. McGraw-Hill Book Co., New York.

Sigman, M., Kopp, C.B., Parmelee, A.H., and Jeffrey, W.E. 1973. Visual Attention and Neurological Organization in Neonates. Child Develop. 44:461-466.

Siqueland, E.R., and Lipsitt, L.P. 1966. Conditioned Head-Turning in Human Newborns. J. Exper. Child Psychol. 3:356-376.

Skeels, H.M. 1966. Adult Status of Children with Contrasting Early Life Experiences: A Follow-up Study. Monogr. Soc. Res. Child Develop., Vol. 31(3), Whole No. 105.

Soule, B., Standley, K., Copans, S., and Davis, M. 1973. Clinical Implications of the Brazelton Scale. Paper presented at the Annual Meeting of the Society for Research in Child Development, March, Philadelphia, Pennsylvania.

Stechler, G. 1964. Newborn Attention as Affected by Medication During Labor. Science 144:315-317.

Steinmann, M. 1975. The Baby-Savers. The New York Times Magazine, May 11, pp. 68-72.

Stern, L. 1973. Critical Comments, pp. 41. In M.H. Klaus and A.A. Fanaroff (eds.). Care of the High Risk Neonate. W.B. Saunders, Philadelphia.

Stone, L.J., Smith, H.T., and Murphy, L.B. 1973. The Competent Infant; Research and Commentary. Basic Books, New York.

Terman, L.M., and Merrill, M.A. 1960. Stanford-Binet Intelligence Scale; Manual for the Third Revision, Form L-M. Houghton Mifflin Co., Boston.

Theorell, K., Prechtl, H.F.R., Blair, A.W., and Lind, J. 1973. Behavioural State Cycles of Normal Newborn Infants: A Comparison of the Effect of Early and Late Cord Clamping. Develop. Med. Child Neurol. 15:597-605.

Tronick, E., Koslowski, B., and Brazelton, T.B. 1973. Neonatal Behavior Among Urban Zambians and Americans. (in press).

Von Noorden, G.K., Dowling, J.E., and Ferguson, D.C. 1970. Experimental Amblyopia in Monkeys: I. Behavioral Studies of Stimulus Deprivation Amblyopia. Arch. Ophthalmol. 84:206-214.

Watanabe, K., Iwase, K., and Hara, K. 1972. Maturation of Visual Evoked Responses in Low-Birthweight Infants. Develop. Med. Child Neurol. 14:425-435.

Weiffenbach, J.M. 1972. Discrete Elicited Motions of the Newborn's Tongue, pp. 347-361. In F. Bosma (ed.). Third Symposium on Oral Sensation and Perception. Charles C. Thomas, Springfield, Illinois.

Weitzman, E.D., and Graziani, L.J. 1968. Maturation and Topography of the Auditory Evoked Response of the Prematurely Born Infant. Develop. Psychobiol. 1:79-89.

Wilson, J.G. 1973. Environment and Birth Defects. Academic Press, New York.

Yarrow, L.J., Rubenstein, J.L., Pedersen, F.A., and Jankowski, J.J. 1971. Dimensions of Early Stimulation: Differential Effects on Infant Development. Paper presented at the Biennial Meeting of the Society for Research in Child Development, April, Minneapolis, Minnesota. Condensed in Merr. Palm. Quart. 18: 205-218, 1972.

Zelson, C., Rubio, E., and Wasserman, E. 1971. Neonatal Narcotic Addiction: Ten Year Observation. Pediatrics 48:178-189.

SOME METHODOLOGICAL CONSIDERATIONS IN THE

STUDY OF ABNORMAL CONDITIONS[1]

Gerald M. Senf

Department of Psychology
University of Illinois
Chicago Circle
Chicago, Illinois 60680

This chapter deals with two aspects of concern in the study of abnormal populations: (1) sample definition and selection, and (2) the assessment of outcome following intervention. The issues discussed are broader than those contained in most of the other chapters which tend to be more substantive in nature. Rather, procedural considerations and research strategy relevant to the study and evaluation of intervention outcomes with abnormal developmental conditions are examined. The focus is primarily on studies with humans, although many of the points made are equally applicable to the study of infrahuman organisms. While I have chosen the childhood malnutrition syndrome discussed by Richardson as my primary example, the comments apply equally to other developmental disorders described in this volume.

I. THE SAMPLE-DIFFERENCE PARADIGM

The basic research paradigm generally adopted for the study of populations exhibiting deviant behavior or deviant developmental characteristics involves the isolation of a target sample which is then compared with a control group selected to illustrate the differential effect of an independent variable or variables upon the organisms' behavioral repertoire. A number of problems attend what I have termed elsewhere this sample-difference approach (Senf, 1975a). The most basic problem is the essentially correlational nature of the sample-difference approach. In utilizing groups that are intact prior to the study, and are constituted by virtue of their abnormal condition, the resulting comparison between the abnormal sample's performance and that of a control group is essentially associational. Rather than assessing the association

of characteristics of the abnormal and normal subjects together
between a predictor variable (or variables) and one or more criterion (dependent) variables, the researcher opts to assign subjects
to abnormal and normal groups and utilize group membership as a
predictor of the dependent variable(s) under study. Though the
structure of this sample-difference approach superficially resembles
more closely designs where the independent variable is manipulated
by the experimenter, the paradigm has no greater interpretive power
over its correlational design counterpart. In fact, by grouping
subjects into two or more groups designated as abnormal or normal,
individual variation within groups which might lawfully relate to
the criterion variables is lost to error variance. Furthermore,
the statistic typically adopted to assess the significance of a
hypothesis such as the $\underline{t}$ or $\underline{F}$ or $\underline{X}^2$ provides only a statement of
the reliability of the finding and not the amount of variance
accounted for by the predictor variable (in this case group membership). Although additional statistical procedures are available to
assess percent of variance accounted for, they are seldom calculated
or reported.

While reasons for adopting the sample-difference approach rather
than a correlational design are many and varied, the central substantive consideration involves the degree to which the character-
istic(s) defining the abnormal group can be scaled. Some group
membership variables such as birthweight are readily scaled and,
hence, amenable to correlational designs, while others such as the
degree of cultural deprivation, minimal brain dysfunction, malnutrition, and the like, are psychometrically difficult to measure.
Research on complex clinical conditions such as these and emotional
disturbance, autism, learning disabilities, and so forth present
even more complex scaling problems such that the sample-difference
approach is preferred to the correlational design.

While studies with infrahuman organisms can typically create
abnormal groups through intervention after random assignment of
subjects to conditions, the intact nature of abnormal human samples
creates the obvious problem that one's criterion variable differences may equally well be accounted for by alternative hypotheses
regarding some other aspect of the pre-existing condition. A
plethora of riches is frequently the result whereby nearly all comparisons between abnormal and normal samples are statistically significant. Minor increments in knowledge result, characterized by
the typical conclusion that the abnormal group performs less well
than the normal control. The fact that the abnormality under study
can frequently not be scaled along a single dimension creates a
need for the sample-difference approach despite its limitations.
The next section of this chapter deals with the issues underlying
sample definition and selection from a number of perspectives:
methodological, theoretical, utilitarian, and philosophical.

II. SAMPLE DEFINITION AND SELECTION

The fact that the sample-difference approach yields essentially correlational information has implications for sample definition and subsequent sample selection within human studies not generally applicable to animal work.

A. Methodological Considerations

1. Sample Comparability. The most basic implication involves the comparability of samples studied by one researcher from time to time and by different researchers at different places and times (Senf, 1975a,b). Though it is obvious that one cannot reconcile an inequivalent result when the subjects under consideration are de-fined and selected differently, it is more often the case than not that samples from study to study are, in fact, defined and selected according to highly disparate procedures. This same problem exists with animal studies where different outcomes are sometimes traceable to different strains of rats in the conflicting experiments (see Greenough et al., this volume) or some variant in the experimental procedure which is sometimes decipherable in the methods section and substantiable through subsequent experiments (see also Walsh and Cummins, 1975). However, these problems are relatively small and generally reconcilable compared to those faced by researchers examining abnormality in human populations.

2. Generalization of Findings. The problems of sample com-parability involve, but are not limited to, the difficulties in scaling the abnormal condition under study as discussed above. The representativeness of one's sample to a broader population needs to be considered as does the construct validity of the assessment pro-cedures used to constitute the abnormal group. The question of sample representativeness and resulting generalizability of findings is a basic issue often overlooked because of the difficulty and expense in obtaining samples whose parent population is known or can be inferred. This and other questions of the utility of results from studies of abnormal subjects are considered below. The pro-cedures of subject selection and their attendant construct validity need further examination.

3. Construct Validity. Typically, an investigator is con-cerned with a rather circumscribed aspect of abnormality such as malnutrition, some facet of emotional disturbance, an aspect of school failure, and so forth. There appears to be a concomitant predominant tendency for the investigator to adopt an operational definition of the subject sample which is both economically feas-ible and convenient (e.g., hospitalization, birthweight below some level). Heavily studied areas of abnormality have evolved measures that meet these requirements, such as the utilization of Conners' scale for hyperactivity among young school-aged children or the

utilization of the 4-9 MMPI profile to operationally define psycho-
pathic deviates. Less researched samples such as the malnourished
have no universally accepted operational definition and, hence,
make comparability from study to study a perplexing undertaking.
In addition, maintaining construct validity across wide age ranges
presents a problem often as psychometrically difficult as that faced
by comparative psychologists. Even when dealing with such basic
variables as birthweight, one must question whether a 1500 g infant
born of a rural Mexican family presents the same degree of "risk" as
does the 1500 g child born of a Caucasian family living in an urban
setting. (Beckwith, this volume, notes the interactions that exist
between birthweight and caretakers' behavior, for example.) This
example represents the most basic of construct validity questions in
scaling the abnormality under question. To utilize the birthweight
example, we are obviously interested more in the etiological causa-
tion and resulting prognosis than in birthweight per se, birthweight
being a convenient index of the degree of prematurity, malnutrition,
etc. We must, however, be extremely careful to assure that the
selection variable eventually to be used as a predictor, whether
through grouping subjects into a category or utilizing the measurement as a variable, is equally appropriate for all subjects in the
study. So it is similarly the case with a subject's record of hospitalization: Many factors impinge on whether a child is or is not
hospitalized for a malnourished condition aside from the malnourishment per se, namely, the facilities available to the parents, their
social knowledge, the parents' attentiveness to the child's condition, and so forth. It is not enough simply to recognize that
the index of abnormality used to define a group of subjects for use
as a predictor variable is a less than perfect measure of the underlying construct which one wishes the group to represent. Because of
the correlational nature of the experimental paradigm, one must be
very certain that factors extraneous to the index of abnormality
are not adding variance that will be wrongly supportive of the hypothesis under question.

     4. Predicted Variance. This concern is especially important
if one wishes to know how much of the variance of the criterion
variable membership in an "abnormal group" accounts for. Finding
differences between subject samples defined by characteristics which
place the abnormal group at "high risk" for poor performance on a
wide range of tasks provides little specific understanding of the
condition under study. Knowledge will accumulate slowly unless the
researcher is very careful to exclude in the selection procedure or
through control groups other factors which might equally well
account for inadequate performance relative to one's "normal" comparison group.

     The construct validity problem in defining abnormal samples
is immensely complicated when univariate dimensions are not available to define the subject sample, such as in conditions of

emotional disturbance, severe learning problems (c.f., Senf, 1973), and the like. In these cases, the reliability of the class principles (Zigler and Phillips, 1962) defining the abnormal condition must be sufficiently well specified, assessed, and reported such that other investigators can be confident that any differences in their results cannot be accounted for by differences in their subject sample. Otherwise, the research endeavor cannot begin to accumulate a knowledge base.

When research is oriented toward isolating significant differences between samples of abnormal and normal functioning individuals on some set of class principles (some definition of abnormality), the key question in my mind is not whether or not a significant difference exists. Rather the question is what percent of the variance in the criterion performance does the group membership or score on the abnormal dimension constitute in predicting the criterion performance? While such a question places much more stringent demands on the experimenter, the knowledge achieved is commensurately greater. It is certainly the case that a replacement of a sole operational definition for any construct of abnormality, whether it be emotional disturbance, learning disability, or malnutrition, is not advisable because of the loss in conceptual power that the retreat to pure operationism represents. Nevertheless, it is important that the defining characteristics of the samples utilized be communicable to other investigators and replicable by them, i.e. that they be reliable indices and that they be demonstrably valid of the construct under study.

The issue of reliability of assessment and that of construct validity are typically ignored in animal studies. However, it is more typically the case with animal studies that the abnormality is experimentally produced and subsequently assessed as, for example, by histological analysis, thereby assuring the "reliability" of group membership. Even here, however, the construct validity issue of the experimental intervention which constitutes the construction of the abnormal versus the normal samples is seldom investigated. Rather, it is assumed to represent an appropriate method of operationalizing the abnormality under study or, at times, even assumed to be an appropriate analogue to some abnormal condition possessed by the human organism. Certainly, these questions cannot be left to the investigator's assumptions. They must be systematically documented, much as one would do were one to construct a formal assessment device (test) of the alleged abnormality. One would be expected to demonstrate that the measure, in fact, relates to other measures of that abnormal condition or to behaviors expected of subjects possessing that abnormal condition aside from the specific behaviors predicted by the hypotheses under study. In short, comparison between the results of animal studies can suffer the same problems as those utilizing humans if: (1) reliability of the abnormality is not assessed, (2) construct validity is not

established, and (3) percent of variance explained is not presented.
Animal studies can be shown to be as suspect as human studies in
these regards despite their noncorrelational "advantage."

5. Summary. To summarize, one must assure oneself as a
researcher that the method of defining the abnormal sample is both
a reliable and valid index of the abnormality under study and that
the degree of relationship between the predictor group and the
criterion is reported. These precautions are seldom taken in
experimental work and their lack has resulted in data whose inter-
dependence and utility are in doubt. This problem is particularly
acute in the case of the more complex and the more recently defined
abnormal conditions such as learning disabilities (c.f., Senf,
1975b). Such a state of affairs may derive from the experimental-
ist's training in sample-difference methodology which teaches him
to believe that the isolation of a difference between groups constitutes an important and interpretable characteristic of the target (abnormal) sample in question. As noted above, such an assumption is extremely tenuous in human studies where the groups are
pre-existing rather than experimentally evolved.

B. Theoretical Issues Involved in Sample Definition

That it is typical for an investigator to be concerned with a
specific area of abnormality is certainly reasonable given the
number and complexity of abnormal conditions. However, a by-
product of the circumscribed concern is frequently a failure to
devote sufficient thought to the relationship between the chosen
operational definition of the construct identifying the abnormal
state and other abnormal conditions. Sample composition is relegated more to a technological undertaking than to a theoretical
consideration of the method's appropriateness. A specific example
from the field of learning disabilities will clarify this point.
Articles on the so-called learning disabled child contain subjects
ranging from black inner-city children performing below national
norms on achievement tests, pediatric and neurology clinic patients,
children attending special schools having already failed at public
school, children referred by public school teachers as not performing up to expectations (sometimes the diagnosis being formalized as
a discrepancy between IQ and achievement indices), and others.
These widely varying subject samples not surprisingly yield very
different results despite similar experimental conditions. Though
it is of value to have a construct defined by more than a single
operation, failure to specify with sufficient clarity the class
principles defining learning disabilities has led to the field's
inability to accumulate empirical knowledge (Senf, 1975a; Senf and
Sushinsky, 1975). These problems of study comparability, as discussed above, are compounded when the procedural section of the
report does not adequately specify the class principles adhered to
when constituting the abnormal group. However, the underlying

problem lies in the lack of consensus regarding the meaning of the
term, in this example "learning disabilities" (c.f., Senf, 1974).
Meaning, in this context, is a consensus on a conceptual level of
what constitutes the abnormal condition from what does not constitute that condition, even though the specific measurement indices
used to select the sample may reasonably vary somewhat from experiment to experiment.

When lack of consensus exists, a field of inquiry finds itself
in a position much like that of the courts in their attempt to
define pornography: Though all definitions seem to fail, many are
willing to claim that they "know it when they see it." I have put
forth the position in another paper (Senf, 1975c) that the specific
concept of abnormality under study represents a part of a larger
theoretical network which is seldom explicitly stated and that this
larger theoretical network regarding the abnormal condition acts to
influence the researcher's choice of operational definitions.
Furthermore, this implicit theoretical structure changes over time.
I have illustrated this temporal change in another paper with
regard to the abnormal condition called learning disabilities (Senf,
1975b), which throughout its short ten-year history has markedly
changed in focus from a medically-oriented construct growing out of
the minimal brain dysfunction work to an educationally-centered
construct concerned with school performance relative to expected
achievement. These changes in definition over time, aside from
making difficult the comparison from study to study, arise from
different theoretical conceptions of the construct of abnormality
in question. If, for example, learning disabilities was considered
part of the minimal brain dysfunction syndrome or synonymous with
it, the research would focus on very different sets of hypotheses
and variables than if it was considered from an educational perspective. Such is, in fact, the case.

The implication of this line of thinking is that the theoretical conception of the abnormal condition under study will influence
the method used to select a sample for study and the results subsequently obtained. New hypotheses regarding the abnormal condition
are typically applied to the subject population which the investigator has previously studied or one similar to it. Thus, for
example, one may derive a new sociological explanation for malnutrition regarding family structure and test it utilizing the same
operational definition that one has used in previous studies despite
the difference of the hypothesis under question. While I have no
argument with such an endeavor per se, what is strikingly missing
in research on abnormality is the application of new hypotheses to
the structure of the conceptual system of abnormal conditions.
Rather, researchers appear to accept conventional definitions of
abnormal states as an acceptable starting point and then employ
research techniques to understand that state. What is lacking, in
my opinion, is the application of new conceptions to the framework

of abnormality itself.

Such an undertaking need not encompass all of abnormality; it can be contained to a more circumscribed domain. An historical example is that of schizophrenia. The traditional categories of Kraepelin have given way through research studies to subcategories which are more empirically-based and for which there now exist more sophisticated measurement techniques (e.g., the MMPI) than the clinical judgement employed to discriminate paranoid, hebephrenic, catatonic, and simple schizophrenics from one another. Similarly, our ideas about other abnormal conditions need to be examined from the point of view of whether the present definition of the abnormal group suits our purposes.

By addressing the question of whether the category of abnormality under study suits one's purposes, one addresses directly the question of whether abnormality has been defined in a way appropriate to the understanding that the researcher seeks. Given that there are an infinite number of ways to conceptualize abnormal conditions and, hence, to constitute abnormal samples, the question becomes how best to group atypical subjects such that the correlates of the group are of a high magnitude and are meaningful with respect to the concerns of the researcher (and to those who wish to change the abnormal condition for the better). Expressed somewhat differently, the question that must be asked about the constitution of abnormal samples is whether the expected class correlates of the abnormal group can reasonably be those in which the experimenter and others are interested.

It thus first becomes a matter of _theoretical_ concern as to whether the group constituted by its particular class principles will have as correlates the behavior which will support the investigator's hypothesis. It can readily be shown, for example, that the child with a learning problem in school is quite likely also to have a lower self-esteem than the average child; self-esteem is not one of the defining characteristics of learning problems but a relatively valid correlate of the condition. If, however, one believes that many learning disabilities are mediated by specific cognitive dysfunctions (e.g. short-term memory) the probability of any given learning disabled child having a short-term memory problem is relatively low because there are so many potential causes for inadequate learning in the early grades. This is not to say that some learning problems are not mediated by short-term memory difficulty but that the class, learning disabilities, is an inadequate predictor of that criterion behavior. Consequently, disentangling the riddle of learning disabilities involves applying one's theoretical conception about the range of problems that might be encompassed to the taxonomic construction of groups, rather than simply to the assessment of whether the presently defined abnormal group possesses one or another particular difficulty. In the latter

case, what is inevitably found is that the relationship between
group membership (learning disabilities) and any particular performance variable is generally low, although usually statistically significant. Little cumulative knowledge is obtained from this type of
research venture.

There are questions here for those working in the area of malnourishment and similar phenomena described in this volume in which
a relatively circumscribed event which damages development is the
object of study. Is malnourishment a unitary concept which can act
as a predictor variable for all of the criterion situations to which
malnourishment might relate? Or, must malnourishment be thought of
as a higher-order construct within which there will be more homogeneous groupings of malnourished individuals; groupings which will
relate highly to certain specific situations though less highly to
others? Specifically, for example, does a child malnourished from
infancy perform in a manner similar to a child not malnourished
until age five? Also, does the malnourished child living in an
otherwise enriched subculture have different affective if not different cognitive correlates of his malnutrition than a child living
in a generally impoverished environment? Researchers in the area of
malnutrition will certainly be able to isolate other variables which
will be useful in systematizing the dimensions within malnourishment
such that there will be a maximization of the relationships between
measurable variables defining group membership in subclasses of the
malnourishment and criterion variables of interest. The general
point is that unless malnourishment truly is a unitary characteristic, error of prediction will result unless one's theoretical
understanding of malnourishment is applied to the structure of the
predictor classes as well as to the selection of criteria with which
to test hypotheses.

C. Utility of Research Results

While the issue of utility is implicitly treated in the fore-
going sections, two additional comments are in order to highlight
its importance. Utility can be thought of as having two aspects:
(1) the degree of relationship between the predictor and criterion
variables, and (2) the practical importance of the criterion variable for the understanding and, hopefully, the amelioration of the
abnormal condition.

Studies which are successful in demonstrating significant
differences between normal and abnormal groups need not necessarily
have satisfied even the first condition of utility. The magnitude
of the relationship, i.e., the variance predicted, may actually be
quite small. Finding statistically significant relationships, even
though of low magnitude, can be defended on basic research grounds
and the present limited state of knowledge. However, I think it is
generally assumed that the funding agencies supporting studies of

abnormality and, by implication, the populus whose tax dollars go
to support those agencies expect that the studies of abnormality
will eventually lead to improved conditions. While journals appear
typically concerned with the statistical significance (reliability)
of a phenomenon, practitioners are concerned with the absolute
degree of predictability. For example, they want to know the number
of false-positives and false-negatives which a test (i.e., predictor
variable) has or be shown some other indicant of the predictor variable's accuracy. For example, to show that learning disabled
children on the average have more short-term memory problems than
normal children is of little surprise to the teacher of the learning
disabled. The teacher's concern is which children have the problem
(if, indeed, the teacher has not already noticed their existence)
and what to do about them.

Utility can be enhanced through the understanding gleaned from
a more thorough analysis of the construct of abnormality under study,
as suggested in the immediate preceding section on theory. To test
a given hypothesis by comparing one sample with another, it is
obviously important to eliminate as many alternative explanations
for the expected result as possible. This can conceivably be done
by equating subjects on variables that would represent alternative
explanations or through the use of control groups. Were one able to
distinguish reliably types of abnormality within broader constructs
such as learning disabilities, emotional disturbance, and perhaps
hormonal dysfunction and malnourishment, one would then gain the
capability of testing one's hypothesis by comparing two or more
groups of abnormal subjects, some expected to show the predicted
outcome and others not. Such an experimental design is far more
powerful than the sample-difference design which compares the
abnormal group with a normal control group, for it equates many of
the historical variables and general self-referent attitudes concomitant with the abnormality, and so forth. For example, it would
be much more useful were it demonstrable that children with visual
learning problems have diminished visual information storage capabilities (Sperling, 1960) relative to a comparison group of children
with auditory learning disabilities than were the comparison group
comprised of nonlearning disabled, "normal" youngsters. In the
former case, it would appear that the target group's disability is
at least specific to the visual sphere, whereas in the latter comparison, inferior performance might just as well be due to some
general test-taking variable, negative self-image, or other general
characteristic correlated with school failure. Furthermore, we may
learn more about malnourishment, for example, by comparing children
with different types of malnourishment or who have become malnourished under different conditions or at different times than
by comparing them with normal controls because the specificity of
our hypotheses can be greater and the possibility of their being
disconfirmed enhanced. In general, it can be expected that the
degree of knowledge obtained is directly proportional to the

probability that the hypothesis under test is disconfirmable.

D. Philosophy of Abnormality

     There appears to this writer an overwhelming tendency on the
part of researchers who study deviance within the perspective of the
psychological profession to make the implicit assumption that the
deviance rests with the individual. Thus, persons are emotionally
disturbed, schizophrenic, neurotic, learning disabled, and so forth.
But deviance is more a social than a statistical judgement, typically
representing an unacceptable degree of behavioral disparity relative
to prevailing cultural values. Deviance can equally well be looked
at as an interaction between the individual and an institution of
society which requires less disparate behavior. I have examined
this proposition at length in other papers (Senf, 1974; Senf and
Sushinsky, 1975). The central question raised was whether learning
disabilities could legitimately be considered as residing within
the child or whether they might be more fruitfully considered as an
interaction between child capabilities, inclinations, and other
characteristics with the demands placed upon the child by the school.
By extension of this thinking the question can be posed within a
statistical framework: What proportion of the variance in the deviant
behavior can be accounted for by child characteristics and how much
by the interaction between the child and the characteristics of the
school system (c.f., also Sarason, 1971). This issue is brought
into bold relief when it is recognized that, despite the inadequacies
many of us have in the realm of singing, there are no singing disabilities in the public school system. Here, it is clear that it is
society not valuing singing among all of its members that prevents
this "disability" from being labeled. On the other hand, society
has a vested interest in developing a populus capable of reading so
that it has a work force suitable to the demands of a technical
society. Hence, schools often label children who perform poorly
in reading relative to their peers as learning disabled.

     Blindness is a case in point which brings us closer to the
issue of malnourishment and other developmental disorders. Although
blindness can certainly be considered an abnormality and a handicap
in which the individual's state statistically accounts for a great
degree of the variance in predicting performance in a variety of
situations, it is the requirement of society that persons learn to
read that gives the blind child particular difficulty in obtaining
information. Were we to have a culture based more heavily on oral
than on visual communication, the blind would not be nearly so handicapped in the educational context.

     While at first blush malnourishment seems most distinctly a
characteristic of the individual, the recognition of the condition
as malnourishment and the steps taken to ameliorate the condition
are certainly influenced by societal variables. The work of the

Black Panthers in this country is a case in point. Thus, for a
thorough understanding of even this condition of abnormality, it
seems necessary to examine more than the psychological impact of
the condition on the individual. One must also recognize and
study its relationship to the social framework in which it occurs.
Such a broadened conception will likely necessitate the generation
of varieties (subgroups) of malnourishment as discussed above.

III. ISSUES IN OUTCOME RESEARCH

Since most of the research in this symposia concerns the basic
principles surrounding rehabilitation, the issue of treatment
effectiveness must inevitably be addressed. In the area of education, and special education particularly, the concern for program
effectiveness has received considerable attention spurred by legis-
lative queries regarding accountability for expenditure of public
funds. While it is not necessarily the case that a thorough understanding of an abnormal condition necessarily will include knowledge
of how to cure or reduce the condition (for it may not be correct-
able), our optimism and sometimes our data do suggest avenues of
intervention.

Outcome research in educational circles has not been particularly kind to the practitioner. Although this writer has not made
any box-score tallies, it is a relatively widely shared impression
that the programs developed to ameliorate the problems of the handicapped child are not demonstrably effective. The word "demonstrably"
must be stressed: Is it the failure of the practitioner to improve
the condition of their charges or is it the imprecision of the
researcher's instruments or the weakness of his experimental designs
and methods which find a lack of significant improvement among
treated abnormal samples? Many of the issues surrounding this
central outcome question are relevant to the area of early malnutrition, low birthweight, hormone dysfunction, and early environmental restriction. After noting some of the basic issues involved
in outcome research, this chapter concludes with an examination of
the problems in defining variables in treatment outcome research.

A. Some Basic Considerations in Outcome Studies

1. Subject Appropriateness. The question of the appropriateness
of the persons selected for examination in an outcome study involves
two groups, the allegedly abnormal sample and the normal control.
Appropriateness, itself, is not a simple notion, being made up of
many specific considerations dependent upon the nature of the abnormality, the specific hypothesis in question, and so forth.
However, some general principles hold. Can it truly be said that
all members of the abnormal group are adequately representative of
the class principles of that abnormal sample? This is another way

of asking the previously discussed question of class principle reliability. Is the treatment under test an appropriate one for all the subjects in the abnormal sample? In studies of educational disabilities, too often children greatly heterogeneous with respect to their educational failure are grouped together under some rubric designating abnormality and administered a treatment procedure which may be theoretically appropriate for only a small subset of that sample. Too often it appears that if the researcher is congenial with the treatment procedure, the subject selection is such that significant differences between the treated and untreated groups are obtained. Without citing specific examples, for such would serve no purpose, it is this writer's opinion that those congenial to the Frostig program for perceptually impaired children (Frostig and Horne, 1964) are more apt to find positive effects of the treatment than those who are less disposed toward so-called "process training." Close examination of these studies often finds that the subjects vary: Those showing favorable results have subjects who were carefully screened and selected by clinicians to be appropriate for the Frostig program while those showing negative outcomes have subjects who were often less carefully selected, frequently being drawn randomly from a group of children receiving additional assistance due to more general learning problems.

Such issues will eventually come to the area of malnutrition and other environmentally-induced deficits. Whether or not the effects of early deprivation can be overcome may be dependent on whether the subsample of deprived children has a long or short history of deprivation or alternatively is deprived at an early or later stage in development. As noted above, there may be various types or patterns of deprivation for which some treatments will prove effective while other varieties may prove intractable. The researcher has to be extremely careful not to let his preconception of the malleability of the condition bias his sample selection in such a way as to assure the results he desires.

2. Treatment Representativeness. While presumably more control will be available in the application of treatments designed to ameliorate the specific conditions described in this volume, treatment within educational circles can be very sloppily and non-professionally administered without such being decipherable in the methods section of the research report. Typically, research on the impact of education programs is accomplished to fulfill thesis requirements at universities (or as a requirement for federal funding). In the former case, the intervention is applied by a relatively untrained and harried experimenter. Whether or not this treatment reflects that given by the practiced professional is a matter of very serious concern in as much as the efficacy of the intervention is thrown into question by a failure to show significant improvement among deviant children in such studies. The issue here is whether those who apply the treatment are representative of

those who in actual practice apply the treatment. More often than
not, those doing the research are not those involved in the clinical
application and so the researcher who does not utilize trained
practitioners and relies instead on graduate students or part-time
assistants may not be adequately assessing the effectiveness of the
treatment in situ. In the latter case, where evaluation is a grant
requirement, the reverse situation holds: The treatment is applied
by representative professionals but the research is conducted with
an inadequate budget, often by inadequately trained individuals, and
within a context highly dependent on "finding" positive effects.
This line of thinking, which contains many critical issues regarding
the appropriate expenditure of research dollars, is tangential to
the present topic.

3. Value of Treatment Not Assessed. An often neglected concern in outcome studies is the value derived by the target individual through association with the helping agent whether or not the
outcome variable shows a significant difference when compared with
that of the control subject's performance. Sometimes the problem
lies in the "control" group. A fact always with us, recognized by
researchers and yet often disregarded in the interpretation of
results, is that there is no vacuum against which to evaluate
effective intervention. Too often, the "untreated" control group,
by virtue of its being identified, receives some additional assistance or benefits by mere attention (the Hawthorne effect). Hence,
what might be impressive gains among the abnormal group are miti-
gated by virtue of disproportionate improvement in the allegedly
untreated control group. While this problem will perennially be
with us, its significance is reduced by focusing on a closer definition of the treatment variables, discussed in a separate section
below.

4. Univariate Approach. Whether the dependent variable
demonstrates that the treatment is effective or not, the appropriateness of the univariate nature of much of our treatment research
must be examined. Animal studies are typically illustrative of
research where the behavior of interest to the experimenter is distilled into a single index called the dependent variable[2]. In the
evaluation of human service programs, the same univariate model
has not served us well for it too often concludes that no good
came from the program despite the expense of many tax dollars. Yet,
were you to talk to the teachers, the child's parents, the school
authorities, and others you might find that the program is highly
thought of, so much so that discontinuation is reacted to with the
same anger afforded the researcher's negative outcome report.
Though research-minded individuals have frequently looked upon such
reactions of practitioners as exemplary of their warmheartedness or
more cynically as their delusional belief in their own impact, it is
very possible that valid program effectiveness lies in areas not
assessed by the researcher's instruments. Hunt's description of the

independence of developmental dimensions in this volume is likely
to apply to the attainment of other formal and informal educational
skills. For example, is a program for the educationally failing
youngster to be discontinued because his rate of progress does not
accelerate despite the fact that the parents attest that the home
situation has markedly improved since the program's initiation? Or
should a program which feeds the malnourished child be discontinued
were it to show that the child's cognitive skills are not measurably
affected? The researcher's failure to take into account the breadth
of dependent measures of interest to others is a critical inadequacy
in an enormous number of outcome studies.

Similarly, univariate thinking on the independent variable side
has fostered a simplistic view of abnormal conditions as present
among animal studies as among those utilizing human subjects. The
large standard error of measurement in psychological research makes
finding lawful relationships of social importance extremely difficult. Richardson's work reported in this volume exemplifies the
strength of a multivariate approach which should be used more often
in my opinion. In this regard, linear regression analyses can be
supplemented by discriminant function analyses and cluster algorithms
(Hardigan, 1975) in order to isolate those subjects on whom the
treatments are effective. This aids the taxonomic effort discussed
above, rather than concluding that the treatment is simply ineffective in general. Multivariate techniques, such as cluster analysis
long under development by biological scientists (Sokal and Sneath,
1963), represent in my opinion a much more productive approach to
outcome evaluation methodology than the univariate models more
common at present.

B. Treatment Variable and Outcome Variable Definitional Concerns

Particularly with a study of human intervention programs, the
definition of the treatment variable is often nearly impossible.
Frequently, a complex of variables are instituted to maximize the
potential positive outcome of the treatment. For scientific purposes, it is obvious that more refined variables, independently
measurable such that they can be looked at in combination and their
impact on one or more dependent variables noted, represent a more
powerful approach to outcome research. Otherwise, outcome research
with successful consequences cannot specify the critically important
variables and, hence, little knowledge is gained toward the goal of
being able to replicate the effective program elsewhere. While it
provides a necessary starting point, the lack of specificity in
such animal research "treatment" variables as "enriched" or "superenriched environments" is a noteworthy analogue to the problem in
human treatment research.

Even when the treatment variables are well specified, their
reliability can be called into question. This problem is equally

true with animal as with human studies. Particularly in infrahuman studies, the <u>reliability</u> of the experimental treatment and the reliability of outcome variables utilized to assess the impact of that treatment are seldom reported. Nor is the relationship between various outcome measures systematically studied. For example, what is the relationship between such variables as trials to asymptotic performance, trials to some performance criterion, errors to some performance criterion, and rate of extinction of a learned response? Different experimenters adopt different performance indices for the same task; study comparability is either unknown or assumed without data which tells us the relationship between these various outcome measures. In the human area, particularly when criterion variables concern academic performance, the plethora of achievement indices available to the researcher make comparability of studies difficult although the situation here is much less serious given that some of the indices used have been previously correlated and are typically normatively scaled.

In summary, the general point urged in this section is that our outcome studies of intervention for abnormal conditions: (1) attend more closely to the measurement concerns surrounding both the intervention and outcome variables, (2) utilize multiple measurement of the treatment and outcome variables, and (3) utilize multivariate designs so that the study will yield greater and more meaningful information. As a consequence of using such procedures, an outcome study will have a much greater probability of yielding information regarding which treatment variables will have the greatest impact on the various outcome measures of interest. Whether discriminant statistics and/or clustering algorithms are chosen by the investigator, the way to accelerate our rate of learning about treating abnormal conditions is to avoid designs which tell us simply that a program (comprised of a complex of intervention tactics) does or does not affect a dependent measure.

C. Utility of Outcome Research

The purpose of outcome research can be examined within research or program evaluation frameworks which traditionally have different value orientations. While research has as its predominant goal the isolation of relationships between antecedent and consequent conditions (though, as discussed before this goal is complicated by the correlational nature of studies with intact abnormal populations), outcome research has sought to evaluate the efficacy of various intervention tactics. It is my opinion that outcome research has adopted implicitly the orientation of basic research in that it too often seeks to establish the statistical reliability of the relationship between two or more variables rather than to contribute directly to the utility of programmatic intervention (Senf and Anderson, 1975). As previously noted, although the concepts of statistical reliability and stability of an individual's score over time are related, the issue in outcome research hinges directly on the probability of a given intervention having the desired effect on a specific individual predicted to benefit from the intervention by virtue of measurable antecedent variables. One way to ask this question statistically is to examine the number of false-positives and false-negatives associated with such a prediction. Another way, prevalent in educational circles, is to assess the degree of improvement in the abnormal individual's behavior by those who take responsibility for the intervention. In both cases, an extremely high relationship (i.e., typically greater than that represented by the .05 significance level) is required in order to make judgements about intervention with specific individuals. If outcome research on human abnormality is ever to become a useful tool for decision making, we are going to have to learn an awful lot more about the specific interactions between individual characteristics and the complexity of treatments that exist in human service settings, these treatments themselves being a complex of variables. Consequently, as urged in the initial section of this paper, researchers are going to have to become capable of grouping abnormal individuals into conceptual categories consistent in their level of abstraction with the variables with which they wish the category grouping to be associated. The study of gross concepts such as emotional disturbance, mental retardation, learning disabilities, and so forth which serve primarily administrative purposes must give way to a more complex conceptual framework atuned to that of the expert practitioner. One would hope that the study of malnutrition and other environmentally-produced deficits would be able to utilize the mistakes of the past (and regretably of the present) in these other areas of abnormality. By using other areas of research as a guide, environmental deprivation work can adopt early on more fruitful research designs which will have utility for the abnormal individual as well as for the researcher seeking knowledge and the rewards accruing to publication of such knowledge.

FOOTNOTES

1. Requests for reprints should be sent to the author at: 1331 E. Thunderhead Drive, Tucson, Arizona 85718.

2. It is to be noted that the authors' work described in the first part of this book is not illustrative in that they typically use a complex of performance assessment situations.

REFERENCES

Frostig, M., and Horne, D. 1964. The Frostig Program for the Development of Visual Perception. Follett Publishing Company, Chicago.

Hardigan, J.A. 1975. Clustering Algorithms. Wiley, New York.

Sarason, S.B. 1971. The Culture of the School and the Problem of Change. Allyn and Bacon, Boston.

Senf, G.M. 1973. Learning Disabilities. Pediatric Clinics of North America 20:607-639.

Senf, G.M. 1974. Learning Disabilities: Child-School Interaction Model. Computer Psychometric Affiliates, Inc., Chicago.

Senf, G.M. 1975a. Future Research Needs in Learning Disabilities, pp. 249-267. In R.P. Anderson and C.G. Halcomb (eds.). Texas Tech Invitational Conference on Learning Disabilities/Minimal Brain Dysfunction. Thomas, Springfield.

Senf, G.M. 1975b. Model Centers Program for Learning Disabled Children: Historical Perspective, pp. 10-26. In R.P. Anderson and C.G. Halcomb (eds.). Texas Tech Invitational Conference on Learning Disabilities/Minimal Brain Dysfunction. Thomas, Springfield.

Senf, G.M. 1975c. Issues Surrounding Classification in Special Education. Under editorial review.

Senf, G.M., and Anderson, D.O. 1975. Program Evaluation Suggestions for Project Initiators. In J.M. McCarthy (ed.). Technical Assistance Manual. Government Printing Office, Washington, D.C. (in press).

Senf, G.M., and Sushinsky, L.W. 1975. State Initiative in Learning Disabilities: Illinois' Project SCREEN. Report II -- Definition and Illinois Practice. J. Learning Disabilities. (in press).

Sokal, R.R., and Sneath, P.H.A. 1963. Principles of Numerical Taxonomy. W. H. Freeman, San Francisco.

Sperling, G. 1960. The Information Available in Brief Visual Presentations. Psychol. Monogr. 74(Whole No. 11).

Walsh, R.N., and Cummins, R.A. 1976. The Open Field Test: A Critical Review. Psychol. Bull. (in press).

Zigler, E., and Phillips, L. 1962. Psychiatric Diagnosis, A Critique. J. Abnorm. Soc. Psychol. 63:607-617.

SUMMARY AND AFTERTHOUGHTS

Robert L. Isaacson

Department of Psychology
University of Florida
Gainesville, Florida 32611

Most of the chapters in this book are related to the theme
that early privation or damage will usually produce reduced
behavioral abilities later in life. Some of these reductions may
be permanent. However, in many cases the premise must be altered
to say that the privation or damage will usually produce altered
abilities. It is not clear whether or not the alteration in abilities is always the same from one individual or species to the next.
Too often the behavioral changes are considered relative to an
assumed "standard" individual or "representative" species, raised
and tested under "usual conditions." The range of treatments presumed to result in altered behavioral abilities include food deprivation, hypoxia, reduced opportunities for movement or for receiving
organized sensory input, trauma, surgical damage to the brain, and
endocrine imbalance. All of these conditions are presumed to overcome the brain's surprisingly effective insulation and resiliency
so as to produce the altered behavioral consequences.

Too often the problems of research in these areas have been
oversimplified. The complexities of animal and human conditions
in the early developmental periods have been distilled into single
dimensions, as have the treatments imposed and the outcomes that
are measured. Senf has pointed out the fallacies behind this
simple-minded approach which, among other things, hides individual
reactions to a particular "treatment." He rightly points up the
need to discover just how much variance can be attributed to one or
another treatment rather than merely to find a significant difference among groups. The need to consider many different groups of
people and their special reactions to environmental conditions is
highlighted by Richardson's demonstration that malnourishment can
lead to different consequences depending on the social and cultural

361

backgrounds of those being studied. Sackett and his colleagues
have shown that the effects of isolation must take into account
differences in genetic endowment of the nonhuman primates: The
pig-tailed monkey does not respond to isolation or emergence from
isolation in the same way as does the rhesus.

A second theme found in the chapters in this book is that
enriched or even "super-enriched" environments can offset or
reduce the structural, functional, or behavioral consequences of
early damage or privation. In general, the bulk of the data
supports the view that subjecting animals to these environments
produces less reduction in abilities or less behavioral alterations
after privation.

On the basis of these reviews and research contributions it
should now be obvious that all stimulation is not alike. To be
effective in altering the behavioral consequences of privation
and brain damage, the sensory input must be organized and not
greatly different from what is anticipated by the subjects being
studied. A variety of experiences seem to be needed (e.g.,
Davenport), but the diversity must not be too great. Infants of
all species are programmed for certain types of sensory input
(see Beckwith) and sensory stimulation must take these dispositions
into account. Flooding the individual with inappropriate sensory
input is like subjecting the individual to noise. It doesn't help
and may even hurt (Hunt). While sensory deprivation is most frequently studied, the importance of motor activity and the sensory
feedback from it for normal development is now recognized (Walsh
and Cummins).

Many of the findings reported underline the caution that must
be exerted before advocating early intervention programs. Merely
increasing the intensity or rate of sensory stimulation to infants
may not produce beneficial results. Both the nature and degree of
sensory stimulation must be considered. It is quite likely that
people (or animals) with diverse endowments and histories will
respond differently to various types of sensory stimulation.

Privation or brain damage will produce different effects when
applied at various times after birth. The most effective times
depend on the species of the animal. There seem to be "critical
periods" for different structures and abilities. At least there
are times in development when stress, or trauma, or deprivation
will produce the most apparent disruptions of structure and function. Yet, many of the reports show that while there may be critical periods for disrupting the developing organism, these effects
may be reversible (Levine and Wiener). Neither malnutrition nor
sensory deprivation produces irreversible and everlasting effects.
On the other hand, intervention in the form of environmental enrichment can produce beneficial effects at many ages, even when

the animals are relatively ancient (Davenport; Walsh and Cummins).

Examining studies of the impaired human infant, many of the
authors exclude from consideration those with hereditary deficiencies (Hunt) or those with real mental deficiencies (Beckwith). I
agree with the authors who do make this distinction. Recently, I
have discussed this matter in a small book about mentally deficient
adults (Isaacson, 1976). By making this distinction, it is likely
that the lives of both the mentally deficient and those with severe
environmental deprivation will be benefitted, even though it may not
be possible to distinguish the mental defective with brain damage
from a person with severe environmental deprivation on the basis of
IQ test scores alone.

This is not to say that the mentally defective cannot benefit
substantially from special training for certain types of skills.
They can benefit from intervention programs. The important message
is that if one wants children or adults to become skillful in certain types of activities, the best procedure is to give them the
specific training which will allow them to do so. The problem with
the Head Start programs and others with similar goals was that they
were not directed toward the attainment of proficiency in academic
areas through a set of appropriate training experiences. As was
pointed out by Hunt, these programs had a mixture of political,
human, and academic goals which diluted the effects of training on
strictly academic skills.

On the other hand, it may be a great mistake to think of programs like Head Start as failures because academic performance was
not greatly improved. It may well be that other aspects of human
life were enriched. Those "other aspects" may not have been
measured (Senf). Quite possibly the changes are subtle and can't
be measured, at least until the children have grown into adulthood.

Throughout many of the chapters I was impressed with the fact
that benefits derived from intervention can only be talked about
as they relate to performances on identified and specific tasks.
However, Davenport does discuss a general improvement in learning
abilities. Yet, I am wary of studies that discuss such general
improvements. Learning and memory abilities exist wherever animal
life exists, despite brain damage and monstrous biologic catas-
trophies. Most studies of abilities at the animal and human level
reveal complex patterns of specific abilities and the behavioral
alterations produced by disruptions of brain development influence
other, more subtle behavioral capacities rather than "learning and
memory" (e.g., Isaacson, 1975).

An important problem for research at the animal level is how
to measure impaired abilities. Sometimes students ask, "What are
mentally retarded animals like?" Often I suggest that they are

those animals that learn our simple laboratory problems the fastest.
This suggestion is based, in part, on the fact that many simple
problems are learned rapidly and remembered well by the mentally
deficient human. The problems that are used in animal laboratories,
almost without exception, are of an absurdly simple nature. Perhaps the classic instance is that of the two-way active avoidance
task. Here animals with extensive brain damage will acquire the
problem faster than intact animals. This suggests that learning
and memory are not being altered. Rather, there are other sorts
of changes in behavioral abilities. The animals may have become
differentially sensitive to environmental change or the effects
of past experience. There may be an inflexibility of behavior. The
point is that it is very difficult to determine just what the criteria for mentally defective or deprived animals should be.

The studies of Burton L. White, reported in the chapter by
Hunt, were of special interest to me. White found that if a child
had well developed competencies by age three, these competencies
more closely resembled those of competent children of age six than
they did of less competent children six years old. Mrs. Tetsuka
Suzuki (1974) found that memory skills of children in the early
grades were very much the same. Children with good verbal memory
abilities in the early grades were more like the children with good
memory abilities at later ages than they were like older children
with poor memory abilities. Therefore, it seems likely that the
development of competencies in educationally relevant tasks is a
pervasive feature of development. Those who fall behind seem to
have their own special problems which usually remain with them.

In schools, the ability to manipulate symbols of various kinds
seems to be a critical factor in achievement. Quite appropriately,
Dr. Lodge talks about these as left hemisphere abilities. The
developmental schedules of the left and the right hemispheres might
be different with the left hemisphere skills lagging somewhat behind.
Adult intelligence is closely associated with left hemisphere skills
while other abilities are based on right hemisphere or subcortical
mechanisms. The lack of reliability of intelligence measures before
the age of three with those measured later on could be due to differences in the development of "intelligences" of separate brain areas,
e.g., left hemisphere IQ, right hemisphere IQ, subcortical IQ, and
the like.

Dr. Beckwith calls attention to the pervasive effects of social
class on the development of the competent infant. She also points
out that poor environmental conditions and low birthweight tend to
augment each other's effects. This seems to be an instance in which
"function-limiting" factors produce additive effects (Walsh and
Cummins). It also calls attention to the role of the environment
in aggravating other disturbances of the individual (see also
Richardson). What is it about the social circumstances of the home

that produces greater or smaller degrees of competencies? What are the specific factors which produce the adverse effects of being born into deprived conditions? What are the mechanisms of deprivation? What is the role of the child itself in stimulating interactions? As a parent, there is no doubt in my mind that children differ in their ability to elicit reactions from their parents. Do male and female children have differential ways of interacting with their parents? The answer is probably "yes" but we know all too little about how this interaction is altered by conditions of environmental privation or by brain damage. Sackett and his coworkers have found the female to be more resistant to the effects of isolation and in many other ways the female seems to be especially hardy (see also Morrison and McKinney).

The effect of the sex of the animal is important in many different aspects of physiology and behavior (e.g., Davenport). In the study of animals with hypothyroidism there are changes in behavior related to the sex of the animal that may be explained by differences in emotionality. Emotionality differences between the sexes is also found in the human. Apparently, it is easier to soothe the female child than it is the male (e.g., Beckwith).

A recent study being completed in my laboratory suggests that the effect of early stress on the development of perseverative qualities may be sex-dependent (Street and Isaacson, in preparation). A preliminary analyses of our data suggests that a relatively minor degree of stress early in the life of the rat produces an increase in perseverative qualities in males but a decrease in the perseverative qualities of behavior in females when they reach adulthood.

From the moment of the union of the egg and the sperm, all subsequent influences are environmental. The interaction between the mother and child begins in the womb. In other work Dr. Sackett has shown that there is something about monkey mothers carrying male offspring that is quite different from similar mothers carrying female offspring (Sackett, Holm, and Landesman-Dwyer, 1975). The differential reactions of other monkeys to the mothers with male or female fetuses may alter the physical environment of the fetus and may change the monkey mothers' reactions to the offspring after birth.

The effects of any treatment or experience can only be evaluated against the species-typical tendencies of the animals. The differences in effects of deprivation on rats and rabbits are a case in point. The rat is a nocturnal animal whereas squirrels are day animals. Not only would one expect that the behavior of the two animals would be different after light deprivation but the neural mechanisms mediating light responsivity in the two species should be altered in different ways as well.

A laboratory event that remains clear in my memory after 20
years is a visit to the laboratory of Dr. Russell DeValois, then
at the University of Michigan. He was recording from cells in
the optic tract and stimulating a dark-adapted cat with flashes
of light. The flash of light produced an abrupt cessation of
activity in these tracts. Until that time I had assumed that
stimulus delivered to the eye, any eye, would produce an increase
in activity rather than a decrease. However, the effect was just
the opposite in a nocturnal animal. In animals that are usually
active during the day, the response of the optic tract to photic
stimulation of the eye is an increase in discharges.

The effect of ambient illumination on the behavior of animals
cannot be ignored. The inhibitory effect of light on exploratory
activity of nocturnal rodents is quite dramatic, but the specific
genetic inheritance of an animal determines the degree of inhibition.

The assessment of the behavioral effects of any manipulation
of the developing organism is difficult. It is not easy to ascertain just how "function-limiting" factors will be expressed in
either animal or human behavior. Many of the technical and procedural problems involved in the study of the malnourished infant
are well covered in the review of Levine and Wiener. They also
exmphasize that all types of malnourishment do not produce the same
consequences, and, further, that correlations between biochemistry
and behavior can be misleading. This same point is made by Morrison
and McKinney. They note that the alterations in steroid levels
after isolation could be secondary to the stress of the situation
and not play a causal role in the abnormal behaviors observed. I
would go even further and say that correlations between anatomical
abberations and behavior are equally dangerous. We can be misled
by correlations into the assumption of causality.

For the most part, the anatomical changes thought to result
from deprivation of sensory experience or from altered chemical
states in the young are based on the assumption of synaptic changes.
These can be a result of altered dendritic branches, terminal bou-
tons, or the spines on the dendrites. The work of Greenough and
his associates (see Greenough, 1975) has been most influential in
this area. However, it should be noted that these dendritic and
bouton changes are correlates of different experiences and conditions. They may, or may not, be the mechanisms through which
behavioral alterations are produced. It is a useful hypothesis
to be sure, but only future research will tell us whether or not
these alterations are the ones producing behavioral change.

The dendritic changes studied by Greenough and others stand
in marked contrast with the much greater differences in the structure of the brain that are produced by accidents or intervention
early in the gestational period or in the first few days of life.

In such cases, aberrant tracts are formed, the number of nerve
cells is permanently reduced, glia cells are produced in great
numbers, and the organization of the cortical areas may be quite
aberrant. These more catastrophic events produce changes that can
be found throughout the brain. In addition secondary reactions can
be found throughout the brain as when an entire hemisphere and
certain subcortical regions are reduced in size after early damage
to a small area of dorsolateral neocortex (Isaacson and Nonneman,
1972). I believe these relatively widespread changes are more
likely to be related to human mental deficiency than are the smaller
changes in the synaptic structure found after early deprivation.

In their chapter, Walsh and Cummins discuss how current ideas
in theory and research have affected therapy. Specifically, they
point to the failure of Western medicine to use anticholinesterases
in the treatment of stroke patients because of the prevalent notion
in the medical community that the consequences of stroke are permanent and unchangeable. They use the term "therapeutic nihilism"
to describe therapeutic measures now employed with stroke patients.

I would agree with Walsh and Cummins' objections to this negative approach. We know far too little about the brain or about the
effects of brain damage to endorse a "nothing can be done" fatalism.
I am also reminded of comments made by my late friend Sidney Jourard.
He pointed out that patients could often sense the attitudes of a
physician. If a physician believed that nothing would help a patient
the patient could know it even if it was not stated. Because of the
persuasive, almost hypnotic, nature of the physician in a white coat,
surrounded with X-rays and test results, this was likely to become a
self-fulfilling prophecy. I am not suggesting that false hopes be
raised, but given our state of relative ignorance about the nervous
system and recovery from damage, patients should be encouraged to
use their own resources to the maximum. At least the physician
should be honest and acknowledge how little is known about the disease mechanisms and the effectiveness of therapies.

A rather unusual type of habilitative therapy has been devised
in the Wisconsin primate laboratories (by Harlow and his associates
in the early 1970s) (Morrison and McKinney). Essentially "monkey
psychiatrists" were assigned to monkey clients with behavioral problems due to some form of isolation procedures. The therapists were
successful in ameliorating the behavioral abnormalities of the formerly isolated monkeys. Again, the specific aspects of the therapist's actions that cause the improvements in the behavior of the
former isolates need to be discovered. In related studies with
pharmacologic agents, chlorpromazine was found to be beneficial for
isolated monkeys as was diazepam which also produced some beneficial
results. The relation of the catecholamines to the isolation syndrome is less than clear, however, since reserpine and alpha-methyl-
para-tyrosine produce behavioral changes that are similar to those in

the "despair stage" of separation while imipramine tends to alleviate the separation syndrome. Why chlorpromazine produces its
beneficial effects also remains to be determined.

Over the past several years, Dr. Barbara Schneiderman Fish and
I have undertaken experiments to find pharmacologic treatments that
would remedy in whole or in part the behavioral deficits found after
bilateral hippocampal destruction. What we have found is that the
lesioned animals show different reactions to various drugs but that
no general alleviation occurs. On some tasks the performance of
the brain-damaged animals improves but this is restricted to certain
tasks on which performance would be improved by the global behavioral
changes induced by the drugs. If the global change is such that the
animals would be impaired on a task, performance is impaired. Therefore, we have not been successful in finding any general remedy or
elixer that benefits the animals with hippocampal damage but rather
have discovered new kinds of task-dependent drug effects.

In his chapter Senf makes a very important point that should
be emphasized. He calls our attention to the changes that occur from
time to time in what people mean by certain terms. "Learning disabilities" is a case in point. Originally it was used to describe
the minimally brain-damaged child, the one who is hyperactive with
poor impulse control. Basically it was a medical, diagnostic expression. Within a relatively short period of time, its use has
turned into an educational direction. It is now used to describe
children who don't do as well as their teachers think they should
or their test scores predict. Usually the evaluation of the under-
achiever is made in reading and mathematics. But Senf points out
that school performance is not only reading and math. Why don't we
hear of under-achievers in singing or dancing? Since I am a singing-
disabled person, this is the comment that instantly commanded my
attention.

Senf's answer is that society is most interested in the development of skilled workers. With an ever-increasing dependence on
technically skilled labor, reading and fundamentals of mathematics
are essential. A person's success is evaluated primarily on the
basis of his educational abilities related to work. Attention and
money are directed toward intervention procedures that have some
likelihood of improving skills related to work but too little
attention is given to those abilities not related to productive
skills. The disabled learner is the potentially disabled worker,
consequently a loss from the viewpoint of the Protestant work ethic.

It seems to me that Senf's comments are an accurate portrait
of the situation. Whether or not the work ethic is as pervasive as
it once was, it still affects our view of the education system.
Perhaps, however, it is time to turn systematic attention to intervention programs for skills and abilities related to personal growth

and fulfillment. There can be no doubt that many of society's problems can be traced to difficulties that go far beyond work and employment.

REFERENCES

Greenough, W.T. 1975. Enduring Brain Effects of Differential Experience and Training. In M. Rosenzweig and E.L. Bennett (eds.). Neural Mechanisms of Learning and Memory. MIT Press, Cambridge, Massachusetts. (in press).

Isaacson, R.L. 1975. Experimental Brain Lesions and Memory. In M. Rosenzweig and E.L. Bennett (eds.). Neural Mechanisms of Learning and Memory. MIT Press, Cambridge, Massachusetts. (in press).

Isaacson, R.L. 1976. The Retarded Adult. Argus Communication, Niles, Illinois.

Isaacson, R.L., and Nonneman, A.J. 1972. Early Brain Damage and Later Development, pp. 29–44. In P. Satz and J. Ross (eds.). The Disabled Learner. Rotterdam University Press, Rotterdam.

Sackett, G., Holm, R., and Landesman-Dwyer, S. 1975. Vulnerability for Abnormal Development: Pregnancy Outcomes and Sex Differences in Macaque Monkeys, pp. 59-76. In N.R. Ellis (ed.). Aberrant Development in Infancy. Lawrence Erlbaum Associates, Hillsdale, New Jersey.

Suzuki, Tetsuko Fujita. 1974. Developmental Changes in the Memory Process. Unpublished M.A. thesis. University of Florida, Gainesville, Florida.

SUBJECT INDEX

A

Abnormality, philosophy of	353, 354
Accomodation	221
Acetylcholinesterase	172, 174, 175, 184
Age	11, 52, 115, 149, 191
Aggression	24, 124, 127, 145, 146
Alpha-methyl-para-tyrosine	150, 154, 155
Amphetamine	34, 35, 184, 185
Anticholinesterase	182, 184, 367
Aphasia	3, 182
Arousal	34, 35, 184, 185
Assessment	6-8, 52, 53, 317-326
Assimilation	221
Attachment	136-140, 215, 216
Auditory system	181
Axon	186, 187

B

Barpressing	86-89, 92
Bayley Infant Scales	318
Birth	313
Birthweight	269, 270, 288-291, 328, 346
Bonding (see Attachment)	
Brain	
Brain anatomy	5, 6, 73, 172-177
Brain chemistry	5, 6, 178
Brain dysfunction	280, 283
Brain physiology (see Electrophysiology)	
Brain weight	172-175
Brazletons Neonatal Assessment Scale	319

C

Caretaker (see also Mother)	236-239, 263, 264, 276-298, 327
Catecholamines	150

V